Planned Change Theories for Nursing

Dedicated to

Joshua James, Jolene June, Jordon Jon,
Benjamin James, Jeremiah Gordon,
Alec Joseph, and Lydia Kathryn.

Their generation makes the joys and pains of
change both necessary and worthwhile.

Planned Change Theories for Nursing

Review, Analysis, and Implications

Constance Rimmer Tiffany
Louette R. Johnson Lutjens

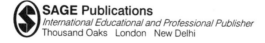
SAGE Publications
International Educational and Professional Publisher
Thousand Oaks   London   New Delhi

For information:

SAGE Publications, Inc.
2455 Teller Road
Thousand Oaks, California 91320
E-mail: order@sagepub.com

SAGE Publications Ltd.
6 Bonhill Street
London EC2A 4PU
United Kingdom

SAGE Publications India Pvt. Ltd.
M-32 Market
Greater Kailash I
New Delhi 110 048 India

Printed in the United States of America

Library of Congress Cataloging-in-Publication Data

Tiffany, Constance Rimmer.
 Planned change theories for nursing: Review, analysis, and
implications / Constance Rimmer Tiffany, Louette R. Johnson Lutjens.
  p. cm.
 Includes bibliographical references and index.
 ISBN 0-7619-0234-1 (cloth : acid-free paper). — ISBN
0-7619-0235-X (pbk. : acid-free paper)
  1. Nursing—Planning. 2. Organizational change. 3. Social
change. 4. Nursing models. I. Lutjens, Louette R. Johnson.
II. Title.
RT89.T54 1998
610.73'01—dc21   97-33801

98 99 00 01 02 03 10 9 8 7 6 5 4 3 2 1

Acquiring Editor:	Dan Ruth
Editorial Assistant:	Anna Howland
Production Editor:	Sanford Robinson
Production Assistant:	Karen Wiley
Typesetter:	Danielle Dillahunt
Indexer:	Julie Sherman Grayson
Cover Designer:	Ravi Balasuriya

Contents

PART III:
PLANNED CHANGE THEORY IN PRACTICE

Preface

We introduce five major areas of thought in this book. First, we present statements of general considerations nurses should take into account when they plan change. Second, we furnish them with expositions of the three planned change theories that nurses use most often. Third, we supply nurses with a more systems-oriented planned change theory than those seen most frequently in nursing literature. Fourth, we provide mechanisms that nurse planners themselves can use to analyze and evaluate planned change theories. Finally, we offer nurses a foundation for open and scholarly dialogue about the relative merits and uses of planned change theories.

This book is divided into two parts separated by an interlude. Part I contains general considerations for nurses who plan change. The interlude provides information that contributes to an understanding of the second part of the book. The second part of the book presents, analyzes, and applies planned change theories and discusses research considerations.

Part I contains eight chapters. After the introductory chapter, three chapters offer information related to the choice and use of a planned change theory. Two of these chapters present the often-neglected but essential topics of social power and ethics. Chapters 5 through 8 discuss diagnosis, innovations (solutions), strategies and tactics, and evaluation of processes and outcomes of a change event.

The interlude offers ideas about worldviews, theory borrowing, and theory sharing. It reviews a nursing theory that nurses might choose, from among many, to combine with a planned change theory.

Part II presents the work of four planned change theorists (Lewin; Bennis, Benne, and Chin; Rogers; Bhola), analyzes their theories, and suggests ways that nurses can access the strengths of each theory and overcome their limitations. Part II also illustrates combinations of the featured planned change theories with a nursing theory. The last two chapters deal with planned change research and nursing research use. Appendixes present learning aids and reference sources.

The fact that this book highlights only four planned change theories does not mean that no other theories merit nurses' consideration; other useful planned change theories exist. We chose three theories because of the frequency of their appearance in nursing periodical literature. The strong systems, dialectical, and constructivist orientation of the fourth theory led to its inclusion. We urge nurse readers to explore planned change literature, to analyze other planned change theories, and to evaluate other theories' usefulness.

The use of the Roy Adaptation Model (RAM) in combination with each planned change theory does not suggest that only the RAM would furnish an appropriate nursing perspective from which to view planned change. We chose the RAM because of our familiarity with the model, its widespread use in nursing, its extensive visibility in the nursing literature, its existing rudimentary extension to social organizations, and the need to keep this book at a manageable length. We encourage nurse readers to examine the fit between a strong planned change theory and the nursing model/theory upon which they base their practice.

Basic Considerations in Planned Change

Introduction

Change is difficult. It helps. It hurts. It helps and hurts at the same time. Change is inevitable. We ignore change at our own peril. Steinbeck (1962) wrote that those who resist change experience sadness: They waste their energy; they feel bitter; they cannot enjoy success.

Change requires activism. Alice Walker said that if she were to remain politically inactive, she would feel like a person who eats a good meal but does nothing to prepare for it or clean up afterward (Dreifus, 1989).

Change invites disaster regardless of whether it is unplanned or planned. Careful planning increases the probability of fruitful outcomes and decreases the likelihood of disaster. Careful planning requires thoughtful study. Planned change theories guide thoughtful study and supply tools for nurse planners.

Social change occurs either unconsciously through the transmission of culture over hundreds or thousands of years or by conscious transformation of culture over a shorter time. Some changes by transformation amount to reaction to outside forces to maintain a homeostatic balance. Other changes by transformation involve anticipatory planning in the form of change directed toward self or change directed toward others (Bhola, 1972). Planners can influence change by transformation much more easily than they can influence change by transmission. Very different kinds of theories describe change by transmission and change by transformation. This book deals with change by transformation. It presents engineering theories that relate to consciously planned change.

Change is one of the most reliably constant phenomena in the world. Environmental factors discourage or encourage social change. Instant communication and rapid transportation modes stimulate change by providing a sense of immediacy. Multiple and competing needs, shifting priorities, diminished or increased resources, and altered care practices signal current changes in health care systems. National and international events (Betts, 1996; Canavan, 1996a; Helmlinger, 1996; Nelson et al., 1996) and scientific discoveries precipitate health care change. This chapter addresses the reasons for studying planned change theories and gives a brief introduction to the four planned change theories featured in the book.

Why Study Planned Change Theories?

This portion of the chapter discusses ways that a thoughtful study of planned change theories helps nurses fulfill nursing's social mandate through either direct or indirect avenues of service. Such study encourages the enlargement of nursing's knowledge base, increases the likelihood of research-based nursing practice, and helps nurses make appropriate selections from among existing planned change theories.

Fulfill Nursing's Social Mandate

Nursing's Social Policy Statement (American Nurses Association [ANA], 1995) provides a framework for understanding the relationship between society and nursing. Society's mandate solicits nursing knowledge and skills. In reply, nurses establish the nature and scope of their practice. Nursing practice responds

> # BOX 1.3
>
> *A major part of health care comes from the hearts, heads, and hands of nurses.*

dynamically to advances in scientific knowledge, political and economic environments, legal conditions, and cultural and demographic patterns. The mandate changes over time with respect to nurses' rights, responsibilities, and accountability.

Nurses, in response to their social mandate, provide a critical part of the world's health care as they creatively map the broad outlines and local details of their practices. In some areas, the majority of health care comes from the heads, hearts, and hands of nurses. When adjustments in health care systems threaten patient safety and nursing practice, nurses must act. Therefore, a great need exists for nurses capable of managing successful change (Canavan, 1996a). Nurses must become part of the policy-making process for a transformed health service (Liddy, 1996; Rispel, 1995); they must "sit at the table" where policy making occurs ("IOM [Institute of Medicine] Issues," 1996); they must use cutting-edge technology (Dreher & Dickenson-Hazard, 1996) not only in clinical matters but in terms of current planned change practices.

Dealing with policy issues requires skill in planning change. Results of the recent *American Journal of Nursing (AJN)* Patient Care Survey (Shindul-Rothschild, Berry, & Long-Middleton, 1996), with more than 7,000 respondents, show that many nurses consider current conditions in health care settings to be dangerous and demoralizing for patients and nurses. According to Sosne (1996),

> There can no longer be any doubt about what the corporatization of health care is doing to patients and the health care workforce. The question at hand is how to make sure that the quality of patient care is not further compromised and that erosions in quality are reversed. (p. 42)

In response,

> nursing must unify its efforts to become a powerful force in assisting the health care field with a thoughtful response to the powerful social changes that are now occurring across the country. We must realign our educational programs, our licensure and certification process, and our clinical delivery systems to transcend the old institutional perspective toward one that spans the continuum of services and broaden the episode-of-illness focus toward the life span of the patient. (Koerner, 1996, p. 42)

To follow Koerner's directive, nurses must have skill in influencing policy making and legislation at all levels as they establish, update, and maintain nurse practice acts and standards for nursing education, licensure, and credentialing. Policy realities that surround nursing create the necessity for nurses to plan change as they negotiate remunerative practices, physical and political space for nursing activities, and professional practice boundaries. Nursing has a continuing need to maintain and coordinate the profession's organizations, not only as viable independent entities but as an organized network of agencies seeking the common good for consumers of care and nurses who provide care.

A strong planned change theory helps nurses to resist change as well as to institute change. When players external to the profession improperly seek to alter the nature and scope of nursing practice or institute measures that call nurses to act as consumer advocates (Canavan, 1996a), their proposals require attention. Internally, nursing's widely divergent and loosely defined professional identity serves as an obstacle to effectiveness in political and policy negotiations (Betts, 1996). Appropriate planned change theories can assist nurses who build coalitions that strengthen the profession. Nurses with a thorough preparation for planning change find that knowledge gives power and strength to the profession (Dickenson-Hazard, 1995). Nurses without a thorough preparation for proactive change planning in the political and public policy domain find themselves handicapped in their efforts to fulfill nursing's social mandate.

Follow Two Avenues of Service

Nursing's Social Policy Statement asserts that nurses fulfill their social mandate through two avenues of service: direct service and indirect service. Nurses perform direct service through interaction with patients; indirect service occurs in a setting removed from the patient. Direct service centers on "person" while indirect service centers on the "environment" of care (ANA, 1995).

Direct service. Recipients of direct service include individuals, groups, families, and communities. Change-oriented phenomena of concern to nurses involve consumers of care in experiences of birth, health, illness, and death. Nurses in both basic and advanced practice collaborate in the development and adjustment of social policies (ANA, 1995). Advanced nursing practice, always clinical in nature, requires both specialization (a limited focus) and expanded knowledge. Advanced practice integrates more theoretical, research-based, and practical knowledge than that required for nursing practice at the basic level (ANA, 1995). Advanced practice nurses function as registered nurses with additional, advanced knowledge, not as substitutes for physicians. They offer consumers something different and often more than what other professions provide (Betts, 1996).

BOX 1.4

Indirect service involves the contextual activities that make direct service possible.

BOX 1.5

"The art of nursing ought to include such arrangements as alone make what I understand by nursing, possible" (Nightingale, 1859/1946, p. 6).

Knowledge of planned change increases the likelihood that an advanced practice nurse will make optimum use of advanced clinical knowledge. Advanced practice nurses, by the very nature of their placement in health care systems, often find themselves less likely than nurses in basic practice to work under administrators who take responsibility for instituting the political and policy changes needed to shelter nursing activities. The study of planned change helps advanced practice nurses create change for purposes of consumer advocacy and in response to the professional practice opportunities and restrictions they face.

Advanced practice nurses need planned change knowledge to skillfully manage and lead practice changes that enhance the profession of nursing and contribute to the well-being of consumers (ANA, 1995). An Institute of Medicine (IOM) committee recognized the value of nurses in advanced practice and recommended an increase in their numbers in acute care settings ("IOM Issues," 1996). The IOM committee, like the ANA, expects advanced practice nurses to provide both direct patient care and clinical leadership. A knowledge of planned change theories strengthens their leadership activities.

Indirect service. Indirect service involves the contextual activities that make direct service possible. Florence Nightingale (1859/1946) wrote that "bad sanitary, bad architectural, and bad administrative arrangements often make it impossible to nurse. But the art of nursing ought to include such arrangements as alone make what I understand by nursing, possible" (p. 6).

When nurses perform indirect service, they deal with barriers that individuals, groups, families, or communities (even countries) encounter in obtaining appropriate care (ANA, 1995). Barriers to the quality of care may include layoffs of health care personnel, the increased use of unlicensed personnel, certain regulatory changes to practice, and proposals such as that for registered care technicians (Canavan, 1996a). Proposed change, such as incentive plans for nurses to cut costs, may have the potential for harm; these call for scrutiny

(Canavan, 1996b), internal professional unity, and the support of the consuming public (Wooden, 1996). Potentially harmful situations require nurses to play an essential role as collaborative planners in health care systems.

Reports of positive results of nurse activism exist. Dodd (1996) cited political and policy techniques through which nurses' influence has helped to halt proposals to weaken Medicare and Medicaid. Nurses also have had a voice in the enforcement of safety and health regulations, obtaining adequate funding for the Nurse Education Act, and securing a place in the federal budget proposal for reimbursement for nurse practitioners and clinical nurse specialists.

The nursing voice is important in policy deliberations. About a decade ago, Knaus, Draper, Wagner, and Zimmerman (1986) and Hartz et al. (1989) conducted research that included examination of supportive and nonsupportive climates for nurses. Results linked such factors as appropriate staffing levels and an appropriate administrative climate that provided nurse input in decisions crucial to the well-being and survival of patients in hospitals. More recently, according to Keepnews (1996), early and increased nursing input in an influential committee might have helped the committee understand the urgency of the problem of inadequate nurse staffing levels. Greater nursing input also might have strengthened recommendations developed by foundation researchers. An earlier development of nursing's seven quality indicators (Canavan, 1996a) might have prevented a great many of the negative effects that have befallen hospitalized persons as the result of the restructuring in the past decade. Fortunately, nurses will have a voice in an upcoming Presidential Advisory Commission on Consumer Protection and Quality in the Health Care Industry (Helmlinger, 1996).

Enlarge Nursing's Knowledge Base

According to the *Nursing Social Policy Statement* (ANA, 1995), nurses have a legal obligation to act in society's best interests. Therefore, nursing, as a profession, commits to self-regulation. One aspect of self-regulation concerns accountability for the development and maintenance of nursing's knowledge base. This knowledge base derives from multiple sources. When nurses generate theories and research findings, the knowledge they develop must fit with nursing values about health and illness. Planned change theories can help nurse researchers working in settings where the conduct of nursing research meets resistance or suffers from inertia.

Move Toward Research-Based Practice

As the knowledge base increases, nurses need ways to incorporate new nursing knowledge into their practices. The introduction of new knowledge often

---

BOX 1.6

As nursing's knowledge base increases, nurses need ways to incorporate new nursing knowledge into their practice.

---

meets resistance. Resistance delays research utilization (Haller, Reynolds, & Horsley, 1979; Horsley, Crane, Crabtree, & Wood, 1983). Planned change theories provide useful ways to meet resistance that comes from psychological, environmental, and social factors. Some of nursing's research utilization models appropriately incorporate planned change theories that offer proactive ways of dealing with resistance.

Choose Appropriate Planned Change Theories

Education, management, and the social sciences most frequently provide the sources of planned change theories. A wide knowledge of planned change theories helps nurses to develop, or select from among them, those that relate best to nursing practice issues and values. The *Nursing Social Policy Statement* (ANA, 1995) details a participative, perceptive mode of nursing practice that fits hand in glove with the characteristics of a high-quality planned change theory. The policy statement asserts that nurses attend to the full range of human experience, whether the need for change arises from feelings of unease, a paradigm shift, or an identified problem. Further, the statement implies that nurses often combine the scientific knowledge they possess with an understanding of the subjective experiences of individuals, groups, families, and communities. Nurses value the full and active participation of patients, clients, and themselves. A change theory based on dialectical and constructivist concepts makes similar recommendations.

Within a caring relationship, nurses make diagnoses, choose treatments, intervene, and evaluate outcomes (ANA, 1995). Some change theories contain similar components: a system for diagnosis, a method for developing or choosing an innovation, a way of selecting and sequencing strategies and tactics, and a means of evaluating both the results of an innovation and the quality of the change processes.

Currently, nurses need accurate information about change theories. Studies demonstrate that despite widespread invocation of planned change theories in nursing literature, nurses seldom have used those theories as accurately or fully as they could be used (Hamel-Craig, 1994; Tiffany, Cheatham, Doornbos, Loudermelt, & Momadi, 1994). Further, nurses seldom carefully evaluate borrowed change theories (Tiffany et al., 1994). Nursing situations contain factors

---

BOX 1.7

Planned change theories provide a conceptual ordering that helps nurse planners choose, develop, and sequence activities necessary to conduct a planned change episode.

---

that nonnursing theories do not consider (Chinn & Kramer, 1991). This circumstance highlights the importance of careful study and evaluation of "foreign" planned change theories for congruence with key nursing concepts such as "person" and "environment" before their incorporation into nursing activities. Such careful study and evaluation could enhance the scope, depth, and quality of the planned change theories and models that nurses currently produce or use.

Planned Change Theories

Planned change theories are engineering theories; they put social science to work in planning change. Change planning theories supply four important intellectual tools that tell nurse planners how to cause change. First, planned change theories picture ways that social change takes place; a comprehensive theory enhances the user's understanding of the dynamics of change. Second, a clear and complete planned change theory tells nurse planners how to work with others in change situations.

Third, planned change theories offer viewpoints from which nurse planners can analyze the context of a change situation. This diverse context includes individuals, groups, economic conditions, resources, climate, and infrastructure. Fourth, planned change theories provide a conceptual ordering that helps nurse planners choose, develop, and sequence activities necessary to conduct a planned change episode. Planned change activities include assessment of social situations in the diagnosis of social problems, development (or selection) of solutions, plans for and implementation of strategies and tactics, and evaluation of change events.

The next seven chapters of this book provide general information regarding important aspects of planned change and tell how four planned change theories relate to each topic. Later sections of the book examine the four featured planned change theories/models (the Lewin microtheories; the change writings of Bennis, Benne, and Chin; the Rogers diffusion model; Bhola's CLER model) and their application in much greater depth.

Summary

This chapter asserts that professional nurses need knowledge of planned change theories to assist them in fulfilling social mandates for their practice. Active professional nurses cannot escape planning change as they provide nursing service, enlarge nursing's knowledge base, and move toward research-based practice. Planned change theories are engineering theories that furnish intellectual tools for analysis of change situations. Nurses should choose planned change theories wisely. Not all change theories fit with nursing situations and purposes. Study of planned change theories assists nurses in making wise theory choices among the many available planned change theories/models, including those featured in this book.

References

American Nurses Association (ANA). (1995). *Nursing's social policy statement.* Washington, DC: American Nurses Publishing.

Betts, V. T. (1996, March). Nursing must be strengthened by its diversity. *American Nurse,* p. 4.

Bhola, H. S. (1972). *Configurations of change: An engineering theory of innovation diffusion, planned change, and development.* Bloomington: Indiana University School of Education.

Canavan, K. (1996a, March). ANA asserts attacks on practice threaten safety. *American Nurse,* pp. 1, 9.

Canavan, K. (1996b, March). Incentive programs for nurses surfacing: Does practice undermine nurse-patient bond? *American Nurse,* p. 8.

Chinn, P. L., & Kramer, M. K. (1991). *Theory and nursing: A systematic approach* (3rd ed.). St. Louis: Mosby Year.

Dickenson-Hazard, N. (1995). Advancing science. *Reflections, 21*(3), 2.

Dodd, C. J. (1996, March 20). [Promotional letter]. (Available from ANA-PAC, 600 Maryland Ave., SW, Suite 100 West, Washington, DC 20024-2571)

Dreher, M. C., & Dickenson-Hazard, N. (1996, January). [Membership letter]. (Available from Sigma Theta Tau International, Inc., 550 West North Street, Indianapolis, IN 46202)

Dreifus, C. (1989). Alice Walker: Active voice. *VIS à VIS: The Magazine of United Airlines, Inc., 3*(11), 92.

Haller, K. B., Reynolds, M. A., & Horsley, J. A. (1979). Developing research-based innovation protocols: Process, criteria, and issues. *Research in Nursing and Health, 2,* 45-51.

Hamel-Craig, M. (1994). *Quality of use of planned change theory in nursing periodical literature.* Unpublished master's research project, Andrews University, Berrien Springs, MI.

Hartz, A. J., Krakaur, H., Kuhn, E. M., Young, M., Jacobsen, S. J., Gay, G., Muenz, L., Katzoff, M., Bailey, R. C., & Rimm, A. A. (1989). Hospital characteristics and mortality rates. *New England Journal of Medicine, 321,* 1720-1725.

Helmlinger, C. (1996, November). Washington watch. *American Journal of Nursing,* pp. 21-22.

Horsley, J. A., Crane, J., Crabtree, M. K., & Wood, D. J. (1983). *Using research to improve nursing practice: A guide.* New York: Grune & Stratton.

IOM issues nurse staffing report. (1996, March). *American Nurse,* p. 8.

Keepnews, D. (1996, January-February). ANA challenges Pew Health Professions' findings. *American Nurse,* p. 3.

Knaus, W. A., Draper, E. A., Wagner, D. P., & Zimmerman, J. E. (1986). An evaluation of outcome from intensive care in major medical centers. *Annals of Internal Medicine, 104,* 410-418.

Koerner, J. E. (1996, November). Aspects of a broader truth. *American Journal of Nursing,* pp. 42-43.

Liddy, K. (1996). Urgent visit nurse practitioners. *ISNA Bulletin, 22*(1), 3.

Nelson, M., Proctor, S., Regev, H., Barnes, D., Sawyer, L., Messias, D., Yoder, L., & Meleis, A. I. (1996). The Cairo Action Plan. *Image: Journal of Nursing Scholarship, 28,* 75-80.

Nightingale, F. (1946). *Notes on nursing: What it is and what it is not.* Philadelphia: J. B. Lippincott. (Original work published 1859)

Rispel, L. (1995). Challenges face nurses in Republic of South Africa. *Image: Journal of Nursing Scholarship, 27,* 231-234.

Shindul-Rothschild, J., Berry, D., & Long-Middleton, E. (1996, November). Where have all the nurses gone? Final results of our patient care survey. *American Journal of Nursing,* pp. 25-39.

Sosne, D. (1996, November). Dangerous experiment with human subjects. *American Journal of Nursing,* pp. 41-42.

Steinbeck, J. (1962). *Travels with Charley: In search of America.* New York: Penguin.

Tiffany, C. R., Cheatham, A. B., Doornbos, D., Loudermelt, L., & Momadi, G. G. (1994). Planned change theory: Survey of nursing periodical literature. *Nursing Management, 25*(2), 54-59.

Wooden, J. M. (1996, March). Nursing unity needed to preserve practice. *American Nurse,* p. 4.

Planned Change Theories
Choose Well, Use Well

BOX 2.2: KEY WORDS AND PHRASES

— **Abstraction**
— **Classical theories of
   change**
— **Constructivism**
— **Dialectics**
— **Diffusion**
— **Diffusion theories**
— **Engineering theory**

— **Espoused theory**
— **Generalization**
— **Level of generality**
— **Macrotheory**
— **Metatheory**
— **Microtheory**
— **Model**
— **Theory-in-use**

People have not always accepted the idea that planned change deserves formal study as a feasible, worthy, and essential activity. Early Calvinists, for example, saw societal order as preordained and nonchanging. Under this viewpoint, planned change cannot occur. Later, rationalist thinking claimed that people who have information about the best way to do things will choose that best way. Under the rationalist system, change is feasible. Planners merely supply information—change follows automatically. In the minds of others, planned change amounts to social tinkering, a wrongful violation of natural law. Currently, advertising, along with other pervasive attempts to plan change, constitutes a prevailing facet of modern life. Casual reading of any newspaper shows a widespread value for planned change (Hornstein, Bunker, Burke, Gindes, & Lewicki, 1971). Some would call planned change essential.

Even though widely accepted, planned change carries drawbacks such as unintended consequences (Rogers, 1995) and inefficiency. This book contends that a sound planned change theory or model appropriate to nursing's purposes helps nurse planners avoid pitfalls and achieve desired changes in an effective and efficient manner. This thesis presents the problem as one of choosing a good planned change theory and using it knowledgeably. Choose a good road map and use it well!

This chapter raises and answers several questions. First, what is a theory? A model? And, more specifically, what is a planned change theory? How can a nurse planner choose a sound and appropriate change theory? Last, what makes up good theory usage?

What Is a Theory?

Theories are idea structures. No one can reach out and touch a theory because theories only represent reality. Theories, built from concepts (a particular kind of abstraction), concern traits that phenomena (items of interest such as molecules of a drug, behavioral reactions, or community customs) have in common. Theories propose relationships (more abstractions) that exist among theory concepts.

According to Kaplan (1964), a theory is a hypothetical, conjectural, symbolic construction, a "device for interpreting, criticizing, and unifying established laws, modifying them to fit data unanticipated in their formulation, and guiding the enterprise of discovering new and more powerful generalizations" (p. 295). Chinn and Kramer (1991) wrote that a theory is "a creative and rigorous structuring of ideas that project a tentative, purposeful, and systematic view of phenomena" (p. 72). Theories come in several forms. A *metatheory* is a theory about theory; a *macrotheory* is a very broad theory that encompasses a wide range of phenomena; a *microtheory* has a narrow range of interest. (See other pages in Kaplan, 1964, and Chinn and Kramer, 1991, for fuller discussions of theory components, characteristics, and uses.)

Generality is a trait possessed by theories. Theories do not refer to any particular case in which an observer examined an item or relationship. Instead, they refer to characteristics that the class of items or relationships generally displays, as a class.

Generalization is a process in which observers look at the characteristics of a sample of a class of items of interest and note what they are like, how they behave, and how they relate. Then observers extrapolate by thinking about how other items of this class, in a similar situation, would behave and relate. When these extrapolations occur in a systematic, scientific manner, the resultant generalizations are called *theory.*

Generalization makes a theory useful because it allows application of theory in any appropriate situation. For example, a theory does not explain what motivates one particular 9-year-old boy to practice the piano. Instead, it explains motivation in a way that users can apply to 9-year-old boys as a class, or to workers in a factory, or to mothers receiving child care instructions.

What Is a Model?

Kaplan (1964) likened models to structural analogies: This thing is like that thing—but only in a limited number of important structural aspects. Either a conceptual model or a physical model comes under the *analog* designation. Models approximate or simplify reality (Fawcett, 1995). In a physical model, the likeness may center on external physical characteristics, which a person can reach out and touch, as in the case of a duck and a decoy. A model may use pictures. It may use words or mathematics. Although models and theories have some characteristics in common, a model differs from a theory. Both clarify, depict, and organize. Models are more abstract than theories (Fawcett, 1993, 1995). Theories, therefore, are "closely tied to particular individuals, groups, situations, or events" (Fawcett, 1993, p. 18). Most of this chapter uses the term *theory* in a generic sense. The chapter very briefly introduces several change theories as examples.

Change Theories

Two basic kinds of change theories exist—theories that help people watch change and theories that help people cause change. Classical theories of change are theories that explain (watch) social changes that span thousands of years (Etzioni & Etzioni-Halevy, 1973). Diffusion theories watch change occur during months, years, or decades. Neither kind of theory aims to cause change. Planned change theories, by contrast, are engineering theories that guide planners (Bhola, 1972) over the short or intermediate term, although a planned change episode may have effects that last for millennia.

A planned change theory is a set of logically interrelated concepts that explain, in a systematic way, the means by which planned change occurs, that predict how various forces in an environment will react in specified change situations, and that help planners control variables that increase or decrease the likelihood of the occurrence of change (Tiffany, 1994; Tiffany, Cheatham, Doornbos, Loudermelt, & Momadi, 1994).

Planned change, in this context, refers to deliberately engineered (not haphazard) change that occurs in groups that vary in size from a small group, such as a family, to an entire society. Those who use planned change theories may work with individuals, but their objective is to alter ways of doing things in social systems.

Planned Change Theories: Choose Well

Analysis involves looking at the way a thing is structured and examining the characteristics and workings of its component parts. Analysis has to precede evaluation. Analysis resembles looking at the characteristics of a thing such as a new car (color, power, engine type, shine, style, size, coordination with self-image, price, and so on). Evaluation of the car and how well it suits the driver proceeds according to criteria. Evaluation starts immediately with a mental rehearsal; it continues during the test drive and later use of the car. People who think they have evaluated something without prior analysis no doubt conducted a covert analysis at an earlier time.

Analyze planned change theories. Zajc (1987) offered an in-depth exploration of issues involved with the analysis and evaluation of models of planned change in education. She developed four perspectives for analysis of planned change models (the nature of the main ideology, the ways people perceive reality, viewpoints about human nature, kinds of scientific methods endorsed). She proposed analysis at four levels (model structure, underlying assumptions about change, suggestions for model use supplied by the model developer, use of the model in the real world). Zajc classified and analyzed 47 planned change models from the discipline of education between the late 1950s and the mid-1980s.

Other schemes for analysis of planned change theories exist. Chin and Benne (1985) characterized approaches toward deliberate changing along a continuum ranging from the least coercive (rational-empirical) through middle ground normative-reeducative strategies, to the most obtrusive (power-coercive). Hornstein et al. (1971) clustered change strategies under headings of individually oriented schemes (designed to reach group-oriented objectives), techno-structural strategies that work through organizational structure (the ways people organize themselves to accomplish work), or technology (the ways that people use knowledge to manage raw materials in the work they do). Hornstein et al. also described data-based strategies (which use information), organizational development (a specific system that uses behavioral science knowledge to renew organizations), violence and coercion, and nonviolent and direct-action strategies such as those employed in the civil rights movement in the southern United States.

Evaluate planned change theories. Tiffany (1994) and Lutjens and Tiffany (1994) considered analysis of planned change theories an essential part of making a choice among them. They used concepts from nursing and nonnursing literature in the development of a procedure designed to measure the quality of a planned change theory both in general terms and in terms of the goodness of fit between a planned change theory and nursing. (See Appendix B.) Just as prospective car owners have to think about the cars they hope to purchase, so those who use the Tiffany and Lütjens procedure need to familiarize themselves with the planned change theories they intend to evaluate. They do this through careful study of reliable literature such as primary sources and the in-depth discussions in this book. The Tiffany-Lutjens procedure (Tiffany et al., 1995) serves as a study guide as planners read change theory literature. Study of a planned change theory enhances the quality of measurement the procedure provides.

Planned Change Theories: Use Well

Hamel-Craig (1994) studied the quality of planned change theory usage in nursing's English-language periodical literature over a two-year period. She found that many nursing periodical articles present, choose, or apply planned change theories improperly. Adequate knowledge precedes appropriate theory choice; appropriate choice precedes efficient and effective use.

Kaplan (1964) wrote that theory must answer to what is in God's world. Theory is of practice—provided that a theory is used properly and its contexts of application are "suitably specified." *Contexts,* in this sense, refers to ideological and practical constraints that surround theory usage. Two major considerations govern the choice of suitable contexts for theory application. These include the nature of assumptions underlying the theory and the level of generality of the theory.

Theory assumptions and theory context. Planned Change theory users should consider the fit between a theory's foundational assumptions and several factors in the practical situation. Theory foundations include general assumptions about the nature of humans and of the world. They also include more specific ideas about knowledge transfer processes, education versus coercion, and proper roles for planners and adopters. Important theory assumptions surround questions of what constitutes proper distributions of power and status, of economic and educational goods. Planners should align theory assumptions with the realities of the local situation. What political realities exist? What personal and professional philosophies do planners hold? How does the practice context coincide with the theory developer's assumptions? These questions deserve study because they pinpoint seemingly small variations that create enormous differences when planners use theories in the real world.

Nurses, for example, value participative decision making, planner-adopter cooperation, and collaboration. According to Macke (1995), collaboration is one of the key skills that nurses need upon entry into the twenty-first century. Transformational nursing processes push collaboration into the forefront as nurses participate in the transformation of the health care system. Thus provision for collaboration between planners and adopters constitutes one of the key concepts that nurse planners will seek in a planned change theory.

Levels of generality. Kaplan (1964) noted that the level of generality of a theory refers to several characteristics, which include theory scope and degree of abstractness. Some planned change theories, especially those founded on systems theory, seem to take in everything in the whole world. As a safety mechanism, a theorist might tell users that they must exclude unessentials to avoid drowning in details. Other theories center on specific processes in well-defined localities. In all instances, planners must harmonize the theory they choose with the organizational component involved. They need to decide whether to include the whole institution or community or a particular segment of it. Theory users locate the origin of the impetus toward change. They also have to determine who constitutes the planning team, and whether or how planners and adopters will change roles. Time spent on accomplishing these intellectual tasks pays handsome dividends.

Theory Combinations?

This book offers several planned change theories and models, variously named. (We have taken at face value the labels that the various theorists gave their systems.) Lewin (1951) called the products of his work "theories." Cook (1986) classed Lewin's formulations as "minitheories"; Kaplan (1964) probably would have named them "microtheories." When Bennis, Benne, and Chin (1985) combined their ideas with those of their invited authors in an edited book, they made no claim to have developed either a model or a theory. Instead, they termed the result of their work a book of "readings." Rogers (1995) and Bhola (1994) developed "models." All presented plans for watching change or for causing it. Blueprints for change vary greatly in origin, level, scope, and degree of completeness; each makes valuable and unique suggestions for planners. Should planners ever combine them? Some say "no," others say "yes."

Purists say, "No." A forced fit used to combine theories bends the theories in question "out of shape." Theories considered for combination may have diverse worldviews, backgrounds, characteristics, assumptions, and levels of generality. One theory's characteristics might fit so poorly with those of another theory that a combination might invalidate one or the other. Further, combinations pose a special danger when users possess only a superficial understanding of the theories in question. Last, two half theories do not necessarily make a whole theory; readers might have trouble creating one congruent frame of reference from them.

Practitioners say, "Yes (but take care)." Wade Lancaster (1982) noted that every planner, consciously or unconsciously, develops models that direct action. Of course, these models are not theories; instead, they are mechanisms for getting a hold on the complex reality that confronts the planner. Humans have no choice but to devise their own realities by using whatever tools (knowledge, experiences, worldviews, and so on) they have on hand.

Even some theorists request combinations of various sorts. Bhola (1982), for example, overtly stated that users of his Configurations (CLER) Model should bring with them as much social science knowledge as they can. He expected planners to find and apply strategies under the umbrella of the CLER Means × Ends element. Lewin's microtheories lack three of the four parts needed for a complete planned change theory. His theories are sophisticated strategies; must planners abandon these useful inventions because of their incompleteness? Probably not.

Argyris and Schön (1985) discussed the differences between espoused theories and theories-in-use. Practitioners who put espoused theories to work find themselves prone to alter the theories. Kaplan (1964) noted the danger of working with too few models, or with models too much alike. Neither did he want to see practitioners belittle entities other than models.

The question should not ask whether, but how. How should planners make combinations? Planners should study a theory, understand its structure, its philosophical base and assumptions, its worldview, its strong and weak points, what it contains and what it does not contain. They should think about what would happen or not happen with various combinations in use. When they consider a combination of a planned change theory with a nursing theory, planners should translate the theory of interest into terms congruent with the nursing theory under consideration, taking care not to warp either theory. Paragraphs that give ideas to consider in several change theory combinations follow the short theory descriptions that appear below. Longer theory descriptions and combinations of change theory and nursing theory appear later in the book.

Characteristics of Specific Planned Change Theories

The choice of three of the four theories featured here (microtheories by Lewin; change writings edited by Bennis, Benne, and Chin; a diffusion model by Rogers) resulted from their popularity among nurses. Researchers (Tiffany et al., 1994) measured popularity by counting the frequency of theory use by nurse authors of change-related articles in nursing periodical literature. The fourth, a model developed by Bhola, is new to most nurses.

Lewin's Microtheories

Lewin's microtheories rank, by far, as the most popular change theories among nurses. What nurse has not heard of "unfreeze, move, (re)freeze"? Yet nurses and nonnurses alike routinely use these theories in a superficial manner scarcely befitting their scientific worth. Lewin's planned change theories are a series of small, closely knit, specific theories that present related, tightly structured strategies. Cook (1986) called them minitheories. Their scope and structure place them in a category that Kaplan (1964) and Chinn and Kramer (1991) called microtheory. Lewin's microtheories contain no system for social system problem diagnosis or for the choice or development of an innovation. They say almost nothing about evaluation of either the processes or the outcomes of change (Lewin, 1951).

Lewin developed all his theories through experimentation, a new method in the field of psychology at the time he worked. The top-down stance of his theories, although widely used in the management world at the time he wrote, runs counter to nursing's values for mutuality. During the last months of his life, Lewin started a program of group dynamics and action research that featured cooperative planning. Lewin, in fact, led the field in proposals for participation, cooperation, and collaboration. Bennis, Benne, and Chin founded many of their ideas about mutuality on Lewin's pioneering efforts. Later authors often credited Lewin for the concepts he was not able to publish.

Lewin's work has suffered from oversimplification by users, perhaps because his language, many formulas, and numerous detailed figures intimidate uninitiated readers. Learning his terminology and studying his formulas and figures would help nurse planners understand his microtheories and use them as sophisticated planned change strategies.

Writings Edited by Bennis, Benne, and Chin (BB&C)

Benne worked with Lewin at the National Training Laboratories before 1947. The cooperative planning evident in Lewin's unfinished work features prominently in the Bennis, Benne, and Chin (1961, 1969, 1985) and Bennis, Benne, Chin, and Corey (1976) books, *The Planning of Change*. Their perspectives emerge from within sections the authors themselves wrote as well as in the sections written by invited authors whose ideas reflected the authors' viewpoints. They did not claim to build a tight, small theory of their own. Instead, they assembled an entire book of readings pertinent to planned change. They tried to meet practical, moral, and ethical challenges by presenting appropriate technologies suitable for educating planners of change.

A general organizational pattern connects the diverse concerns presented in the 1985 edition of the Bennis, Benne, and Chin book. Some book sections give very abstract theoretical material; others have a specific outlook. These editors advocated planner-target cooperation and offered specific ways to implement it. They or their invited authors addressed the matter of problem diagnosis and the choice or development of innovations in a number of places in their book. They also emphasized strategy, while evaluation received less attention. The section on moral and ethical issues addresses practical concerns as well as moral and ethical matters that planners face in the conduct of change. Some readers feel intimidated by language in some parts of the BB&C books and the BBC&C book but many other sections give easy access to ideas. Some of the sections contain material now outdated.

The Rogers Diffusion Model

Research concerning the spread of agricultural innovations under development in Iowa influenced the work of Rogers. Rogers expanded the idea of an adoption frequency curve, which appeared both in 1903 and later in a Ryan and Gross (1943) study of the diffusion of hybrid seed corn. The Rogers model traces the diffusion, over time, of an innovation in a social unit. It offers many implications for planning change. In a tightly structured, linear, time-oriented sequence, it deals with the specifics of prior conditions, characteristics of innovations and adopters, and adopter decisions.

Rogers attempted to put organizational variables into his model but the 1983 and 1995 versions showed no essential change from the earlier stance. His model gives almost no attention to social problem diagnosis. It places major emphasis on characteristics of innovations. The model features communication (mainly one way) almost to the exclusion of other strategies. The Rogers model pays major attention to evaluating the outcomes of adoption of innovations; this is one of the model's strengths. Evaluation of strategies centers mainly on communication strategies.

The Rogers model advocates cooperative interaction between planners and adopters mainly by implication. Users find the Rogers writings informative, integrated, and easy to read. The model lends itself well to descriptive diffusion research that pictures the spread of new practices among members of a particular population.

Bhola's Configurations (CLER) Model

Bhola's Configurations, Linkages, Environment, and Resources (CLER) Model shows the influence of his eclectic background in physics, mathematics, English literature, education, and literacy. The evolution of CLER began when Bhola accepted the task of organizing a set of more than 300 cards bearing statements about planned change. Interested both in planned change and in theory, Bhola worked on what he then called an engineering theory. His work resulted in a systems-oriented planned change model that attends to the complexities of modern change situations. The CLER model aims to cause change. It contains all four parts necessary for a planned change theory and operates at a high level of generality.

Bhola linked model concepts together in a large and logically integrated structure founded on systems, dialectical, and constructivist theories. This model requires very high levels of collaboration between planners and targets of change; no one who uses it properly devises an autocratic, top-down change sequence. Bhola provided practical steps to guide model users as they plan a change episode. The unfamiliar language of this model has intimidated first-time nurse readers, who often become converts after they achieve familiarity with model concepts.

Combinations of Planned
Change Theories and Models

The following sections compare and contrast the various theories and models highlighted in this book and present some factors users will want to think about if they consider combining them.

Lewin's Microtheories
and BB&C's Writings

The foundational assumptions of these two systems differ greatly: Lewin proposed top-down change; BB&C mandate high levels of adopter participation. (Lewin's theories do not prohibit participation—they simply do not mandate it. Judging from Lewin's last, unfinished work, planner-adopter cooperation eventually would have filtered into his theories.) Levels of generality also differ: Lewin provided microtheories; BB&C, a collection of diverse essays. Planners who use this combination will need to make reasoned choices from among the very diverse ideas in the BB&C book sections and add them to the Lewin theories to structure practical strategies.

Lewin's Microtheories and
the Rogers Diffusion Model

The Lewin theories and the Rogers model have similar foundational assumptions; both deal with top-down change. Lewin causes it; Rogers watches it (but furnishes implications for planners). Both systems virtually omit diagnosis and offer little content regarding evaluation of change processes. The Lewin microtheories occupy a more specific level of generality than does the Rogers model; planners could use them as strategies within the Rogers model.

Lewin's Microtheories
and Bhola's CLER Model

Lewin's theories do not incorporate CLER assumptions about participation but neither do they rule out participation. Any Lewin-CLER combination would include collaboration. CLER, a model with all four parts essential to a complete change theory, operates at a very high level of generality; Lewin microtheories would help make CLER practical if planners can devise ways to measure forces in what CLER calls the "environment." CLER easily accommodates information from outside itself if that information coincides with CLER's basic assumptions (foundational theories) of systems, dialectics, and constructivism.

BB&C's Writings and
the Rogers Diffusion Model

The BB&C writings stress participation and ethics to a much larger extent than does the Rogers model. The Rogers model deals with innovations more thoroughly than do the BB&C writings. The Rogers model is geared more to watching change than to causing change; the BB&C ideas aim to cause change.

The BB&C system operates at a much more general level than does the Rogers model. Planners who combine the two systems might find the task difficult because the two systems possess such different assumptions.

BB&C's Writings and
Bhola's CLER Model

Because the BB&C and CLER systems share many basic assumptions, planners might be able to combine them profitably. Planners could follow the pragmatic framework given by CLER as an organizer more easily than they could develop a specific course of action from the whole of the diverse BB&C writings. Specific sections in the BB&C books offer many practical ideas and insights that would lend themselves well to formation of the specific strategies that CLER expects planners to choose or develop. The BB&C system also contributes specific ideas about ethics.

The Rogers Diffusion Model
and Bhola's CLER Model

The basic assumptions of these two models differ widely. First, the Rogers model watches diffusion, and CLER is a model designed specifically for causing change to occur. Further, CLER mandates planner-adopter interaction; the Rogers model addresses the issue by implication. CLER is the more general of the two models. In a combination of the two models, the Rogers model would contribute specific ideas about innovation and population characteristics. A researcher might use the Rogers model to track diffusion that was planned and carried out under the CLER framework.

Summary

In times past, people thought that planned change was impossible or wrong. Society now accepts planned change as a usual event, and scholars have developed many planned change theories.

A theory is an idea structure, an abstraction. It makes general statements that explain and predict how a certain class of phenomena operate in the real world. Application allows theory users to control the circumstances encountered in research or practice.

A model is an analogy that (through a physical structure, a narrative, mathematics, a picture, or the like) draws parallels between the structure of the model and what the model represents. A model helps model users plan a course of action for dealing with a situation at hand.

A planned change theory is a theory that explains how change occurs. It predicts the results of certain classes of change strategies and tactics. A planned change theory should have four parts: a system for diagnosis of social problems, a means for selecting or developing an innovation, a way to choose and implement strategies for causing change, and methods for evaluation of outcomes and processes.

Nurse planners would do well to study, analyze, and evaluate the planned change theories they intend to apply in real-world situations. They can use the procedure developed by Tiffany et al. (1995) for this purpose. It will serve as both a study guide and a vehicle for theory evaluation.

For high-quality planned change theory use, planners must make an appropriate fit between the assumptions of a theory and the characteristics of the real-world change situation. They also should consider the fit between the level of generality of the theory or model and the level of the unit targeted for change.

Planned change theories and models differ in scope and intent. Planners who decide to combine theories and/or models should give careful consideration to their characteristics so that they can make logical and useful combinations and avoid ill-fated mutations. They need an adequate fund of knowledge about the theories in question before they attempt to combine them. As examples, the chapter gives short summaries of several planned change theories and suggests benefits and pitfalls that might result from theory combinations.

References

Argyris, C., & Schön, D. A. (1985). Evaluating theories of action. In W. G. Bennis, K. D. Benne, & R. Chin (Eds.), *The planning of change* (4th ed., pp. 108-117). New York: Holt, Rinehart & Winston.

Bennis, W. G., Benne, K. D., & Chin, R. (Eds.). (1961). *The planning of change: Readings in the applied behavioral sciences* (1st ed.). New York: Holt, Rinehart & Winston.

Bennis, W. G., Benne, K. D., & Chin, R. (Eds.). (1969). *The planning of change* (2nd ed.). New York: Holt, Rinehart & Winston.

Bennis, W. G., Benne, K. D., & Chin, R. (Eds.). (1985). *The planning of change* (4th ed.). New York: Holt, Rinehart & Winston.

Bennis, W. G., Benne, K. D., Chin, R., & Corey, K. E. (Eds.). (1976). *The planning of change* (3rd ed.). New York: Holt, Rinehart & Winston.

Bhola, H. S. (1972). *Configurations of change: An engineering theory of innovation diffusion, planned change, and development.* Bloomington: Indiana University School of Education.

Bhola, H. S. (1982). Planning change in education and development: The CLER model in the context of a mega model. *Viewpoints in Teaching and Learning, 58*(4), 1-35.

Bhola, H. S. (1994). The CLER model: Thinking through change. *Nursing Management, 25*(5), 59-63.

Chin, R., & Benne, K. D. (1985). General strategies for effecting change in human systems. In W. G. Bennis, K. D. Benne, & R. Chin (Eds.), *The planning of change* (4th ed.) (pp. 108-117). New York: Holt, Rinehart & Winston.

Chinn, P. L., & Kramer, M. K. (1991). *Theory and nursing: A systematic approach.* St. Louis: Mosby Yearbook.

Cook, S. (1986). An overall view. In E. Stivers & S. Wheelan (Eds.), *The Lewin legacy: Field theory in current practice* (pp. xi-xiv). New York: Springer-Verlag.

Etzioni, A., & Etzioni-Halevy, E. (1973). *Social change: Sources, patterns, and consequences* (2nd ed.). New York: Basic Books.

Fawcett, J. (1993). *Analysis and evaluation of nursing theories.* Philadelphia: Davis.

Fawcett, J. (1995). *Analysis and evaluation of conceptual models of nursing* (3rd ed.). Philadelphia: Davis.

Hamel-Craig, M. (1994). *Quality of use of planned change theory in nursing periodical literature.* Unpublished master's research project, Andrews University, Berrien Springs, MI.

Hornstein, H. H., Bunker, B. B., Burke, W. W., Gindes, M., & Lewicki, R. J. (1971). *Social intervention: A behavioral science approach.* New York: Free Press.

Kaplan, A. (1964). *The conduct of inquiry: Methodology for behavioral science.* Scranton, PA: Chandler.

Lancaster, W. (1982). Model building and the change process. In J. Lancaster & W. Lancaster (Eds.), *Concepts for advanced nursing practice: The nurse as a change agent.* St. Louis: Mosby.

Lewin, K. (1951). *Field theory in social science.* New York: Harper.

Lutjens, L. R. J., & Tiffany, C. R. (1994). Evaluating planned change theories. *Nursing Management, 25*(3), 54-57.

Macke, E. (1995, August). President's message: Professional collaboration imperative. *S.T.A.T.: Start Taking Action Today (District One, Indiana State Nurses Association).* (Newsletter available from ISNA District 1, 1710 W 100 N, Angola, IN 46703)

Rogers, E. M. (1983). *Diffusion of innovations* (3rd ed.). New York: Free Press.

Rogers, E. M. (1995). *Diffusion of innovations* (4th ed.). New York: Free Press.

Ryan, B., & Gross, N. C. (1943). The diffusion of hybrid seed corn in two Iowa communities. *Rural Sociology, 8,* 15-24.

Tiffany, C. R. (1994). Analysis of planned change theories. *Nursing Management, 25*(2), 60-62.

Tiffany, C. R., Cheatham, A. B., Doornbos, D., Loudermelt, L., & Momadi, G. G. (1994). Planned change theory: Survey of nursing periodical literature. *Nursing Management, 25*(7), 54-59.

Tiffany, C. R., Lutjens, L. R. J., Dwyer, L., Watson, C., Wietor, B., & Willison, S. (1995). Development and initial assessment of the Tiffany/Lütjens Planned Change Theory Evaluation Instrument. *Nursing Administration Quarterly, 19*(2), 75-76.

Zajc, L. (1987). Models of planned educational change: Their ideational and ideological contexts and evolution since the late 1950s. *Dissertation Abstracts International, 48,* 05A. (University Microfilms No. AAC87-17840)

Power

Fuel for Your Engine

BOX 3.1: LOOKING AHEAD

Chapter 3: Power: Fuel for Your Engine
Ways to View Power
Power in Planned Change Theories
Power for Nurse Planners

BOX 3.2: KEY WORDS AND PHRASES

— **Collaboration**
— **Destructive power**
— **Doctor-nurse game**
— **Economic power**
— **Force field**
— **Integrative power**
— **Levers of nurse power**
— **Power as ability**

— **Power as compliance**
— **Power-coercive strategies**
— **Power field**
— **Power trap**
— **Sacrifice trap**
— **Space allocation**
— **Threat power**

If nurse planners wish to achieve success, they must think of social power as an integral component of planned change. Gilbert (1995) reproved those who write or speak about empowerment without first defining *power*. This chapter first defines *power* before it tells how planned change theories view power. It then discusses power in the context of planned change in nursing.

BOX 3.3

Social change is "the creation of new power experiences for individuals and new power relationships among individuals, groups, and structures" (Bhola, 1975, p. 22).

Ways to View Power

This section describes three ways of looking at social power. The first way views power as an inherent ability that every person has. The second focuses on compliance. The third sees power as having three faces. Views of power deserve consideration because of the essential nature of power, but not all views of power have equal utility in the planning of change. Further, nurse planners' ideas about power shape the direction and the chances for success of the change activities they propose and direct.

Power as Ability

Under the ability viewpoint, power is more than a relationship between two actors. All living persons, thus all nurses, have power. People vary in the amounts of power they possess. Two people in the same power transaction at the same time may experience power in different systems. Both can win because each marches to a different drummer (Bhola, 1975). Hawks (1991), who used the Walker and Avant (1988) system of concept analysis, saw this kind of power as "power to."

The ability perspective claims that certain procedures (i.e., inclusion of individuals in decisions that affect them) increase commitment. Under this view, the power bucket can expand and the enlarged bucket can hold more power than the smaller bucket. An increase in commitment harnesses increased amounts of power. Hoarding power decreases it and weakens the organization (Tannenbaum, 1968). Increased commitment enlarges the total amount of power and makes more power available for change planners to use. This increase enhances the likelihood of successful change planning if planners use the available power wisely. (See Figure 3.1.)

Nurse planners who operate under change theories that coincide with the ability view of power will take care to give members of their planning team and of the adopter population a stake in decisions that affect them. These planners will tend to choose change theories that provide for ample collaboration by means of dialogue and shared decision making.

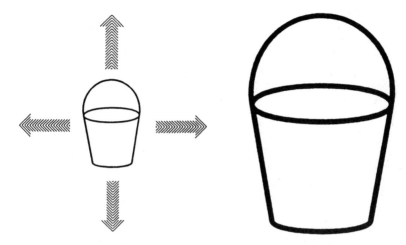

Figure 3.1. Collaboration Fosters the Commitment That Expands the Power Bucket

Figure 3.2. The Compliance View of Social Power Describes Power as Similar to a Fixed Quantity of Water in a Rigid Bucket

Power as Compliance

The compliance view of power requires at least two people. This view defines power as one actor's ability to influence another person to do what the first actor wants (Etzioni, 1961; French & Raven, 1959). Hawks (1991) called this "power over." The compliance definition finds expression in the common belief that social power is like water in a rigid bucket; the bucket can't expand and it contains a fixed amount of water. Therefore, power allocation gives limited amounts of power to individuals (or they grab it!). (See Figure 3.2.) The 1960s saw popular definitions of power that featured compliance of one person with the wishes or demands of another. Several compliance definitions appear in Table 3.1.

Nurse planners who view power as the compliance of one person with the wishes or demands of another will tend to choose change theories that suggest or mandate strong persuasion or coercion. They will look favorably upon theories that make no provision for collaboration among change planners or between planners and adopters.

Three Faces of Power

Boulding (1989) saw the compliance view as unnecessarily restrictive and proposed a larger perspective. He wrote that power has three faces: (a) threat

TABLE 3.1 Compliance-Oriented Definitions of Social Power

In *expert power*, others think the "expert" has superior knowledge about and tells the truth about very specific areas. Some "halo effect" may exist (French & Raven, 1959). Well-educated nurses illustrate expert power.

Coercive power depends on the severity of threatened punishment and the probability of punishment (French & Raven, 1959). Threatened punishment takes the form of restricted movement, denial of satisfaction of needs, or pain, deformity, or death (Etzioni, 1961). Superiors who can hire and fire wield some coercive power.

Reward power concerns the allocation of such rewards as money and nonmonetary fringe benefits, services, and so on. (Etzioni, 1961; French & Raven, 1959). Superiors who can adjust wages and benefits have reward power.

Legitimate power stems from internalized values that say that persons in certain positions must influence lower participants who, in turn, must comply (Etzioni, 1961). Nursing instructors have legitimate power.

Referent power stems from values about attractiveness and the desires of some to identify with those they consider attractive (French & Raven, 1959). Popular entertainment and sports personalities have referent power.

Normative power exists when leaders control symbols that allocate rewards such as prestige, public esteem, and acceptance (Etzioni, 1961). Superiors such as directors and administrators have normative power.

Option power rests on the number and attractiveness of options available to an actor (Thibaut & Kelly, 1959). A young nurse whose nurse manager wants to keep her or him on the job and who has won a scholarship to enter a graduate program has option power.

power (destructive elements), (b) economic (exchange) power, and (c) integrative power (love). Integrative power transcends the other types. No one type exists in isolation from the others; all three exist simultaneously in varying amounts. They interact in complex ways. For example, political power, with a large threat element, needs some kind of monetary input, often in the form of campaign contributions. It also must have some integrative power that inspires a measure of respect for political leaders. Collaboration, a concept analyzed by nurse authors Henneman, Lee, and Cohen (1995), acts as a universal survival strategy that unconsciously produces integrative power.

Nurse planners who view power through the Boulding descriptions will choose change theories that allow for a complex interplay among the various forces found in a change situation. They will consider what kinds of power are necessary to the change effort at each stage of the change episode and will plan to develop the most appropriate face of power at the most opportune time.

Power in Planned Change Theories

Some change theories almost ignore power concerns. Others see power as a multifaceted, inherent, and important characteristic of living persons. Others view power in compliance terms. The following paragraphs present power from the perspective of the four planned change theories highlighted in this book.

Lewin's Microtheories

Lewin wrote a great deal about force fields and very little about power. In his theories, a power field and a force field possess separate conceptual dimensions. Power refers to the likelihood that one person will induce forces on someone else (compliance model). Conversely, a force field is the total of the influences toward change or toward nonchange present in the physical and social environment of an individual or group. These influences come from people and other entities in the field (Lewin, 1951).

Bennis, Benne, and Chin's Writings

Bennis, Benne, and Chin (BB&C) and their invited authors (1985) dealt with a great many power concepts. Their chart of change strategies (pp. 44-45) devotes about one fourth of its space to power-coercive strategies of deliberate change. For BB&C, power-coercive strategies fall into the compliance category and do not fit requirements of present-day society. They do not advocate the use of power-coercive change strategies.

The BB&C book takes readers beyond the compliance viewpoint into the power-as-ability camp. One of their invited authors (Snyder, 1985) provided a discussion of levers of organizational power that include a participative, collaborative management style; a strong "people orientation"; and a loose organizational structure. Kennedy (1985) wrote about the incredible value of human beings in getting things done. Mason and Mitroff (1985) described a power-oriented theory of strategy that centers on cooperation among organizational participants. None of these essays ignores the compliance aspects of power but all three reason from a power-as-ability viewpoint. The essays also have an implicit relationship with the ideas found in Boulding's (1989) three faces of power.

The Rogers Diffusion Model

The 1983 and 1995 editions of the Rogers book do not index the word *power.* The *structure* of the Rogers diffusion model makes no provision for power and little provision for collaboration between planners and adopters but this does not mean that the Rogers model lacks attention to power. The model approaches power issues from an another perspective. For example, Rogers and Shoemaker (1971) connected the compliance concept of power with ethical concerns surrounding collective adoption decisions, power distributions in society, and the distribution of "Good" among people in various socioeconomic levels. Both the 1983

BOX 3.4

Knowledge of power and how to use it is no luxury in today's nursing world.

---

and 1995 editions of the Rogers book expand upon the idea of social equality or inequality, and thus power balances, as an outcome of an adoption decision.

Bhola's Configurations (CLER) Model

Bhola definitely used an ability viewpoint of power in his CLER model. He wrote that "to *be* is to be power*ful*" (Bhola, 1975, pp. 6, 7). He defined power as an active principle, an inherent characteristic of every living person. Inequality of power within and among groups and institutions makes possible such societal work as social change. Groups are power fields with multiple power transactions and controls among and between individual members. CLER requires planners to identify and work with centers of social power as part of planning and intervention processes.

Berle's (1969) five natural laws of power and Bhola's (1972) corollaries to them state that power fills any social vacuum created by chaos; the absence of power breeds anarchy, not freedom. Only individual persons possess power; there is no such thing as, for example, class power. Power always stems from ideology and depends on institutions. Responsibility invariably accompanies power. Bhola (1975) noted that equating power with coercion and force generates a narrow and negative position.

Power for Nurse Planners

Social power is the electricity that brings social change planning to life; no change occurs without power. Therefore, nurse planners must learn how to obtain and use power. Bhola (1975) wrote that civilization would be impossible if power did not exist or were not used in responsible ways. Thus the study of power forms an essential part of any educational program. Studying power helps nurses employ power and equips them to deal with power distributions in civilized ways.

For example, knowledge of power network languages empowers nurses, as occurs when nurses use institutional dialects to negotiate appropriate space allocations for nursing activities. Lack of knowledge of power and failure to use available power networks weakens nurses. For example, clinically competent and beloved nurse manager who did not understand accounting language could

---

BOX 3.5

Education at its best is education in power (Bhola, 1975).

---

not read financial printouts. This manager did not detect the sabotage efforts of a finance person who inserted misplaced financial charges designed to ruin the manager's reputation as a financial conservative. As a result, she lost her position.

Nurses who consult with one another form networks that strengthen them individually as well as collectively. A study (Hofling, Brotzman, Dalrymple, Graves, & Pierce, 1966) in which nurses were not allowed to converse with one another regarding a bogus prescription for a medication overdose showed that 95% of nurses in the sample would have given a spuriously prescribed drug overdose. When Rank and Jacobson (1977) repeated the study in two hospitals, they reasoned that networking among nurses is the norm, not the exception. They allowed their nurse subjects to network as usual. Noncompliance with the bogus order reached 90% in one hospital and 88% in the second. When their study results refuted the findings of the earlier study, Rank and Jacobson reasoned that networks helped the nurse subjects resist practices harmful to themselves and to others.

The following subsections discuss sources of power for nurse planners, the relationship between monopolies and (nurse) power, abstention from power, and the use and misuse of social power.

Sources of power. The most important power source for nurse planners is the power they already have. Labelle (1986) cited existing levers of nurse power that have close connections with the public good. Nurses work at many levels of the health care system—primary, secondary, and tertiary. They practice nursing in diverse settings and constitute the largest group of health care providers in most countries of the world. Nursing organizations exist in many thousands of communities and in states, provinces, and countries; nurses form professional associations easily. Nurses contact consumers directly; they often put consumers in touch with other health care and illness-care professionals. Nurses possess and control vast amounts of information. They have knowledge, competencies, and skills from scientific training. Not only do nurses access communication channels regularly, they vote.

Monopolies. Like other professions, nursing is a monopoly. States have licensing laws for nurses; licensing laws create monopolies and prevent competition. Not only do they protect the public, professional monopolies generate power for professions. For example, many registered nurses and allied health professionals have sufficient knowledge and skill to function safely in independent (or interdependent) roles and to serve as entry points into the illness-care system. But physicians often have legal control over the sale of hospital services, prescription drugs, the services of registered nurses and allied health professionals, and medical devices.

Nurses in advanced practice should remember that some checks and balances among professions exist. Krause (1977) reported a 1968 Supreme Court ruling that said the people provide professions with a mandate for practice and the people can take it away. Charles F. Rule (1988), speaking for the Antitrust Division of the federal government, warned the House of Delegates of the American Medical Association that physicians do not have the right to override competition from other professions (this includes nurses in advanced practice) by whatever means they choose. To break antitrust rules could result in loss of personal freedom (i.e., jail terms). Physicians may not, among themselves, conspire to restrict consumers' preferences.

Abstention from power. Powerlessness and abstention from power deserve differentiation. Powerlessness involves lack of capacity; abstention entails a decision. Boulding (1989) wrote that the renunciation of power involves the freest exercise of human will. Conversely, striving for greatness equals folly because striving erodes integrative power and causes economic impoverishment. Kanter (1983) described managers who give their original ideas to their teams and take care not to claim credit. They increase the total power supply when they let the team harvest the rewards of developing the idea.

Power use and misuse. Power is neutral, neither good nor bad. Power does not corrupt; power misuse does. Power misuse destroys power by making it unavailable for constructive purposes. The resultant vacuum creates powerlessness. In Boulding's (1989) terms, each of the threat, exchange, and love faces of power contains destructive, productive, and integrative characteristics, but in different proportions. He contends that the destructive elements of threat power consume such large amounts of energy that little good results from threat. Lack of power, like poverty, is evil; it prevents individuals from realizing their potentials. Kanter (1978) wrote that persons operating in environments of powerlessness pay a great deal of attention to rules, guard their domains, and dominate others. Their weapon of choice is holding everyone else back.

Nurses must learn to identify themselves and their opinions, to respect themselves and what they think. They must trust self and trust potential partners. Nurses must learn to work with other professionals as colleagues rather than as servants (Hassenflug, 1977).

Nurses can combat some of the negative effects of power misuse and powerlessness by adopting a proactive stance. A good planned change theory will help them identify centers of power and will give them guidelines for dealing realistically with situations where otherwise they might succumb to powerlessness.

Nurses need to identify power traps. These include the doctor-nurse game (Stein, 1967; Stein, Watts, & Howell, 1990), "sweet suffering" (Shainess, 1984), the sacrifice trap (Boulding, 1989), lack of knowledge of essential topics such as space allocation policies and accounting, and courtesy that disguises ulterior motives.

Nurses cannot afford permanent disenchantment. They have important, critical, and enduring work to do. Nurses have the respect of others as a result of their social commitment and highly specialized knowledge. Nurses should remember that they do hold power in their hands. Nurses face a new challenge to increase their power by combining self-regard with their deep interest in others (Donley, 1989).

Summary

This chapter presented three views of social power: power as ability, power as compliance, and power as an entity with three faces that Boulding called threat power, economic power, and integrative power. The discussion summarized views of power taken by four planned change theories: Lewin's microtheories (compliance), Bennis, Benne, and Chin's planned change writings (power as ability), Rogers's diffusion model (compliance), and Bhola's CLER model (power as ability). The section on power and nurse planners considered sources of power for nurses. Nurses must confront power in a personal way. They may abstain from use of certain kinds of power to prevent power misuse by themselves and by others. One challenge for nurses lies in the area of avoiding power traps. Only by combining healthy self-regard with the tradition of caring that has distinguished nursing for centuries can nurses maintain hope for the future.

References

Bennis, W. B., Benne, K. D., & Chin, R. (1985). *The planning of change* (4th ed.). New York: Holt, Rinehart & Winston.

Berle, A. A. (1969). *Power.* New York: Harcourt, Brace, & World.

Bhola, H. S. (1972). Notes toward a theory: Cultural action as elite initiatives in affiliation/exclusion. *Viewpoints, 48*(3), 1-37.

Bhola, H. S. (1975). *Power: The anchor of stability, the lever of change.* Bloomington: Indiana University, School of Education. (ERIC Document Reproduction Service No. ED 117 828)

Boulding, K. E. (1989). *Three faces of power.* Newbury Park, CA: Sage.

Donley, R. (1989). A coming home. *Reflections, 15*(4), 10.

Etzioni, A. (1961). *Complex organizations.* New York: Free Press.

French, J. R. P., & Raven, B. H. (1959). The bases of social power. In D. Cartwright (Ed.), *Studies in social power* (pp. 150-167). Ann Arbor, MI: Institute for Social Research.

Gilbert, T. (1995). Nursing: Empowerment and the problem of power. *Journal of Advanced Nursing, 21,* 865-881.

Hassenflug, L. W. (1977). Resocializing the nursing role. In *Use it or lose it* (pp. 1-5). New York: National League for Nursing.

Hawks, J. H. (1991). Power: A concept analysis. *Journal of Advanced Nursing, 16,* 754-762.

Henneman, E. A., Lee, J. L., & Cohen, J. I. (1995). Collaboration: A concept analysis. *Journal of Advanced Nursing, 21,* 103-109.

Hofling, C. K., Brotzman, E., Dalrymple, S., Graves, N., & Pierce, C. M. (1966). An experimental study of nurse-physician relationships. *Journal of Nervous and Mental Diseases, 143,* 171-180.

Kanter, R. M. (1978, April 6). Powerlessness. *New York Times,* p. 21.

Kanter, R. M. (1983). *The change masters.* New York: Simon & Schuster.

Kennedy, A. A. (1985). Ruminations on change: The incredible value of human beings in getting things done. In W. G. Bennis, K. D. Benne, & R. Chin (Eds.), *The planning of change* (4th ed., pp. 325-335). New York: Holt, Rinehart & Winston.

Krause, E. A. (1977). *Power and illness: The political sociology of health and medical care.* New York: Elsevier.

Labelle, H. (1986). Nurses as a social force. *Journal of Advanced Nursing, 11,* 247-253.

Lewin, K. (1951). *Field theory in social science.* Chicago: University of Chicago Press.

Mason, R. O., & Mitroff, I. I. (1985). A teleological power-oriented theory of strategy. In W. G. Bennis, K. D. Benne, & R. Chin (Eds.), *The planning of change* (4th ed., pp. 215-223). New York: Holt, Rinehart & Winston.

Rank, S. G., & Jacobson, C. K. (1977). Hospital nurses' compliance with medication overdose orders: A failure to replicate. *Journal of Health and Social Behavior, 18,* 188-193.

Rogers, E. M. (1983). *Diffusion of innovations* (3rd ed.). New York: Free Press.

Rogers, E. M. (1995). *Diffusion of innovations* (4th ed.). New York: Free Press.

Rogers, E. M., & Shoemaker, F. F. (1971). *Communication of innovations: A cross-cultural approach* (2nd ed.). New York: Free Press.

Rule, C. F. (1988, December). *Antitrust enforcement and the medical profession: No special treatment.* Remarks presented at the interim meeting of the American Medical Association House of Delegates, Dallas, TX.

Shainess, N. (1984). *Sweet suffering: Woman as victim.* New York: Pocket Books.

Snyder, R. C. (1985). To improve corporate innovation, manage corporate culture. In W. G. Bennis, K. D. Benne, & R. Chin (Eds.), *The planning of change* (4th ed., pp. 164-176). New York: Holt, Rinehart & Winston.

Stein, L. I. (1967). The doctor-nurse game. *Archives of General Psychiatry, 16,* 699-703.

Stein, L. I., Watts, D. T., & Howell, T. (1990). The doctor-nurse game revisited. *New England Journal of Medicine, 322,* 546-549.

Tannenbaum, A. S. (1968). *Control in organizations.* New York: McGraw-Hill.

Thibaut, J. W., & Kelly, H. H. (1959). *The social psychology of groups.* New York: John Wiley.

Walker, L. O., & Avant, K. C. (1988). *Strategies for theory construction in nursing* (2nd ed.). Norwalk, CT: Appleton-Century-Crofts.

The "High Ground"
in Social Change

BOX 4.2: KEYWORDS AND PHRASES

— Blame the victim
— Directive role
— Innovation
— Innovation-decision process
— Normative-reeducative strategy
— Persuasion
— Unaffiliated mode

Social change hurts as well as helps. It disrupts usual ways of doing things, infringes on comfort zones, and threatens self-concepts. Should nurses, therefore, renounce the planner role? This book declares that nurses properly claim their traditional activist role; instead of abandoning it, nurses should take the "high ground" as they fulfill their social mandate.

The study of planned change should create a strengthened concern for responsibility and commitment to duty because planners seldom can promote the good of one segment of society without diminishing the good of another. For example, the turn-of-the-century introduction of death control in developing countries, through immunization and antimalarial campaigns, without simultaneous acceptance of birth control produced massive overpopulation. Misery in later generations may surpass what would have existed without earlier death control attempts.

In dealing with the "high ground," this chapter first discusses several operating modes that planners might assume. Then the discussion turns to the place of moral and ethical issues in four planned change theories.

Operating Modes in Planned Change

Zaltman and Duncan (1977) would ask whose values a change program should serve and by whose standards planners should make diagnoses and choose solutions. What the planners and the affected group define as problems could differ widely. Planners, clients, and adopters must state values and clarify goals. According to Bermant and Warwick (1985), diagnostic words such as social system *health* or *illness* keep weaker groups in passive roles. From another perspective, perhaps weaker groups can be strengthened through the conscientious collaborative efforts of planners and group members to restore social system "health."

Even in evaluation procedures, planners should think about the primacy of various groups as they employ values as standards for evaluation. Should the group with higher stakes in the outcome have the most say in evaluation? Who in a group should define the interests of the group? Who should control evaluation when more than one set of group interests emerges? If planners recognize the validity of one viewpoint, should a parallel or opposing view also have consideration?

Accepting responsibility for planning change. Planners get responsibility for planning change in two ways. Either they accept responsibility from someone else or they assume responsibility themselves without assignment. Regardless of the way planners obtain responsibility for planned change, they have several accompanying duties. These concern the planners' personal preparation for the task at hand—keeping promises and telling the truth, doing no harm, and improving the condition of the adopter population (Ross, 1930). Bermant and Warwick (1985) wrote that planners themselves should consider their own competence, choice of interventions, truth telling, and confidentiality; planners also should make clear statements about accountability and openly disclose prior commitments and loyalties.

TABLE 4.1 Planner Responsibility and Affiliation Modes

		Ways of Obtaining Responsibility	
		Assigned	*Assumed*
	Affiliated	I	II
Modes of Affiliation			
	Unaffiliated	III	IV

Zaltman and Duncan (1977) doubted claims for value neutrality. They wrote that planners always have value positions; planners themselves should examine and state these openly. They questioned whether planners should work for clients with value systems different than their own. For example, what should a nurse planner with antiabortion values do if the hospital where he or she works starts offering abortion services? A question also arises about the proper course for a nurse planner who is asked by administration to make a change that cannot succeed under the values the administrators currently hold. Such questions introduce the matter of whom the planner serves—the persons who hired her or him, the entire organization, or the final recipients of the change. Can the planner drop out of the change effort if insurmountable problems appear? Who will deal with the problems caused by change—the planner, or someone else?

Affiliation modes. Planners operate in either the affiliated or the unaffiliated modes described by Hornstein, Bunker, Burke, Gindes, and Lewicki (1971). Affiliated planners work through a more or less formalized agreement, such as an employer-employee or administrator-consultant relationship. Unaffiliated planners have no formal ties with the social system that absorbs their attention; they always assume responsibility for making change. Their stance may be *unlegal* (which differs from *illegal*).

Certain types of assignments, especially those involving advocacy, deny access to the affiliated mode. Moving from the affiliated mode to the unaffiliated mode destroys admission to the forum in which the planner may have spoken previously. This nullifies whatever connection the planner had with the social system and may destroy opportunities for planning change. Conversely, the unaffiliated mode sometimes provides liberty to speak in effective ways. Whether the planner will work in the affiliated or the unaffiliated mode depends partly upon planner and client goals. (See Tables 4.1 and 4.2.)

TABLE 4.2 Thinking About Planner Responsibility and Affiliation

1. Can you envision a situation that could fall into Cell III in Table 4.1? If so, describe the situation.
2. Can you picture a change situation with several adopter populations (social systems to which a change effort is directed)?
3. Could client (i.e., hiring agency) and adopter population (i.e., employees) groups differ in Cell I? In Cell II? Cell IV?
4. Do people in an adopter population always know they are the objects of change? Should they know?
5. How can the planner balance her or his obligations to client and adopter populations in Cells I, II, and IV?
6. Does the planner owe primary allegiance to the client or to the adopter population in Cell I (II, IV)?
7. How do planners move from Cell II to Cell I? From Cell IV to Cell I? Be specific.
8. How can planners in Cell IV establish checks and balances for the propriety of their own operations?
9. How can planners in Cell IV stay focused enough to avoid wasting society's resources?
10. Describe a Cell IV nursing situation.

Self-help or other-help? Should help for social problems come from an agent internal to the social system (the family, group, institution, governmental jurisdiction, society) that experiences the problem or from a source (external agent) outside the social system? Brickman et al. (1985) supplied a set of four models of helping and coping that describe the attribution of responsibility for both problems and solutions. Their models represent situations that range from individual therapy to social action programs. In the Moral Model (Cell I), society holds the person or social system experiencing a problem responsible for both the cause of and the cure for the problem, a traditional blame-the-victim outlook. In the Enlightenment Model (Cell II), society holds persons internal to the problem-prone system responsible for causing the problem but allows outside helpers to provide a solution. (See Tables 4.3 and 4.4.)

The Compensatory Model (Cell III) places responsibility for the problem outside the troubled person or group but lets the person or group find an internal solution. The Medical Model (Cell IV) gives responsibility for both the cause (or discovery) of the problem and its cure to those outside the afflicted area. Planners find descriptions of these cell positions useful because they raise valid moral and ethical questions. People in real life seldom are entirely responsible or wholly lacking in responsibility for either the causes of their problems or the solutions to them. The real world is messy.

Each cell carries inferences worth mentioning in the context of planned change in nursing. The Cell I position implies the competence of the affected

TABLE 4.3 Accountability for Problems and Solutions

		Responsibility for Finding and Implementing Solution	
		Internal Agent(s)	*External Agent(s)*
Responsibility for Causing Problem	Internal Agent(s)	I Moral Model	II Enlightenment Model
	External Agent(s)	III Compensatory Model	IV Medical Model

SOURCE: Adapted from "Models of Helping and Coping," by P. Brickman et al. (1985). In W. G. Bennis, K. D. Benne, & R. Chin, (Eds.), *The planning of change* (4th ed.), p. 291. Copyright 1985 by Holt, Rinehart & Winston. Adapted with permission.

population to diagnose and treat their own problems when, in fact, they might not have the necessary resources for either diagnosis or solutions. Other cells present similar problems.

Rogers and Shoemaker (1971) offered a chart that describes the sources of problem recognition and solution generation. (See Table 4.5.) This chart, which resembles the Brickman et al. (1985) chart, provides a useful look at categories of social change and raises questions about practical and ethical issues raised by the Rogers model and Lewin microtheories for planning change. In Cell I of the Rogers and Shoemaker chart, both the diagnosis of problems and the solutions

TABLE 4.4 Thinking About Accountability for Problems

1. Into which cell in Table 4.3 does a blame-the-victim viewpoint fit best?

2. Which cell gives the most autonomy to adopters?

3. Which cell requires adopters to possess the most resources?

4. Which cell is the most like modern advertising?

5. What must adopters do in Cell IV?

6. Until recently, only 1 of the 50 U.S. states did not use tax money to finance medical fees for collection of evidence against the crime of rape. In that state, the victim had to pay. In which cell would the (prior) situation in the 50th state fall? (The 50th state changed its law in 1995.)

7. In which cell does mass suicide in a cult fit?

8. Can an adopter population (Cell III) always correct the wrongs done to them by others? If so, how long does the process take? (Think of former slave populations.)

9. Does Cell III, with its avoidance of blame for adopters, foster human dignity? (Later in the chapter, compare Table 4.3 with other tables.)

10. Which cell gives the most "humane" position?

TABLE 4.5 Planning and Implementation Modes

		Origin of Solution	
		Internal Agent(s)	External Agent(s)
Origin of Problem Recognition	Internal Agent(s)	I. Immanent* (totally internal change)	II. Selective contact change
	External Agent(s)	III. Induced immanent change	IV. Directed contact change

SOURCE: Rogers and Shoemaker (1971, p. 8). Reprinted with the permission of The Free Press, a division of Simon & Schuster, from *Communication of Innovations: A Cross-Cultural Approach, Second Edition,* by Everett M. Rogers with F. Floyd Shoemaker. Copyright © 1971 by The Free Press.

NOTE: *Indwelling* is a synonym for *immanent.*

for them come from persons internal to the social system experiencing a problem. In Cell IV, both the diagnosis and the solution come from outside the social system; Cells II and III demonstrate interim positions. Table 4.6 has a sample of moral, ethical, and practical questions that arise from these four positions.

The contrast of other-help with self-help reminds nurses of advocacy. Advocacy suggests the fidelity and beneficence that improve the condition of others through such strategies as education. The putting together of the ideas of other-help and self-help suggests respect for autonomy (i.e., informed consent) and beneficence (no harm, prevention of harm, removal of harm, and promotion of good, as in the case of a registered nurse who prevents an inebriated physician

TABLE 4.6 Thinking About Planning and Implementation

1. What assumptions about the location of ability, knowledge, and resources needed for change does a Cell I (Cell II, III, or IV) situation carry?

2. What are the moral and ethical responsibilities of a competent professional in a Cell I (Cell II, III, or IV) situation?

3. Which two cells have the most (least) likelihood of an appropriate fit between the problem diagnosed and the solution chosen or developed?

4. Do benefits and liabilities balance out in each cell?

5. Which cell situation offers the greatest likelihood of producing long-lasting change? Which offers the least likelihood of long-term change?

6. Which cell position gives the most (the least) autonomy to the adopter population?

7. In what kind of nursing situation would the Cell IV position be the most useful?

8. Which cell position most closely resembles the medical model?

9. Where would Lewin's change theories fit best? BB&C's writings? The Rogers diffusion model? CLER?

TABLE 4.7 Another Planning and Implementation Mode

		External Agent(s)	
		Recognize(s) problem	*Do(es) not recognize problem*
Internal Agent(s)	Recognizes problem	I. Cooperative mode (probably not 50-50)	II. Active internal agent; inactive external agent
	Do(es) not recognize	III. Inactive internal agent; active external agent	IV. Abdication of responsibility by both internal and external agents

NOTE: Although this diagram refers only to problem recognition, nurse planners could adapt the ideas it presents for use in many stages of the change planning process.

from performing surgery). It also suggests justice, in which the nurse treats all persons fairly but differently, according to their needs.

Planning and implementation modes. Planned change always involves manipulation of social forces. Manipulation may have the mild face of education or the bold face of coercion. According to Zaltman and Duncan (1977), planners can organize their affairs to avoid the more onerous forms of manipulation (lying, innuendo, presentation of opinion as fact, deliberate omission, or implied obviousness done with an intent to deceive). Planners should know about the parties involved and provide as many realistic alternatives as possible. They should give reasons for the solution and the strategies they advocate and work out a system of responsibility for possible negative consequences.

Bermant and Warwick (1985) suggest freedom as a safeguard. Adopters must have the capacity to choose. This capacity involves their ability to understand the implications of choices; planners should supply information appropriate to the level of understanding possessed by adopters. Freedom also involves the availability of information under circumstances without coercion; even positive rewards exert pressure. Thus safeguards include the provision of understandable and accessible information, participation through negotiation and informed consent, and empowerment that enlarges the abilities of the weak.

Another planning and implementation mode. Table 4.7 uses some of the same components (column headings, row stubs) found in Table 4.5 but assembles them differently. The changed heading and stub positions yield divergent results inside the cells. (See Tables 4.7 and 4.8.) Cell I provides for the collaborative planning considered morally right and ethically sound by several authors. Benne (1985)

TABLE 4.8 Thinking About Cooperative Planning and Implementation

---

1. What assumptions does each cell position in Table 4.7 make about the ability and responsibility of planners and adopters?

2. Which cell(s) in Tables 4.5 and 4.7 best fit(s) your own personal style?

3. Which cell(s) in Tables 4.5 and 4.7 provide(s) the climate most advantageous to planner learning? To adopter learning?

4. Describe a clinical or administrative situation that would fit in Cell II (Cell III) of Table 4.7.

5. Describe a situation that would fit in Cell IV. What helpful course of action, with long-term benefits, might a nurse planner take in such a situation?

6. Where do each of the four planned change theories discussed in this chapter fit best in Table 4.7?

7. In which cell in which table (4.3, 4.5, 4.7) does advocacy fit?

8. Is the Cell I planner in Table 4.7 a neutral agent or a biased advocate?

9. How does the planner working in Cell I (Cell II, III, IV) deal with resistance?

10. Do planners working in Cell I situations earn their keep? How much skill do they need?

11. Which cell situation most resembles that of a family with two alcoholic parents?

---

called this collaboration "social interdependence"; Bermant and Warwick (1985) termed it "participation"; and Zaltman and Duncan (1977) named it "goal clarification," "openness," and "freedom of choice." Note that a Cell I position does not necessarily call for a 50-50 division of planning activities between planner and adopter groups. Instead, it provides for flexibility, which allows planners and adopters to collaborate in ways commensurate with their abilities.

Moral and Ethical Issues
in Planned Change Theories

Planned change theorists concern themselves mainly with the development of theories that reflect what exists in the real world of change rather than with the presentation of moral and ethical principles. Nevertheless, change theories address moral and ethical concerns by design, by omission, or by implication. The following sections discuss the place of moral and ethical issues in four planned change theories.

Lewin's Microtheories

The tenor of Lewin's (1948) writings about the proper rearing of children, the restoration of war-ravaged nations to world citizenship, and the righting of wrongs in society demonstrates the scope of concern he had for the well-being of individuals and populations. Lewin did not write overtly about ethics, so readers must infer what stance he took as they read his work.

Lewin (1951) developed his microtheories through experimentation, a novelty in the psychology of his day. In these experiments, the diagnosis of the social problems was always done by someone other than the planner or adopter, perhaps by a government dietitian or a plant manager. Moreover, some "higher authority" provided a solution, such as orange juice for babies or increased production in a manufacturing plant. The planners' job entailed the manipulation of forces in the psychological environment (field) in ways that would cause change to occur. Cooperative planning did not exist; not even the planner had a say in diagnosing problems or selecting solutions. The lack of cooperative planning coincided with the norms of the World War II culture that existed when Lewin developed his theories as part of the war effort. (He escaped Nazi Germany with little but his life and family; his mother died in a gas chamber in spite of his rescue efforts.) The acceptability of the top-down assumptions that underlie Lewin's experiments depends at least in part upon the cultural and moral/ethical viewpoints of readers. Nurse planners who use Lewin's theories will wish to evaluate them in light of their own personal and professional standards and change situations.

Lewin's microtheories cover only strategy; this restricts their time scope in the change process and gives planners an opportunity to consider combining the theories with perspectives that permit adopters' involvement in change decisions. Nurse planners will remember that Lewin's microtheories make a useful contribution by asking them to look at multiple forces in the change environment. Furthermore, a planner may find him- or herself the member of a change team who must implement change mandated from above, like the situations in Lewin's examples.

Bennis, Benne, and Chin's Writings

Bennis, Benne, and Chin (1985) put a series of essays, mainly written by others, into several editions of their book of readings. Their stance on moral and ethical issues emerges from the nature of writings they supplied or solicited. These authors openly rejected power-coercive strategies of change as inappropriate for modern society. Instead, they opted for the normative-reeducative strategies that feature high levels of participation and cooperation. The normative-reeducative strategies inherently impose duties of self-improvement, beneficence, and fidelity. Quite a number of the Bennis, Benne, and Chin (BB&C) essays recognize the value of human ingenuity and propose organizational systems that emphasize human rights and the duty of improving the condition of other human beings. The writings they collected differ from the three theories/models in this series by presenting formal and scholarly discussions of morality and ethics. A drawback exists in the fact that the BB&C writings come from so many diverse sources that the issues remain somewhat poorly synthesized. Nevertheless, the BB&C books provide valuable reference sources.

The Rogers Diffusion Model

Rogers (1995) did not index such terms as *morality, ethics,* or *social responsibility.* His description of the innovation-decision process leaves little room for adopters to influence problem diagnosis or innovation choice. Nevertheless, Rogers did attend to moral issues. He expressed concern about the unintended consequences of innovations that might harm adopters, cautioned planners about undue influence (coercion) in situations involving collective decisions, and provided for some adopter education in the persuasion process. The Rogers diffusion model relates more to persuasion (as found in advertising) than to informed decision making. The model centers on the role of the expert planner who has adopters' interests at heart as she or he persuades adopters to choose and use a particular innovation. In 1971, Rogers and Shoemaker lamented the directive role that most planners assume and noted that effective intervention most often occurs through massive programs of directed change in which adopters have little input about either the identification of the problem or the generation of solutions. They hoped that in the future a more sophisticated populace would use planners as consulting experts rather than directors of change projects, thus educating people and moving them toward the capacity to both identify and solve problems within their own societies.

The Rogers diffusion model looks at multiple adopter populations and considers them in a time-oriented, linear fashion ordered by socioeconomic strata. Rogers paid serious attention to the fact that the adoption of "modernizing" innovations often widens the socioeconomic gap between the rich and the poor.

Bhola's Configurations (CLER) Model

Bhola confronted moral and ethical questions early in the development of his Configurations, Linkages, Environment, Resources (CLER) Model (1972) by writing that society should allow competent planners to plan change if they work toward the common good and if their mandate comes from the people who will experience the change. Established procedures to remove incompetent or ill-willed planners from their positions must exist, and individual adopters must have the freedom not to adopt the innovations that planners offer. Later, Bhola (1994) used the theoretical foundations of dialectics and constructivism to mandate collaborative planning of a most fundamental kind at every stage of the planning and implementation process. These theoretical foundations require the kind of participation that Bermant and Warwick (1985) called a safeguard for the freedom of the adopters. A third CLER foundation, systems theory, instructs planners to consider input from all groups concerned in the change situation. Targets of change become planners during the change process. Planners who use the dialogue mandated by dialectical theory and the collaborative planning required by constructivism will, at the least, avoid the perils of coercion as they deal with involved groups.

Summary

Because social change always hurts someone, somewhere, nurse planners should take care to make change in an ethical manner. In addition to illness care, nurses' professional responsibilities include health promotion and disease prevention; these activities often require planned social change. Careful making of change necessitates consideration of moral and ethical issues in several areas. These issues relate to ways of obtaining a mandate for change, types of affiliations with organizations, ways of assigning accountability for problems and solutions, modes of planning and implementation of change projects, and matters of cooperative planning.

Some models of accountability for problems and solutions blame victims of inequities and/or expect victims to find and implement their own solutions to problems perpetrated by others. Other modes of accountability neither blame the victim nor expect self-help from the victim. A collaborative planning mode provides safeguards against abuse by recognizing the interests of both planners and adopters.

The four planned change theories discussed in this book differ in their treatment of ethical issues. Although Lewin did not address ethics in any overt way in his change theories, he propounded moral and ethical principles in his more general writings. Bennis, Benne, and Chin overtly discussed moral and ethical issues. Rogers's work contains a number of discussions that imply attention to moral concerns. Bhola's CLER model finds its foundation in dialectical theory and constructivism, which mandate collaboration between planners and adopters to help to safeguard the well-being of both.

The real world of planned change is a complex and confusing place. Not all change theories offer equal help to nurse planners; all offer useful implications and suggestions. A systems theory foundation enables a planned change theory to confront some of the complexity of conflicting interests in the real world. Planned change models that mandate collaboration have some likelihood of alignment with moral and ethical principles. According to Zaltman and Duncan (1977), ethics has been a neglected topic in the study of social change. Nurse planners will find the study of ethics in planned change a fruitful area of exploration.

References

Benne, K. D. (1985). Moral dilemmas of managers. In W. G. Bennis, K. D. Benne, & R. Chin (Eds.), *The planning of change* (4th ed., pp. 471-579). New York: Holt, Rinehart & Winston.

Bennis, W. G., Benne, K. D., & Chin, R. (1985).*The planning of change* (4th ed.). New York: Holt, Rinehart & Winston.

Bermant, G., & Warwick, D. P. (1985). The ethics of social intervention: Power, freedom, and accountability. In W. G. Bennis, K. D. Benne, & R. Chin (Eds.), *The planning of change* (4th ed., pp. 449-479). New York: Holt, Rinehart & Winston.

Bhola, H. S. (1972). *Configurations of change: An engineering theory of innovation diffusion, planned change, and development.* Bloomington: Indiana University School of Education.

Bhola, H. S. (1994). The CLER model: Thinking through change. *Nursing Management, 25*(5), 59-63.

Brickman, P., Karuza, J., Cohn, E., Rabinowitz, V. C., Coates, D., & Kidder, L. (1985). Models of helping and coping. In W. G. Bennis, K. D. Benne, & R. Chin (Eds.), *The planning of change* (4th ed., pp. 287-311). New York: Holt, Rinehart & Winston.

Hornstein, H. H., Bunker, B. B., Burke, W. W., Gindes, M., & Lewicki, R. J. (1971). *Social intervention: A behavioral science approach.* New York: Free Press.

Lewin, K. (1948). *Resolving social conflicts: Selected papers on group dynamics.* New York: Harper.

Lewin, K. (1951). *Field theory in social science: Selected theoretical papers.* Chicago: University of Chicago Press.

Rogers, E. M. (1995). *Diffusion of innovations* (4th ed.). New York: Free Press.

Rogers, E. M., & Shoemaker, F. F. (1971). *Communication of innovations: A cross-cultural approach* (2nd ed.). New York: Free Press.

Ross, W. D. (1930). *The right and the good.* Oxford: Oxford University Press.

Zaltman, G., & Duncan, R. (1977). *Strategies for planned change.* New York: John Wiley.

A Problem

Says Who? (Diagnostics)

BOX 5.2: KEY WORDS AND PHRASES

— Action research
— Applied research
— Criterion-referenced
   standards
— Dialogic relationship
— Growth-oriented standards
— Hypothesis
— Matrix of discovery
— Measurement method
— Need creation
— Need recognition
— Nomenclature

— Normative standards
— Objective approach
— Organizational behavior
— Qualitative approach
— Quantitative approach
— Standard
— Subjective approach
— Successive approximation
— Technology
— Triangulation
— Unit of analysis
— Utilitarian standard

A diagnosis is a name for a problem. This name has meanings that refer to related factors and to defining characteristics (Gordon, 1987). Social systems, as truly as physiological and psychological systems, have related factors and exhibit defining characteristics. In a social change situation, diagnostic statements include defining characteristics that indicate deviations from standards for social system functioning; deviations signify either actual or potential dysfunctions. An accurate diagnosis provides the basis for all subsequent steps in the change process. Planning a change episode without making a thoughtful diagnosis resembles giving an answer without hearing the question.

Some disciplines house their diagnoses in well-developed nomenclatures. Planners of change do not. Lack of precision in labeling social problems in an established nomenclature does not invalidate the worth of the diagnostic process or of a particular diagnosis. This chapter addresses several aspects of the diagnostic process in social situations and tells how four major planned change theories relate to the matter of diagnosis.

The Diagnostic Process

The term *diagnosis* has two meanings (Gordon, 1987). One meaning refers (as above) to the name of a problem. The second meaning refers to the process of naming the problem. A nursing diagnosis has three essential structural components: the name of the problem, the related factors, and the defining characteristics of the problem. Related factors are described as "antecedent to, associated with, related to, contributing to, or abetting" the problem (North American Nursing Diagnosis Association, 1992). Although initially developed to diagnose problems in human systems, nurses have used nursing diagnoses to name problems in communities and organizations. The problems occurring in social systems, similar to human systems, have factors relating to the characteristics that define and describe the problem.

The diagnostic process recognizes standards, assesses the current situation of the social system and measures deviations from standards, and analyzes those deviations. The process employs a series of successive approximations that repeatedly propose and rule out diagnostic hypotheses (plausible diagnoses) in the search for a workable diagnosis. Box 5.3 furnishes sources of information regarding diagnostic reasoning processes in any kind of situation. Box 5.4 provides examples of resources that explain the diagnostic process as applied in organizations.

Looking at Standards

Nurse planners commonly make diagnostic judgments that range from simple (i.e., identifying a lack of immunization for a specific geographic area of a city) to complex (identifying political and social problems responsible for low immunization rates). Such judgments always involve comparison of the actual

BOX 5.3: EXAMPLES OF ESSAYS ON DIAGNOSTIC REASONING PROCESSES

Carnevali, D. L., Mitchell, P. H., Woods, N. F., & Tanner, C. A. (1984). *Diagnostic reasoning in nursing.* Philadelphia: J. B. Lippincott.

Cartwright, D. (1951). Foreword. In K. Lewin (1951). *Field theory in social science* (pp. vii-xv). Chicago: University of Chicago Press. (See pp. ix-xi.)

Guskin, A. E., & Chesler, M. A. (1973). Partisan diagnosis of social problems. In G. Zaltman (Ed.), *Processes and phenomena of social change* (pp. 353-376). New York: John Wiley.

Walker, L. O., & Avant, K. C. (1988). *Strategies for theory construction in nursing* (2nd ed.). Norwalk, CT: Appleton-Century-Crofts.

Willis, D. P., & Parris, S. V. (Eds.). (1989). Framing disease: The creation and negotiation of explanatory schemes. *Milbank Quarterly, 67*(Suppl. 1), 1-152.

Zaltman, G., & Duncan, R. (1977). *Strategies for planned change.* New York: John Wiley. (See chap. 12 and see "diagnosis" in index.)

BOX 5.4. EXAMPLES OF LITERATURE THAT DEALS WITH DIAGNOSIS IN GROUPS AND ORGANIZATIONS

Dalziel, M., & Schoonhover, S. C. (1988). *Changing ways: A practical tool for implementing change within organizations.* New York: American Management Association.

Egan, G. (1988). *Change agent skills B: Managing innovation and change.* San Diego, CA: University Associates. (See chaps. 1 & 2.)

Harrison, M. I. (1987). *Diagnosing organizations: Methods, models, and processes.* Newbury Park, CA: Sage.

Kilmann, R. H., & Mitroff, I. I. (1979). Problem defining and the consulting/intervention process. *California Management Review, 21*(3), 26-33.

Lippitt, G. L., Langseth, P., & Mossop, J. (1985). *Implementing organizational change.* San Francisco: Jossey-Bass. (See chaps. 1 & 6.)

London, M. (1988). *Change agents: New roles and innovation strategies for human resource professionals.* San Francisco: Jossey-Bass. (See chap. 9.)

Nadler, D. A., & Tushman, M. L. (1980, Autumn). A model for diagnosing organizational behavior. *Organizational Dynamics,* pp. 35-51.

Porras, J. I. (1987). *Stream analysis: A powerful way to diagnose and manage organizational change.* Reading, MA: Addison-Wesley.

Zander, K. (1985). Analyzing your workplace. In D. J. Mason & S. W. Talbot (Eds.), *Political action handbook for nurses* (pp. 227-239). Menlo Park, CA: Addison-Wesley.

NOTE: Computerized databases that index business literature and nursing and nonnursing needs assessment literature show many sources of ideas about measurement in groups, organizations, and communities.

situation (i.e., existing immunization rates) with an "ideal" (i.e., optimum immunization rates).

Sources of standards. According to Chinn and Kramer (1991), the term *paradigm* concerns those worldviews or ideologies that persons use to find meaning and coherence for what they see in the world. Additionally, the term "implies standards or criteria for assigning value or worth to both the processes and products of a discipline" (p. 76). Thus a paradigm serves as a source for the standards by which nurse planners consider a situation deviant and, therefore, a problem. When a paradigm changes, standards also change.

Under any paradigm, or worldview, specific standards used by nurse planners come from a variety of sources. Personal standards reflect the planner's age and her or his familial, religious, and cultural background. The planner's professional practice domain strongly influences standards. Professional education may (or may not) supply standards from social science about development of social systems over time, the ways that social systems operate, technology and structural relationships, and functioning of people in social settings. Standards come from mandates such as health care organizations' mission statements or from government regulations. At a more general level, war and/or revolution can produce new health care standards very quickly.

Kinds of standards. Kinds of standards relate to what "the crowd" does, to absolute reference points, or to growth, utility, or personal wants. Kinds of standards also relate to maintenance of the status quo or a search for a different level of group functioning.

Normative standards use performance of a particular group as a reference point. Normative standards often introduce competition. People at the lower end of the scale might feel discouraged; those at the higher end may not feel the need to operate at potential. Under normative standards, division of scores into "good" and "bad" categories relates to the performance of the group that furnished the norms. Planners who apply normative standards must question the extent that the target group resembles the normative group and whether the "norming" process used a representative sample. Planners also ask about the application of statistical processes.

Criterion-referenced standards use an "absolute" reference point furnished by external standards, not norms. Performance relates to a cutoff point arbitrarily established for "passing." Professional associations often use this kind of standard. The use of normative and criterion-referenced standards occurs so often in society that planners may not look beyond them to different views of reality that could energize a social system.

Growth-oriented standards plot one individual's or group's past and present achievement "growth points" over time. These standards do not consider others' performance. Pronouncements of "official" organizations do not matter. Growth-oriented standards serve a useful purpose in the measurement of groups who might experience discouragement when compared with peers or an absolute standard. The lack of a reference point outside the individual or group hampers the use of this kind of standard in professions or industries.

According to Taylor (1986), utilitarian standards ask whether or not a practice works, and how well it works. Utilitarian standards confront questions of safety, effectiveness, and efficiency. They work when people in a social system cannot meet a normative or a criterion-referenced standard developed in a more favorable situation. Utilitarian standards have the advantage of promoting innovativeness and creativity.

Personal wants might influence planners to use inappropriate standards in diagnosing the need for planned change. Zaltman and Duncan (1977) cited the case of officials in a drug company who bemoaned the company's lower-than-desired sales revenue. They decided to launch an advertising campaign to link decreased social isolation with antidepressant drug use. The Federal Trade Commission discovered and stopped the scheme.

Robert and Weiss (1988) discussed the difference between the maintenance of the status quo (problem solving) and a move to a different level of functioning (innovating). Problem solving occurs when planners simply desire to monitor a situation and to correct deviations from existing standards; no new standards come into play. Innovating occurs when planners consider the usual standard of performance unacceptable; new standards are the order of the day. (See Figure 5.1.)

Measuring Deviations
From Standards

Early questions in the diagnostic process locate the problem and identify the persons who will deal with it. Planners choose a unit of analysis such as corporation, wing, unit, village, shift, work group, class, committee, or team. Standards suggest what planners should assess and/or measure but planners must decide which factors relate to the problem and what kinds of relationships exist. For example, in a rural African village, the problem that appears as dysentery might relate to poor sanitation, malnutrition, overpopulation, overgrazing, desertification, or a combination of factors (Dettwyler, 1994). In early stages, planners take care to assess all reasonably connected factors. Box 5.5 gives ideas about kinds of variables and instruments nurses might use in diagnosing social problem situations.

Planners who take an objective approach value quantification, measurement, and statistics. They emphasize observable and measurable aspects of social functioning and organizational behavior. The quantitative diagnostician makes

PROBLEM SOLVING

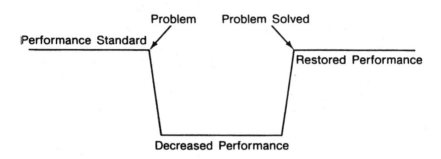

In *problem solving*, you can only be as good as you used to be.

INNOVATION

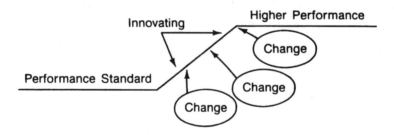

In *innovating*, you can achieve new levels of performance, return, etc.

Figure 5.1. Problem Solving Versus Innovation
SOURCE: From "The Innovation Formula: How Organizations Turn Change into Opportunity,"
by M. Robert and A. Weiss, 1988, p. 12. Copyright © 1988 by Ballinger. Reprinted by
permission.

frequent use of institutional records, time and motion studies, and detailed
observations. These planners choose instruments considered reliable and
valid.

In the subjective, qualitative approach, planners use observations and interviews extensively and stay attuned to their own subjective experiences. Planners

---

BOX 5.5: EXAMPLES OF VARIABLES AND INSTRUMENTS USEFUL IN PLANNING SOCIAL CHANGE

Blalock, H. M. (1989). *Power and conflict: Toward a general theory.* Newbury Park, CA: Sage.

Champion, V. L., & Leach, A. (1989). Variables related to research utilization in nursing: An empirical investigation. *Journal of Advanced Nursing, 14,* 705-710.

Flarey, D. L. (1991). The social climate scale: A tool for organizational change and development. *Journal of Nursing Administration, 21*(4), 37-44.

Funk, S. G., Champagne, M. T., Wiese, R. A., & Tornquist, E. M. (1991). The barriers to research utilization scale. *Applied Nursing Research, 4*(1), 30-45.

James, I., Milne, D. L., & Firth, H. (1990). A systematic comparison of feedback and staff discussion in changing the ward atmosphere. *Journal of Advanced Nursing, 15,* 329-336.

Mager, R. F., & Pipe, P. (1970). *Analyzing performance problems: "You really oughta wanna."* Belmont, CA: Fearon.

Moos, R. (1987). *The Social Climate Scale: A user's guide.* Palo Alto, CA: Consulting Psychologists Press.

Moos, R. (1994). *Work Environment Scale manual* (3rd ed.). Palo Alto, CA: Consulting Psychologists Press.

Moos, R., & Spinrad, S. (1984). *The social climate scales: An annotated bibliography 1979-1983.* Palo Alto, CA: Consulting Psychologists Press.

Price, J. L., & Mueller, C. W. (1986). *Handbook of organizational measurement.* Marshfield, MA: Pitman.

Smith, M. C., & Barton, J. A. (1992). Technologic enrichment of a community needs assessment. *Nursing Outlook, 40,* 33-37.

Stamps, P. L., & Piedmont, E. B. (1986). *Nurses and work satisfaction: An index for measurement.* Ann Arbor, MI: Health Administration Press Perspectives.

Turnipseed, D. (1990). Evaluation of health care work environments via a social climate scale: Results of a field study. *Hospital Health Services Administration, 35,* 245-262.

Walczak, J. R., McGuire, D. B., Haisfield, M. E., & Beezley, A. (1994). A survey of research-related activities and perceived barriers to research utilization among professional oncology nurses. *Oncology Nursing Forum, 21,* 710-715.

---

use historical records and accounts of everyday incidents. They search for meaning in the broad scope of the situation. Nurse planners who combine quantitative and qualitative perspectives when making diagnoses in social systems will find the result useful.

Analyzing Deviations
From Standards

Formal data interpretation begins with the clarification of unsupported or conflicting information. Double checking of inferences that tempt toward premature closure occurs through triangulation (such as the use of instruments from diverse measurement modes). For example, planners might diagnose an unsuccessful patient-education class by a combination of a return demonstration, a class evaluation, and a paper-and-pencil test. Meaning emerges as planners compare data with standards. Information that represents critical indicators of social system ills deserves selective attention.

Moles (1964) proposed a scientific method called the matrix of discovery. A matrix is a chart of rectangular cells framed by column head and row stub designations usually supplied by planners. Each cell represents the situation that results when the factors described by its own column head and row stub designations interact. Every cell represents a different combination of factors and, therefore, a unique situation. Nurse planners fill cell spaces with notes pertinent to the interaction of column head and row stub factors for each cell. As the planners fill in the cell spaces, they note relationships they did not imagine before. Some cells indicate harmful or useless relationships or, perhaps, no relationship at all. (See Table 5.1.)

Gordon (1987) suggested rechecking questionable data, considering the logic of possible/probable diagnoses, obtaining feedback, evaluating the adequacy of sample size, and appraising measurement error. Nurse planners look at situations from the adopters' points of view and take care to verify data in ways that cause as little alienation as possible. Every client report merits respectful consideration.

Exploration of many alternative diagnoses takes priority because planners cannot choose a correct diagnosis that is absent from the list of alternatives; a diagnosis must exist if it is to be included in those under consideration. In an effort to expand the scope of their search for a correct diagnosis, planners could make a second or third matrix with an altogether different framework (such as that supplied by psychology, microbiology, chemistry, or sociology) to search for the problem. A high incidence of nosocomial infections, for example, might stem from a careless attitude on the part of caregivers, from a change in housekeeping procedures, or from bacterial contamination in the factory that supplies goods supposed to be sterile. (See Table 5.2.)

As a last step, planners eliminate the least likely diagnoses and choose the most likely ones as guides for their actions in producing social change. Even then they prepare to reformulate diagnoses and subsequent plans if the need arises.

TABLE 5.1 A Simple Matrix of Discovery

Key Indicators	Unit 1	Unit 2	Unit 3	Unit 4
Standard 1 Med Error Rate Low	__/100 doses	__/100 doses	__/100 doses	__/100 doses
Standard 2 Falls Rate Low	__/100 patient days	__/100 patient days	__/100 patient days	__/100 patient days
Standard 3 Decubiti Development Rate Low	__/100 patient days	__/100 patient days	__/100 patient days	__/100 patient days
Standard 4 Plans of Care Current	__/100 plans current	__/100 plans current	__/100 plans current	__/100 plans current

NOTE: Planners devise column headings and row stubs that apply to the local problem and problem situation. They also develop units of measurement as needed so that comparisons remain comparable across cells. This table lists the number of occurrences per 100 cases.

Four Theorists' Views of the Diagnostic Process

Some developers of planned change theories and models say little about the diagnosis of social system problems; others carefully discuss diagnosis. The following paragraphs summarize four theorists' views about diagnosis.

Lewin's Microtheories

Although he did not used the term *paradigm* in connection with values and the formation of standards, Lewin made important contributions to an understanding of the ways that paradigm shifts occur. He discussed sources of group standards and the ways they change in his individual-group relationships microtheory. He stated that individuals have cognitive, affective, and motoric experiences that provide a background for their values. Individuals strengthen their values within the context of the group interactions where values become

TABLE 5.2 A Matrix of Diagnostic Discovery

| Variables | *Sources of Explanations for Defining Characteristics* | | | |
	Psychology	*Microbiology*	*Chemistry*	*Sociology*
Type(s) of patients				
Location of affected unit(s)				
Incidence over time				
RN/LPN/CNA ratios				
and so on				

NOTE: Planners devise column headings and row stubs that might apply to the local problem and problem context. They relate these headings and stubs as they come together in the various cells. This helps them brainstorm regarding factors possibly related to the defining characteristics of the local problem.

group standards. Standards develop into power fields that exert pressure toward conformity to group standards. Individuals set goals that reflect those group standards.

In spite of the development of his individual-group relationships microtheory, in his experiments Lewin (1951) left the diagnosis of social problems to higher authorities somewhere else. Later, after Lewin's death, Chin and Benne (1985) noted that Lewin had advocated collaboration among researchers, educators, and activists in the identification of needs for change. Action research that included participation of adopters occupied Lewin in the last months of his life, but reporting this work fell to his team members. Their findings influenced the development of the Bennis, Benne, and Chin writings.

Bennis, Benne, and Chin's Writings

Freud, in addition to Lewin, influenced the development of the normative-reeducative strategies for change advocated by Bennis, Benne, and Chin (1985). Freud contributed ideas concerning the unconscious and preconscious foundations of human behaviors. His perspectives set the stage for the dialogic relationship between planners and adopters included in the normative-reeducative outlook. Standards concern values, norms, and relationships in social systems. Mutual interaction between planners and clients forms a broad basis for problem diagnosis.

The Rogers Diffusion Model

Rogers and Shoemaker (1971) bemoaned the directive role that planners often take. Diagnosis in the Rogers (1995) diffusion model usually assumes that planners recognize problems or needs. Political processes can produce need recognition, which, according to Rogers, comes from any one of a number of value perspectives (such as blame the individual or blame the system). Basic or applied research might reveal solutions before the public senses a "need." In such instances, planners might attempt to create needs for new goods through information campaigns that could include advertising. Rogers reported that researchers debate whether need recognition or invention of an innovation comes first.

Bhola's Configurations (CLER) Model

Bhola's (1994) CLER model takes planners on a cognitive journey; it provides a theoretical framework (systems, dialectical, and constructivist theories) that suggests rational steps for planning (1991). Planners {P} diagnose problems and develop subsequent objectives {O} jointly with adopters {A} in a series of planning and replanning sessions ({P} $\times$ {O} $\times$ {A} ensemble). Diagnoses incorporate social system knowledge supplied by adopters and technical knowledge supplied by planners.

Summary

This chapter defines *diagnosis* as a name for a problem. This name refers to related factors and defining characteristics. Social change planning owns no established taxonomy of diagnoses. The diagnostic process, which has utility in social change, consists of a series of successive approximations in which planners compare existing social conditions with standards. Several types of standards exist. Normative standards compare individual or group behaviors with the achievement or behaviors of a "normal" group. Criterion-referenced standards use a more or less arbitrary cutoff point set by an "official" organization or a person in a position of authority. Growth-oriented standards plot performance against the performer's own record. Utilitarian standards ask whether a situation serves safety, efficiency, and effectiveness. Some persons use their own wants as standards. A system maintenance viewpoint preserves the status quo; an innovative approach calls for new standards.

Standards govern what planners measure; the choice of a quantitative, qualitative, or combined approach suggests measurement methods. As planners analyze deviations from standards, they generate and rule out many possible/probable diagnoses in a series of successive approximations. They think alternately of the whole situation and of details within it. They also may use a matrix to help them recognize alternative explanations for the deviations they see. Planners revise diagnoses if the need arises.

Although Lewin did not directly address the matter of problem diagnosis in his microtheories, he did discuss the formation of group standards. Bennis, Benne, and Chin advocated a cooperative behavioral science approach in the determination of problems. They valued a people-oriented technology. The Rogers diffusion model recognizes the impact of political processes and provides for diagnoses by planners without major adopter input. Bhola's CLER model requires cooperative action between planners and adopters in the diagnostic process.

References

Bennis, W. G., Benne, K. D., & Chin, R. (1985). *The planning of change* (4th ed.). New York: Holt, Rinehart & Winston.

Bhola, H. S. (1991, December). *Designing from the heart of an epistemic triangle: Systemic, dialectical, and constructivist strategies for systems design and systems change.* Paper presented at the Third Annual Conference of Comprehensive Systems Design of Education organized by the International Systems Institute, Asilomar Conference Center, Monterey, CA.

Bhola, H. S. (1994). The CLER model: Thinking through change. *Nursing Management, 25*(5), 59-63.

Chin, R., & Benne, K. D. (1985). General strategies for effecting changes in human systems. In W. G. Bennis, K. D. Benne, & R. Chin (Eds.), *The planning of change* (4th ed., pp. 22-45). New York: Holt, Rinehart & Winston.

Chinn, P. L., & Kramer, M. K. (1991). *Theory and nursing: A systematic approach.* St. Louis: Mosby.

Dettwyler, K. A. (1994). *Dancing skeletons: Life and death in West Africa.* Prospect Heights, IL: Waveland.

Gordon, M. (1987). *Nursing diagnosis: Process and application* (2nd ed.). New York: McGraw-Hill.

Lewin, K. (1951). *Field theory in social science.* Chicago: University of Chicago Press.

Moles, A. (1964). Le contenu d'une méthodologie appliquée: Un essai de recensement des méthodes [The content of an applied methodology: An attempt at reviewing methods]. In R. Caude & A. Moles, *Methodology: Toward a science of action* (pp. 45-82). Paris: Gauthier-Villars. (Selected portions of the text translated by F. Augsberger, 1976, for Tiffany)

North American Nursing Diagnosis Association. (1992). *Nursing diagnoses: Definitions and classification.* St. Louis, MO: Author.

Robert, M., & Weiss, A. (1988). *The innovation formula: How organizations turn change into opportunity.* Cambridge, MA: Ballinger.

Rogers, E. M. (1995). *Diffusion of innovations* (4th ed.). New York: Free Press.

Rogers, E. M., & Shoemaker, F. F. (1971). *Communication of innovations: A cross-cultural approach* (2nd ed.). New York: Free Press.

Taylor, R. (1986). *Christian concepts: Core of professional nursing practice.* (Available from the Department of Nursing, Andrews University, Berrien Springs, MI 49104)

Zaltman, G., & Duncan, R. (1977). *Strategies for planned change.* New York: John Wiley.

Solutions That Fit

Choose the Right Path

BOX 6.1: LOOKING AHEAD

Chapter 6: Solutions That Fit: Choose the Right Path

Standards Suggest Innovations
Characteristics of Innovations
Stages of Innovation Development and Dissemination
Innovation Consequences
Innovations in Planned Change Theories

BOX 6.2: KEY WORDS AND PHRASES

— Adopter
— Innovator
— Protocol
— Resources
— Task analysis
— Technology cluster

Innovations are new solutions to problems. They don't have to be new inventions, they merely have to be new to the adopter population. Merriam-Webster's *Collegiate Dictionary* (1990) defines *innovation* as a new idea, method, or device. Bhola (1965) mentioned three domains (cognitive, affective, psychomotor) familiar to teachers. These classify an innovation as a concept, attitude, or tool (with psychomotor skills) introduced in a social group that had not fully used it before. The innovator does not necessarily invent the innovation; she or he might introduce something developed by someone else. An innovation could consist of a product or new way of using a tool. It will involve relationships in the form of programs, projects, institutions, restructured roles, or even the capacity to alter roles, relationships, or practices.

This chapter deals with standards that suggest innovations, characteristics of innovations, and stages of innovation development and dissemination. It ends with discussions of innovation consequences and of the place of innovations in four planned change theories.

Standards Suggest Innovations

Formal standards come from people's worldviews (paradigms), as expressed in such societal mandates as nurse practice acts, official definitions of nursing, accreditation requirements, and institutional mission statements. Informally, a person's beliefs and cultural background provide standards so that even "what the Joneses do" furnishes standards.

Standards (values) serve as yardsticks against which to measure (diagnose) a problem situation. Standards also beget goals (objectives) for the solution of social problems. Planners and adopters choose or develop innovations (solutions) that they expect will meet goals. Thus standards (values) lay a foundation for diagnoses and they also suggest goals, direct planners and adopters toward particular innovations, link innovations to problems, tie problems and innovations to strategies, and infer evaluation procedures.

Standards always carry the personal and professional biases of their owners. Biases should get the recognition and public exposure that encourage negotiation among the parties involved in the change episode. Planners must consider whose standards shall be recognized in the choice or development of an innovation. In other words, who "calls the shots" in deciding which solution best fits a social problem?

Characteristics of Innovations

Every innovation consists of a combination of parts and relates to particular basic assumptions. Each has a specific magnitude, possesses technical characteristics, and requires resources for its use. Bhola (1984) advocated the "unpacking" of innovations to reveal as many social and technical implications as possible in advance of innovation use.

G. U.P.

Component parts. Every innovation has *conceptual, attitudinal, psychomotor* (Bhola, 1994), and *relational components.* Each component, sometimes with the exception of the psychomotor skills component, appears to a certain extent in every innovation.

The conceptual component of an innovation relates to the ability of humans to think. It concerns the ideas and logic that an innovation contains. The conceptual component can range from simple to extremely complex. Attitudinal components relate to the ability of humans to emote. They concern the values for which people feel attachment and what people "feel" should happen. Psychomotor skills, such as those needed to administer an injection, use a computer keyboard, or insert a nasogastric tube involve human abilities to act.

Relational components of innovations stem from the human ability to associate. Relationships vary in intensity, complexity, and length. They occur in combinations as small as a dyad or as large as a society; they range from casual meetings to deep involvements. Organizational relationships (structures) may assume a lean, flat, decentralized form or they may consist of multiple layers of authority figures. Some organizational relationships last for centuries; others are transient.

Basic assumptions. The basic assumptions of an innovation implicitly or explicitly state what people expect the innovation to accomplish and how they expect it to work. Neither planners nor adopters ever recognize all the assumptions of an innovation. Because many assumptions do not resemble reality or form a logical basis for an innovation, planners and adopters should identify assumptions as early as possible. Naive planners who expect innovations to function reliably and without harmful consequences may not find their expectations validated in real life.

Magnitudes. Innovations vary in magnitude in terms of characteristics such as the number of people affected and the size of the packaging of the innovations. Some innovations involve individual adoption; others require group adoption. The cultivation of coca as a cash crop provides an example of aggregate individual decisions that have produced widespread social changes. These changes have so altered the economies of certain countries that the collapse of the coca trade without a massive substitute would cause economic collapse of an unprecedented scale. At the other end of the spectrum, the fluoridation of a community water supply represents innovations that require a group decision.

The size of an innovation package sometimes affects people in dramatic ways. Rogers (1995) recounted the story of a tomato-picking machine in California. The manufacturer had the choice of producing machines in one of several sizes. The company opted to make large machines. The choice separated small farmers from large farmers and put 3,200 small farmers out of business and 32,000 hand pickers out of work.

Technical characteristics. The social aspects of an innovation do not emerge without adequate exploration of its technical characteristics. Rogers (1995) gave three kinds of questions that adopters ask: What is the innovation? How does it work? Why does it work? He classified needed knowledge as how-to knowledge and principles knowledge. *How-to knowledge* tells the adopter how much of the innovation to secure and how to use it correctly. Complex innovations require more knowledge than do simple innovations. While Rogers's advice lends itself well to tangible products, it applies also to the less tangible goods and services of health education and health care. When, for example, should a person take a particular medication? How much (two pills every four hours, or four pills every two hours)? How often should clinic checkups occur?

Principles knowledge tells how and why an innovation works. It explains the germ theory that underlies vaccinations and latrines and reveals the fundamentals of human reproduction so that people understand how birth control methods work. In one example, people in a Third World country who had heard no explanation about the ways that vitamin A works for vision problems ground the pills and put the powder into their eyes, with disastrous results. Lack of how-to and principles knowledge before adoption of an innovation often leads to inappropriate and/or discontinued use.

Task analysis helps planners provide information about an innovation. Task analysis is the examination of a task to delineate the underlying assumptions and relevant elements of the task. It categorizes, prioritizes, sequences, and relates these elements in a fashion that will appear logical to the uninitiated person who must carry out the task. Task analysis done early in the innovation development process helps pinpoint needed aspects of redesign. It takes into account human and environmental elements and lays the foundation for future teaching when the innovation comes into use.

Task analysis occurs best from the user's point of view. It assumes particular importance in nursing because nurse educators constantly instruct nurses and nursing students in the details of new technologies; nurse managers direct the operation of nursing units and departments; and clinicians educate individuals, families, and groups in the fine points of their own care. Many tasks carry enormous potential for harm if error occurs.

Resource requirements. Every innovation requires resources for its development, adoption, and continued use. Resources involve much more than money. Resources also include time, land, buildings, goodwill, knowledge, political connections, legal mandates, water, soil, space, and so on. According to Bhola

(1972), "resources are material, conceptual and psychological abilities and capacities of innovators to cause diffusion and of adopter systems to absorb the innovations; and the time available to them both for playing the change episode" (p. II-7).

Stages of Innovation Development and Dissemination

Innovation development and dissemination take time. Rogers (1995) reckoned that a major technological breakthrough takes about 20 years from basic research to marketing of the innovation. Only rarely and by accident do complete and polished innovations appear. Even innovations that planners appropriate from other sources demand adaptation. The process of innovation development has several stages: inquiry of some sort, product design, fabrication, and packaging. The development process provides an opportunity for the cooperative planning that makes an innovation acceptable and useful to adopters; collaborative planning turns adopters into planners. Planners should remember that innovations such as policy changes and new management methods require development as surely as tangible goods do.

Inquiry. Whether the inquiry needed for innovation development takes the form of trial-and-error planning, sophisticated research, or something between depends upon many factors. The intensity of needs, the state of the art, and the level of difficulty of the problem and solution all pertain.

Product design. Whether innovations come from trial-and-error methods, basic research, or a point somewhere between, they need a number of experimental runs. Each successive approximation comes closer to the objectives (goals) established through attention to the standards specified for the product. For many innovations, safety considerations suggest small trials in which only a few persons experience risk. Small trials also involve less expense than large trials, which is the reason that hospitals often use a pilot unit when they try a new machine, a different method of care delivery, or an innovative approach to documentation.

Fabrication and packaging. Fabrication translates research results into usable products. The CURN research utilization model (Haller, Reynolds, & Horsley, 1979; Horsley, Crane, Crabtree, & Wood, 1983) describes ways to close the gap between research results and practice applications. After they emphasized the importance of choosing high-quality research for application, these authors outlined ways to develop practice protocols that make research findings usable. Each protocol states the need for change, describes the proposed innovation, gives a summary of research, and provides guidelines for implementation. The protocol also plans for evaluation of outcomes and supplies educational materials for users. The development of a protocol does not end the fabrication process. Before final packaging for use, experiments in the form of clinical trials assess safety, feasibility, and costs.

When innovations form clusters of related technologies (Rogers, 1995), planners must make decisions about the timing of the release of the parts. Pressures from outside agencies might urge quick release of all cluster components, when, in the opinion of planners, only certain parts merit early release or use.

Planners should think about the time needed for distribution of the innovation and time that people will need for learning about it. Not all innovations work quickly. Just as some medications require a priming dose or an extended period of time for therapeutic drug levels to accumulate, so an adequate accumulation of effects of innovations may take time. For example, health education campaigns do not produce healthy populations overnight. Neither do commitments always develop quickly and, according to Bhola (1972), the level of needed commitment varies at each stage. As they plan packaging, planners should foresee and work to counteract the possibility that an innovation with delayed results will provide naysayers an opportunity to downgrade its reputation.

Innovation Consequences

All innovations have consequences. Nurse authors have noted this and have written about the desirable and undesirable impact of innovations. Pillar, Jacox, and Redman (1990) advocated more nurse involvement in evaluation of new technologies for safety, efficacy, cost, benefits, and social impact. They challenged the notion that new technologies always represent progress.

Seldom can planners separate the desirable and undesirable consequences of an innovation. Neither can they foresee and eliminate all unintended negative effects. Just as pain relievers addict, antibiotics kill normal flora as well as pathogens, and antineoplastics kill normal cells in addition to tumor tissue, so innovations harm as well as help.

Whether people in a social system judge results of innovations as harmful or helpful depends upon the standards they apply. Rogers (1995) maintained that every social system has qualities, such as family bonds and respect for life and for individuals, that enhance life and therefore prove functional for the system. This does not mean that every organization should survive but, instead, that humanitarian aspects of a system deserve preservation.

Direct and indirect consequences. Innovations have indirect as well as direct consequences. Bhola (1972) described an iceberg effect—an iceberg reveals only a small part of its total mass above water. Only a few results of an innovation are visible before its adoption. For example, the education of women about child care might increase their awareness of the importance of literacy for girl children, which could empower a future generation of women. Again, good nursing care not only enhances the well-being of the recipients, it sometimes inspires onlookers toward entering the nursing profession.

Unintended consequences. Unintended consequences are effects of innovations other than those envisioned by planners. Rogers (1995) provided a generalization, stating that "undesirable, indirect, and unanticipated consequences of innovations usually go together" (p. 421). The most advanced innovations produce the most unintended consequences.

In an example of unanticipated results, pregnant teens cared for by midwives maintained their own health and had healthy babies, but some of them also repeated unwed pregnancies so that they could receive the nurturance they craved and could obtain only from the midwives. Planners cannot avoid uncertainty about consequences.

Unequal consequences. Not every social group receives equal benefit from a particular innovation. Rogers (1995) wrote that the adoption of modernizing innovations may widen the gap between high and low socioeconomic groups. Planners favor adopters with high levels of education because advanced education often combines with the innovativeness associated with high rates of adoption. This leads planners to give early adopters advance notice of new things and thus greater opportunity than persons in lower socioeconomic groups to evaluate the ways that an innovation provides benefit. The advance notice and increased understanding linked to education help early adopters avoid risks associated with adoption. The more educated persons also have more unencumbered money to use in their experiments with innovations and to make innovation use profitable. The sobering facts cited above pinpoint the importance of ethical considerations in the making of social change. These facts also show the importance of the collaboration of adopters with planners in the choice or development of innovations.

Innovations in Planned Change Theories

Some planned change theories ignore the matter of innovations; others consider the topic important. The following paragraphs present the matter of innovations and of who chooses or develops them from the perspective of the four planned change theories highlighted in this book.

Lewin's Microtheories

Lewin (1951, 1958) proposed numerous innovations in child care, social concern, the rehabilitation of nations, research methods, and other issues important to society. But he did not address the matter of innovations as an integral part of his planned change microtheories. In the examples that illustrate these theories, he simply accepted the solutions to problems that "higher" authorities advocated. Reports of his experiments show that he did not question the nature of innovations used in his experiments. For example, during World War II, he compared methods used to persuade homemakers in groups of Red Cross volunteers to use "unattractive" cuts of meat so that the "better" meats could go to overseas troops. The innovation (cuts of meat) received no attention whatsoever. All research emphasis centered on methods of persuasion. The same held true for whatever innovation (higher production levels in a factory, diets involving orange juice, evaporated milk, cod liver oil, and so on) the government or some other authority proposed.

Bennis, Benne, and Chin's Writings

Ideas presented at the outset of this chapter claimed that an innovation might be a concrete object such as a tool or device or a new way of using a tool. It also could be a new way of relating (a new role, a new institution, new management practices). These ways of looking at innovations cover the work of Bennis, Benne, and Chin (1985). They did not highlight innovations, the second part of a complete planned change theory. Instead, they combined the second and third change theory components (innovation and strategy) under social science methods for renewing organizations. In a sense, this makes organizational renewal both the innovation (the solution, outcome, goal) and the strategy (the process for reaching the goal). Under this viewpoint, renewal enables people in the organization to do what needs to be done to create organizational health. Their emphasis on restructuring and renewal resembles organizational development (OD) concepts.

The Rogers Diffusion Model

Rogers's (1995) writings on innovations rate among the strongest in the field of social change. Although Rogers did not openly discuss the place of standards in the choice of innovations, he did address standards indirectly when he noted that planners often carry a proinnovation bias. He said that most diffusion researchers seldom make their biases public; they simply imply that an innovation should be diffused in a social system without questions concerning its suitability and without alteration. Rogers considered lack of recognition of one's own biases dangerous in an intellectual sense as well as in an ethical sense. Bias leads planners to ignore alternative solutions, deny adopter collaboration, thwart people's discontinuance of hurtful innovations, and equate change with improvement. Rogers also addressed ethical concerns connected with group decisions as well as the unintended, latent consequences of innovations.

Rogers made an important contribution to diffusion knowledge when he described the attributes of innovations as relative advantage, compatibility with the local social situation, complexity (difficulty of use), trialability (the extent that adopters can try out the innovation without adopting it), and observability. (The section that presents the Rogers diffusion model in a later part of the book provides more detail about his views on innovations.)

Bhola's Configurations (CLER) Model

Like Rogers's work, Bhola's early monographs (1965, 1972) highlighted the idea of innovations as solutions to problems. He characterized an innovation as a concept, an attitude, or a tool (with skills) new to a particular population. The innovator might not be the inventor. Every innovation requires resources for its adoption and use. Planners should "unpack" innovations by considering the hidden requirements and implications linked to their conceptual, attitudinal, and psychomotor components. They should look at innovations as collections of many smaller innovations that require multitudes of adjustments by adopters. Adjustments involve the area of values, attitudes, and emotions, and may require the learning of new psychomotor skills. Relationships may change. The need for time, money, and physical resources may increase.

In his later work, Bhola (1991) addressed the matter of standards in the process of choosing innovations in an indirect way. He based his CLER model on a foundation that includes systems theory, dialectics, and constructivism. This foundation mandates the collaboration of planners and adopters. Under this model, adopters become planners. Collaboration increases the likelihood that innovations will include both the social knowledge possessed by adopters and the technical knowledge furnished by planners. It encourages recognition of the values of all participants as standards for the choice or development of innovations.

Summary

Innovations are solutions to problems. These solutions are not necessarily new in the world, but they are new to the social system that adopts them. All innovations have conceptual, attitudinal, and relational components; some also have skills (psychomotor) components. The innovator who introduces them is not necessarily the inventor.

All innovations relate either to consciously claimed or to unconsciously held standards. Standards relate to worldviews (paradigms). The same standards that served in diagnosis of the problem act as foundations of the innovation, provided, of course, that the people who make the diagnosis also choose or develop the innovation. Every innovation carries both explicit and implicit assumptions about the ways it will operate and what it will accomplish once adopted. Expectations based on assumptions might not hold true in real life. Innovations vary in size according to the number of people affected and the number of social system members who make adoption decisions.

Adopters often ask questions about why and how innovations work. Planners should furnish explanations so that adopters can understand both the principles and the specific details of innovation use. In task analysis, planners look at an innovation from the adopters' viewpoint. All innovations require resources of time, money, knowledge, energy, and so on for their development and use.

Innovations might be tangible goods or might be as abstract as new ways of relating. Innovation development and dissemination take time. Inquiry that ranges from trial and error, through applied research, to basic research precedes innovation development and fabrication for all kinds of products. Test runs determine what problems might arise after adoption. Nursing has a research utilization model (the CURN model) that has specific procedures for transforming research findings from the research mode to innovations suitable for the practice mode.

Adoption of innovations does not always benefit adopters; sometimes refusal to adopt an innovation better suits adopter needs. Innovations have indirect and direct consequences, unintended consequences, and, sometimes, unequal consequences that widen gaps between rich and poor.

Lewin did not write about innovations as integral parts of the change process. In the reports of the research that he did to develop his change theories, he accepted solutions supplied by someone else. Bennis, Benne, and Chin wrote little about innovations. In essence, the innovations they presented were methods for renewing organizations. These methods, like those of organizational development (OD), represent both innovation and strategy. Rogers characterized attributes of innovations as relative advantage, compatibility with the existing situation, complexity, trialability, and observability. Bhola defined the conceptual, attitudinal, and psychomotor skills components of innovations. He founded his CLER model on collaboration so that planners and adopters, together, make decisions about the nature and amount of the innovation for their particular situation. This outlook incorporates the social knowledge possessed by adopters and the technical knowledge furnished by planners. It helps to include the values of both adopters and planners in the development of solutions to social problems.

References

Bennis, W. G., Benne, K. D., & Chin, R. (1985). *The planning of change* (4th ed.). New York: Holt, Rinehart & Winston.

Bhola, H. S. (1965, November). *Innovation research and theory.* Preconference document for the Conference on Strategies for Educational Change, Columbus, Ohio State University School of Education.

Bhola, H. S. (1972). *Configurations of change: An engineering theory of innovation diffusion, planned change, and development.* Bloomington: Indiana University School of Education.

Bhola, H. S. (1984, November). *Tailor-made strategies of dissemination: The story and theory connection.* Paper presented at the Seventh Annual Vocational Education Dissemination Conference of the National Center for Research in Vocational Education, Columbus, OH.

Bhola, H. S. (1991, December). *Designing from the heart of an epistemic triangle: Systemic, dialectical, and constructivist strategies for systems design and systems change.* Paper presented at the Third Annual Conference of Comprehensive Systems Design organized by the International Systems Institute, Asilomar Conference Center, Monterey, CA.

Bhola, H. S. (1994). The CLER model: Thinking through change. *Nursing Management, 25*(5), 59-63.

Haller, K. B., Reynolds, M. A., & Horsley, J. A. (1979). Developing research-based innovation protocols: Process, criteria, and issues. *Research in Nursing and Health, 2,* 45-51.

Horsley, J. A., Crane, J., Crabtree, M. K., & Wood, D. J. (1983). *Using research to improve nursing practice: A guide.* New York: Grune & Stratton.

Lewin, K. (1951). *Field theory in social science.* Chicago: University of Chicago Press.

Lewin, K. (1958). Group decision and social change. In T. M. Newcomb & E. L. Hartley (Eds.), *Readings in social psychology* (pp. 197-211). New York: Holt.

Pillar, B., Jacox, A. K., & Redman, B. K. (1990). Technology, its assessment, and nursing. *Nursing Outlook, 38,* 16-19.

Rogers, E. M. (1995). *Diffusion of innovations* (4th ed.). New York: Free Press.

Webster's ninth new collegiate dictionary. (1990). Springfield, MA: Merriam-Webster.

Action Plans to Get You There

Strategies and Tactics

BOX 7.2: KEY WORDS AND PHRASES

— Affiliated change agent
— Channel
— Channels microtheory
— Data-based strategies
— Data-based strategies with initiatory aims
— Data-based strategies with pragmatic aims
— Dialectical theory
— Force field analysis microtheory

— Gantt chart
— Linking-pin concept
— Program Evaluation and Review Technique (PERT)
— Rational-empirical strategies
— Resistance
— Segmentation
— Social structure
— Strategy
— Tactic
— Technostructural strategy

A fter planners have diagnosed a social system problem and have chosen or developed a solution, what can they do to make sure the innovation that they selected gets used? How will they reach desired objectives?

This chapter starts with descriptions of strategies and tactics that help people in social systems reach their goals. Next, the chapter discusses the combination and sequencing of strategies. At the end, it tells how several strategies would fit with four planned change theories and summarizes the ways the theories would deal with resistance to planned change.

A *strategy* is a plan of action developed in terms of a particular theory or model (Goodman, 1977) and designed to accomplish the aims of a plan for change. Strategies promote the adoption of an innovation (solution). A strategy is less comprehensive than a change theory or model but more comprehensive than a tactic. A *tactic* is a particular maneuver that furthers the aims of a particular strategy (Goodman, 1977). A tactic is not merely a task; a task accomplishes a planning detail necessary for efficiency (an example is paying a routine electric bill).

Planners avoid problems when they use strategies that have basic assumptions congruent with the theory or model under which they do their planning. Likewise, they should choose tactics in keeping with the strategies they use. Education and persuasion serve as examples of strategies. Tactics could include getting an uncommitted accountant onto a planning committee, isolating a working team, reserving a classroom, or sending a representative to a city council meeting.

Planned Change Strategies

The following description of change strategies starts with the most neutral strategy and ends with the most coercive. Each description represents a family of strategies, all related, but each different. They are described in general terms. Each supplies examples of tactics that might align with the strategy presented in the subsection.

Educational Strategies

An educational strategy is a strategy that provides relatively unbiased presentations of fact intended to serve as a rational justification for action. Education does not necessarily tell learners what choices to make. Instead, educational strategies assume that people have rational qualities and can learn to adjust their behaviors to benefit themselves and others when they acquire the information needed for making decisions. Education takes a great deal of time. Used in advance of other strategies, it helps people adjust to rapid, forced change.

Planners who use education need knowledge resources, teaching skills, long-term financial and human resources, and long-term commitment. They need media skills and access to instructional media. Adopters need the intelligence and cultural experiences that permit comprehension of the information presented. They also need the time and the money resources that education demands. Because it supplies knowledge and skills necessary to self-help, education amounts to a type of facilitation.

Education helps adopters see problems and develop skills. It works well with complex innovations and lowers resistance to "modernization." Recidivism diminishes with a sufficient quality and quantity of education. Education works poorly when factual ambiguity exists, when an innovation involves the ego, under conditions of very active opposition, and when adopters either do not have or do not want the knowledge and skills they need to evaluate information. It does not do well in large-scale efforts over a short time period. Benne (1985), Schein and Bennis (1985), and Zaltman and Duncan (1977) wrote about educational strategies. (The work of Zaltman and Duncan, 1977, provided much of the material for this section of the chapter.)

Tactics appropriate to education include the hiring of teachers with philosophies that match change objectives, developing publicity for educational offerings, securing physical facilities for instruction, and arranging accreditation for offerings.

Facilitative Strategies

Facilitative strategies ease the implementation of change by providing resources critical to change. Facilitative strategies assume that the adopter group recognizes a problem, agrees to the appropriateness of remedial action, and exhibits a willingness to accept help. They assume that people are good, that they know quite a lot about how to solve their own problems, but that they simply don't have the resources they need to meet appropriate goals. Facilitation requires a definite, unhurried timetable for publicity and for planning resources. Planners cannot give what they do not have, so they must prepare to end the effort when they have expended available resources. Provision for long-term resource procurement may have to shift to a funding agency.

Planners who use facilitation must organize; they must develop multiple approaches; and they must connect the need with the innovation. They often require administrative support. They must have commitment and communication skills. Adopters have to perceive the need for change and must see the connection between the problem and the proposed solution. Adopters lack resources, may feel handicapped, and might have decreased motivation. The greater the concern about means and ends among the adopter group, the greater the success of the strategy.

Facilitation does not create openness. It cannot work in a hurry. It does not work when general resistance exists, and it will fail if the system cannot maintain the innovation after planners have gone. The maximum facilitation possible does not always help adopters; it may remove the incentives that adopters need. Cowen (1985), Kennedy (1985), and Zaltman and Duncan (1977) wrote about facilitation.

Tactics vary according to the types of resources needed for facilitation. They include resource procurement, advance publicity campaigns, arrangements for maintenance activities, and information sessions to help planners and adopters clarify objectives, assess available and needed resources, and establish goals.

Technostructural Strategies

Technostructural strategies are planned change strategies that alter technology to access social structure in groups or that alter social structure to get at technology. The social groups involved vary in size from dyads to societies. Technostructural strategies sometimes use physical structure such as color, lighting, or alignment or assignment of space to alter social structure or technology. They assume a three-way interaction among technology, structure, and physical space. Technology and the physical environment both influence organizational structure but do not fully determine its form. Most important, for each technology an optimum social structure exists. Technostructural strategies take considerable time, from months to decades or more. Planners must understand relationships between technology and structure. They need placement in the social system that allows them to make the necessary changes in structure, technology, or physical space. Adopters may have to learn new skills; at the least they will have to maintain flexible attitudes.

Planners need to consider social status differences that might yield to technostructural strategies only with great difficulty. Ignoring prevailing cultural beliefs can cause failure. Technostructural strategies thus might need to be combined with other strategies. Hornstein, Bunker, Burke, Gindes, and Lewicki (1971), Lynch (1974), and Woodward (1965) wrote about technostructural strategies.

Tactics appropriate to technostructural strategies could include hiring an architect to make plans for altered space, connecting work groups with the use of Likert's (1967) linking-pin concept, shifting one's worldview about cause and effect (Senge, 1990), introducing new machines, or changing an interior space design or furniture arrangements.

Data-Based Strategies

Data-based strategies are those strategies that collect and use data for purposes of making social change. Data-based strategies come in two varieties—those with initiatory aims and those with pragmatic aims.

Data-based strategies with initiatory aims. Data-based strategies with initiatory aims are strategies that develop and maintain a problem-solving climate in a social system. They use maximum participation of social system members. These strategies assume that people make decisions based on nonrational factors. They also assume that both the data and the collection and processing of data can help people identify problems. Participants may take into account subtle factors that planners, by themselves, might miss. The discussions involved can have more value than the data collected. This strategy precedes any action program.

Data-based strategies with initiatory aims require considerable time for data collection and for discussion. Planners need skill in facilitation of group processes. They need integrity to follow through in solving problems that participants identify, and they must have affiliation with the organization in question to gain access to the organization's members. Therefore, unaffiliated planners (change agents) cannot use this strategy.

A data-based strategy with initiatory aims works best when organizational "families" exist so that discussion occurs easily. Also, participants need hunches about the nature of problems. One weakness resides in the fact that the strategy itself does not provide a rational basis for choosing a particular solution to a problem. Further, the strategy provides no basis for generalization of results to another setting. Benne (1985), Hornstein et al., (1971), Schein (1985), and Schön (1985) wrote about data-based strategies with initiatory aims.

Tactics used with data-based strategies with initiatory aims include many kinds of data collection methods, arrangements for group discussion meetings, the use of flip charts to record participants' ideas, and careful listening to comments.

Data-based strategies with pragmatic aims. Data-based strategies with pragmatic aims seek to find the best innovation for solving the problem at hand. The data depict environmental conditions, demonstrate the value of alternative solutions, and provide people with a rational, scientific basis for choosing a particular innovation. These strategies assume that people are rational and able to recognize and respond to truth, and that planners can ask the "right" questions. They assume that planners can present data in understandable ways so that people can make reasoned choices. All data-based strategies require time for data collection and analysis; all precede action programs. Under pragmatic aims, planners need research-type skills not only in data collection but also in data analysis and presentation.

Unaffiliated planners may use a data-based strategy with pragmatic aims to act on intermediaries, such as lawmakers, who will act on a third party. Unaffiliated planners must use dramatic, comprehensible, and credible data. They might use mass media for dissemination of data. Little cooperation, perhaps even a noncooperative stance, exists between planners and the target group in such instances. The target group must understand data presentations and come to trust the planners if this kind of planned change is to be effective (Hornstein et al., 1971).

Tactics used depend in part upon the affiliation of the planners. Both affiliated and unaffiliated planners will use scientific data collection and data analysis procedures. Affiliated planners may schedule data collection and information meetings. They secure permission for their activities and may have participants sign informed consent forms. Unaffiliated planners will gather information from public records, use concealed surveillance, gain the cooperation of credible public figures such as scientists and clergy, and conduct interviews among an aggrieved population.

One of the problems with data-based strategies with pragmatic aims lies in the fact that people can identify a problem more easily than they can find a "right" solution. Also, data are easily contaminated, which makes precision difficult to achieve. For example, either too much or too little participation can contaminate data. The complexity of some problems makes them difficult to define. Nevertheless, planners sometimes can generalize results from data-based strategies with pragmatic aims.

Communication Strategies

Communication strategies are planned change strategies that spread information, over time, through channels in a social system. A communication strategy assumes that communication networks of various types exist in the adopter population. Communication requires time for messages to spread. It requires study of social system characteristics and careful message preparation that may entail many steps. Planners may make use of many communication channels and networks, such as the mass media.

When they segment the adopter population, planners determine which part of the population will adopt early and which will adopt later. Persons with more than the average amount of money and education often adopt innovations earlier than adopters with less money and education. Opinion leaders among potential adopters are active only with respect to some innovations. Nonleaders do not necessarily follow in any direct sense, so planners need to remember not to use overly simplistic models of communication networks. They also should present media messages in terms that adopters can understand and accept. Messages may be so persuasive that adopters make decisions before carefully weighing all the advantages and disadvantages of the innovation. Communication strategies use all kinds of media presentations (print, video, movie, computer networks, telephone, megaphone, word of mouth, radio, and so on). Each message requires thoughtful preparation as well as sending and receiving (Rogers, 1995).

Tactics in communication strategies include analysis of adopter populations as in a community survey or poll. Planners must secure the means of transmission of messages, plan preparation and spread of messages, and prepare to evaluate the effectiveness of messages.

Persuasive Strategies

Persuasive strategies attempt to produce change through reasoning, urging, and inducement. Planners usually base these strategies on rational appeal, but they sometimes attempt to produce change partly through bias in the structure and presentation of the message. Persuasive strategies assume that behavior that is rewarded is continued; once people try something new, they probably will continue to use it. They do not assume total rationality. They assume the propriety of some distortion and moderate amounts of persuasion.

In persuasion, the fewer the resources available to planners, the faster change must occur. These strategies find use during the legitimation stage of an innovation or when planners cannot sustain coercive methods. Planners who use persuasive strategies obtain their power from knowledge of adopter value systems and direct or indirect control over resources valuable to adopters. Adopters might not feel a need for or have a commitment to the innovation offered by planners. Planners use persuasive strategies for purposes of controlling resistance or when the innovation seems ambiguous or has no clearly defined advantage for adopters. Persuasive strategies work only when adopters possess resources needed for adoption; persuasion does not work when planners have no attractive resources. (One cannot wring blood out of a turnip!) Exaggerations about benefits and minimization of risks often backfire. Because persuasion may create resistance, even those planners who condone its use will find it works against sustained change (Zaltman & Duncan, 1977).

Tactics under persuasive strategies might include offers of positive incentives such as commodities and services or negative incentives that withhold goods and services. Planners might use recruitment, job advancement, urging, inducement, and rational and/or emotional appeals. They might produce and present emotionally charged movies or radio programs. They could arrange debates, rallies, and citizen forums or employ newspaper editorials and articles.

Coercive Strategies

In coercive strategies, there exists some kind of obligatory relationship between planners and adopters. Adopters find themselves dependent upon planners for satisfaction of some kind of goals or needs. Dependency flows from the nature and desirability of goals controlled by planners as well as the availability and cost of alternatives. The strength of the strategy relates directly to the degree of dependency that exists.

Coercive strategies assume that coercion constitutes an appropriate means of producing social change. They also assume that power usage will produce change, and that people will not conform unless made to do so. Coercive strategies, in addition to persuasive strategies, do things *to* people rather than *with* people. This might imply that planners do not value adopters.

When protracted decision making delays action for a long time, planners might use coercion. They find the strategy useful when they have little time and change must occur rapidly, or when only one segment of a population is opposed to change. Coercion works best before resistance arises. Planners control rewards and punishments and need the assets for weathering retaliation and for sustaining surveillance, sometimes over a long time period.

In coercion, adopters exhibit a low level of commitment to change. The more options adopters have, the less power planners have. Coercion does not work well when adopters do not have the resources necessary for adoption or when planners cannot monitor the situation over time. Coercion often leads to suboptimal implementation of an innovation and it may create problems other than the ones planners intended to solve (Bakan, 1985; Hornstein et al., 1971; Zaltman & Duncan, 1977).

Coercive tactics often include economic threats. They frequently employ elements of surprise. Realistic threats, perhaps backed by weapons, predominate. Imprisonment may occur. Starvation and other denials of basic needs may serve as tactics.

Evaluating, Combining, and Sequencing Strategies

Zaltman and Duncan (1977) urge conscientious strategy choice, cautious strategy combination, and prudent strategy sequencing to prevent planned change from becoming planned disaster. Throughout, organization is essential. Detailed newsmagazine accounts of a presidential election in the United States furnish many positive and negative examples of strategy and tactic choice, combination, and use.

Choosing strategies. Planners, ideally, work under the umbrella of a planned change theory. They should think about the assumptions a theory makes and consider whether these assumptions cohere with the assumptions of the strategies under consideration, with nursing values, and with their own professional or personal values. They consider the amount of time required for a particular strategy to work. Other questions involve the availability of resources such as knowledge, money, and infrastructure elements. Every strategy introduces problems. For example, a certain strategy might conflict with the innovation under consideration. Planners consider whether they and adopters can overcome the problems that a particular strategy entails.

Combining strategies. Strategy combinations require care because strategies can cancel or augment one another as occurs when the extreme anxiety created by coercive strategies cancels educational strategies by creating conditions under which learning almost certainly cannot occur. On the other hand, technostructural strategies might function well when associated with normative-reeducative strategies that help members of a work group understand one another's values as related to the job situation.

Sequencing strategies. Mager and Pipe (1984) provided an excellent example of combining and sequencing educational and persuasive activities. They reasoned that efforts to persuade employees to produce excellent work would prove ineffective if the employees did not have the requisite knowledge and skills. Therefore, they provided for education, with practice, before the persuasion that would occur with such tactics as performance reviews, pay increases, or pay cuts. They also provided escape hatches, such as job transfer for employees not able to profit by educational offerings or redesign for jobs with impossible requirements.

Getting organized. Planners can increase the quality of strategizing and the likelihood of remaining organized throughout a change episode with the use of a Program Evaluation and Review Technique (PERT) chart (Archer, Kelly, & Bisch, 1984; Bhola, 1973) or its forerunner, the Gantt chart (Marriner-Tomey, 1992). These time-oriented charts range from simple ones that concern a few people to complex compendia of tasks and assignments, performance standards and regulations, expected outcomes, and dates and costs for everything. This is the place where planners make a time line for the tactics they intend to use. In real life, planners take care not to set PERT or Gantt charts in concrete because the change situation will require many adjustments. As they strategize, planners develop blueprints for contingencies and devise possible responses to resistance.

Strategies in Planned Change Theories

The following subsections discuss the ways that four change theories relate to strategies and provide ideas about the ways that the theories would deal with resistance to change. Readers might wish to refer to the theory presentation, critique, and application chapters found later in the book.

Lewin's Microtheories

Lewin's (1951) microtheories fit this chapter's definition of strategies. These microtheories can combine with other strategies in ways that enrich both the Lewin theories and the other strategies. For example, the psychological aspects and techniques of education in shaping group norms received much attention from Lewin in his individual-group (I-G) relationships microtheory. This emphasis suggests that most of his theories can be used with educational strategies. Further, data-based strategies with initiatory aims would fit well with the small groups that Lewin proposed for changing group standards through educational sessions (I-G microtheory).

Data-based strategies with pragmatic aims resonate with the Lewin examples that accept an innovation from an outside authority without involvement of adopters, an approach that produces a "doing-*to*-people" effect. Data-based strategies would assist in the measurement of forces needed for Lewin's force field analysis. Additionally, the I-G microtheory explains how some persuasive strategies work. Concepts in the channels microtheory, which looks at gatekeepers and the passage of new ideas into and through organizations, relate easily to technostructural and communication strategies. Facilitation, if used to increase forces pointing toward adoption of "favorable" group standards, fits with the I-G relationship microtheory. Coercion does not readily find a place with Lewin's microtheories.

Lewin's microtheories, by analyzing and manipulating forces in a field, place major emphasis on dealing with resistance to the development of a new equilibrium (change). He would measure current forces for and against change, and would work to augment those favoring change and diminish those retarding movement toward the new equilibrium. Lewin also would intervene in ways designed to stabilize a changed social system and thus achieve permanence of the new level of functioning.

Bennis, Benne, and Chin's Writings

Bennis, Benne, and Chin (1985) divided deliberate strategies of changing into three categories: rational-empirical, normative-reeducative, and power-coercive. Their inclusion of a wide variety of strategies under these three headings shows that they recognized many kinds of strategies. They expressed a preference for normative-reeducative strategies by stating that this family of strategies is the "most appropriate to the conditions of contemporary life and to the advancement of scientific and democratic values in human society" (p. 13). They predicted that continuing social science scholarship would extend the use of normative-reeducative strategies throughout society.

Bennis, Benne, and Chin (BB&C) definitely would use facilitative and technostructural strategies. They would recommend data-based strategies with initiatory aims and would look carefully at the environment by means of data-based strategies with pragmatic aims. They would favor communication in planned change programs. For them, reeducation would include tactics oriented toward reaching emotions as well as intellect. They would employ persuasion with great caution and would not choose coercive strategies or tactics. These authors would work with adopters in a manager-employee or teacher-student type of relationship.

Bennis, Benne, and Chin, through an invited author (Klein, 1985), considered resistance to change extremely valuable from both ethical and practical points of view. Resistance protects the integrity of the adopter system. In their view, the planner has a preponderance of technical knowledge but would work cooperatively with adopters, inviting their participation. BB&C would survey the environment to determine its nature and would go about creating norms favorable to renewal. They also would reeducate adopters so that they could use an innovation to their own advantage. Accountability, ethics, and participation of adopters assume importance in the BB&C writings.

The Rogers Diffusion Model

Rogers (1983, 1995) spent a great deal of his professional time thinking about communication. This gives a communication flavor to his model. Rogers would use education to inform adopters about characteristics of innovations. Persuasion would enter the scene because Rogers's decision-making sequence allows little adopter input in product development. Data-based strategies with pragmatic aims would help planners discover the nature of the adopter population and would influence the formulation of advertising messages.

If Rogers used facilitation, it might take the form of innovation improvements or incentives designed to make an innovation attractive to potential adopters. Because the Rogers model does not include adopters in problem diagnosis, data-based strategies with initiatory aims probably would not make the roster. Although the Rogers model has a definite communication and advertising slant, nothing about the model suggests the employment of coercion as a strategy. Rogers's later work incorporated some organizational behavior concepts that did not affect the 1983 or 1995 core statements of his model, which remained almost unchanged from earlier editions. The Rogers model provides a beneficent "doing-*to*" effect.

The Rogers diffusion model would call resistance "rejection" and give it a major place by explaining how and why it occurs and preparing planners to observe resistance and report its dynamics. The planner who uses the Rogers model would cope with resistance by avoiding and/or providing for cultural pitfalls, technological barriers, and communication errors.

Bhola's Configurations (CLER) Model

Although Bhola's (1994) CLER model does not, of itself, contain planned change strategies, it does mandate the use of strategies from other social science sources. CLER definitely embraces education. Facilitation relates closely to *resources*—the "R" in CLER and one of the model's four main elements. Configurations (C), linkages (L), and environment (E), the other three main CLER elements, relate to technostructural strategies. Data-based strategies with initiatory aims correspond to CLER's dialectical theory foundation. Data-based strategies with pragmatic aims would help planners in their analyses of organizations and social systems (C, L, and E) and resources (R). Bhola defined linkages (L) as communication. If planners employed persuasion while using CLER, they would not implement those strategies that tend toward coercion. Coercion itself would not appear on a roster of CLER-approved strategies.

CLER circumvents resistance by treating adopters as partners in planning. Planners, with their technical expertise, provide important input. Adopter input, geared to the social aspects of the situation, assumes equal importance. Collaboration (dialogic action) is the name of Bhola's game. He would work together with adopters to develop objectives, along with innovations designed to meet those objectives, and strategies that assure their realization.

Summary

A strategy is an overall plan of action developed in terms of a particular model or theory of change and designed to meet a specific objective. Tactics are particular maneuvers dictated by strategy. Strategies presented here include education (which provides information resources crucial to change), facilitation (which provides other resources critical to change), technostructural strategies (based on integral relationships between organizational structure, technology, and the physical structure of surroundings), and data-based strategies (that depend on data to produce change). The section also includes discussions of communication strategies (which stress media, networks, channels, and so on), persuasion (designed to produce change through inducement), and coercion (designed to produce change through force).

The section on combining and sequencing strategies stresses the importance of asking questions about the basic assumptions held by the theory-in-use and how these relate to the assumptions that accompany strategies. Further questions help planners predict whether or not strategies will cancel one another. Tactics must possess assumptions congruent with the strategies they implement. Planners can use Program Evaluation and Review Technique (PERT) or Gantt charts for assistance in sequencing strategies and tactics and in organizing associated tasks. Data-based and facilitative strategies fit easily with Lewin's microtheories. Bennis, Benne, and Chin would stress strategies and tactics that fall under the normative-reductive umbrella. The Rogers model lines up well with communication and persuasive strategies. Bhola's CLER model embrace education, communication, and facilitation. None of the four theorists espouses violence and coercion.

References

Archer, S. E., Kelly, C., D., & Bisch, S. A. (1984). *Implementing change in communities: A collaborative process.* St. Louis: Mosby.

Bakan, D. (1985). The interface between war and the social sciences. In W. G. Bennis, K. D. Benne, & R. Chin (Eds.), *The planning of change* (4th ed., pp. 382-392). New York: Holt, Rinehart & Winston.

Benne, K. D. (1985). The process of reeducation: An assessment of Kurt Lewin's views. In W. G. Bennis, K. D. Benne, & R. Chin (Eds.), *The planning of change* (4th ed., pp. 272-283). New York: Holt, Rinehart & Winston.

Bennis, W. G., Benne, K. D., & Chin, R. (1985). *The planning of change* (4th ed.). New York: Holt, Rinehart & Winston.

Bhola, H. S. (1973). *Planning, programming, and administration of functional literacy.* Bloomington: Indiana University. (ERIC Document Reproduction Service No. ED 091 555)

Bhola, H. S. (1994). The CLER model: Thinking through change. *Nursing Management, 25*(5), 59-63.

Cowen, E. L. (1985). Help is where you find it. In W. G. Bennis, K. D. Benne, & R. Chin (Eds.), *The planning of change* (4th ed., pp. 311-324). New York: Holt, Rinehart & Winston.

Goodman, G. (1977). An application of educational change theory to a Christian education innovation. *Dissertation Abstracts International, 38*(04), 2018A. (University Microfilms No. 77-221010)

Hornstein, H. H., Bunker, B. B., Burke, W. W., Gindes, M., & Lewicki, R. J. (1971). *Social intervention: A behavioral science approach.* New York: Free Press.

Kennedy, A. A. (1985). Ruminations on change: The incredible value of human beings in getting things done. In W. G. Bennis, K. D. Benne, & R. Chin (Eds.), *The planning of change* (4th ed., pp. 325-335). New York: Holt, Rinehart & Winston.

Klein, D. (1985). Some notes on the dynamics of resistance to change: Some notes on the defender role. In W. G. Bennis, K. D. Benne, & R. Chin (Eds.), *The planning of change* (4th ed., pp. 98-105). New York: Holt, Rinehart & Winston.

Lewin, K. (1951). *Fields theory in social science.* Chicago: University of Chicago Press.

Likert, R. (1967). *The human organization: Its management and value.* New York: McGraw-Hill.

Lynch, B. P. (1974). An empirical assessment of Perrow's technology construct. *Administrative Science Quarterly, 19,* 338-356.

Mager, R. F., & Pipe, P. (1984). *Analyzing performance problems: Or "You really oughta wanna."* Belmont, CA: Lake.

Marriner-Tomey, A. (1992). *Nursing management* (4th ed.). St. Louis: Mosby-Year Book.

Rogers, E. M. (1983). *Diffusion of innovations* (3rd ed.). New York: Free Press.

Rogers, E. M. (1995). *Diffusion of innovations* (4th ed.). New York: Free Press.

Schein, E. (1985). Process consultation. In W. G. Bennis, K. D. Benne, & R. Chin (Eds.), *The planning of change* (4th ed., pp. 283-287). New York: Holt, Rinehart & Winston.

Schein, E., & Bennis, W. G. (1985). Laboratory education and reeducation. In W. G. Bennis, K. D. Benne, & R. Chin (Eds.), *The planning of change* (4th ed., pp. 335-351). New York: Holt, Rinehart & Winston.

Schön, D. A. (1985). Conversational planning. In W. G. Bennis, K. D. Benne, & R. Chin (Eds.), *The planning of change* (4th ed., pp. 247-253). New York: Holt, Rinehart & Winston.

Senge, P. M. (1990). *The fifth discipline: The art and practice of the learning organization.* New York: Doubleday/Currency.

Woodward, J. (1965). *Industrial organization, theory, and practice.* London: Oxford University Press.

Zaltman, G., & Duncan, R. (1977). *Strategies for planned change.* New York: John Wiley.

Did It Work?
(Evaluation)

BOX 8.2: KEY WORDS AND PHRASES
— Formative evaluation
— Goal-based evaluation
— Goal-free evaluation
— Individual-blame bias
— Pro-innovation bias
— Summative evaluation

Evaluation examines the degree to which the conduct and outcomes of a planned change event coincide with the values of people involved in it. Evaluation of a change episode can address the validity of the diagnosis; the impact of the innovation; the goodness of fit between the theory, strategies, and tactics and the change situation; and the effectiveness of the application of the change theory, strategies, and tactics.

87

Analysis is evaluation's twin sister. It precedes evaluation and identifies the underlying themes and component parts of the change situation; it tells planners what to evaluate. Analysis asks questions about what exists; evaluation asks about success in terms of such characteristics as effectiveness, appropriateness, consistency, suitability, and relevance (Tiffany, 1994).

Evaluation differs from monitoring. Monitoring looks at current functioning in terms of deviations from standards without questioning the standards. In evaluation, nothing gets excluded from scrutiny. Monitoring cannot lead to a higher overall purpose, but a thorough evaluation can, because evaluation asks fundamental questions about the appropriateness and direction of the operation itself, with no holds barred. Evaluation can ask such an outrageous question as whether a system or organization should exist at all. (See Figure 5.1.) Thus evaluation of a change episode can ask whether or not that episode should have happened in the first place.

This chapter discusses the reasons evaluation should occur, considers the timing of evaluation, who should evaluate, what should be evaluated, and approaches to evaluation. It ends with a summary of the viewpoint each of four planned change theories holds with respect to evaluation.

Why and When to Evaluate

In a well-conducted change event, evaluation at least partially justifies the pain of change endured by persons involved in the event. It also helps to justify the considerable expenditure of societal resources necessary to almost any planned change venture. A thorough evaluation of an unsuccessful change event pinpoints and clarifies problems in ways that permit planners to learn from negative incidents and erroneous viewpoints.

Preparation for evaluation starts early. The components of a planned change episode suggest phases of an evaluation process. Evaluation begins with the first of the successive approximations employed in problem diagnosis and continues throughout the change process. Evaluation procedures differ according to their time phases. Formative evaluation occurs during the development and conduct of the change event; summative evaluation follows completion of the change episode. Formative evaluation can suggest adjustments to plans for change before finalization of the effort. Summative evaluation can make judgments that relate to future plans.

Who Should Evaluate

Planners, of course, should evaluate. But evaluation by planners alone produces results biased toward planners' interests and might not represent the opinions of other groups. Collaboration with the hiring agency (client), adopters (if these differ from other groups), the aggrieved population, and other involved persons or groups enriches evaluation findings. Inclusion of "unofficial" participants in evaluation processes strengthens any kind of evaluation.

What to Evaluate

Evaluation should *judge the basic intent and outcomes of a change episode.* When planners evaluate, they might question whether the change episode should have happened. Perhaps the event should have had a stronger client focus that more plainly contributed to the betterment of the nation's health care situation. Maybe the change effort should have preserved an institution vital to community interests.

Planners also should *evaluate* their own *planned change theory choices.* They should make an appropriate theory choice and give reasons for it. They draw parallels between the theory's basic assumptions and the practice situation. Hamel-Craig (1994) wrote about the evaluation of planned change theory application. First, the choice of a planned change theory includes a comparison of several theories and an examination of their previous use. Planners verify the need for change theory application. They familiarize involved persons with the change theory and apply the theory in a way that agrees with nursing purposes. They also might use the theory to explain, predict, or generalize to another situation. After completion of the change episode, planners tell how the theory influenced the change process and compare their results with those achieved by previous theory users. They ask how the level of adopter satisfaction compares with that found under change methods usual for this situation; they include recommendations for future theory use; and they evaluate the potential impact that this theory application could have on future theory development. When appropriate, they provide a report to the theorist.

In evaluation, important questions also concern the *validity of the diagnosis,* the *choice of an innovation,* the *choice and conduct of strategies and tactics,* and the evaluation itself. Planners ask if the initial diagnosis focused on the under-lying causes of the problem or if it reflected only superficial characteristics. They question whether the diagnosis described a social problem accurately in terms of its nature, size, and location.

Evaluation assesses the innovation with respect to its suitability and results. The innovation must fit both the diagnosis and the social situation. If the nature of the innovation forced adoption by unwilling persons (as in the fluoridation of a community water supply), planners take this into account. They question whether the innovation was too expensive in terms of available resources. They ask about the likelihood that it will produce the intended outcome or whether it might have adverse unintended effects in the future.

Evaluation also looks at choice of strategy and tactics to see whether these fit with the theory and the situation. Strategies and tactics must not demand unavailable resources. Change planners should recognize the value of humans in the application of strategies and tactics. They judge the effectiveness of strategies and tactics and decide whether planners sequenced them appropriately.

A thorough evaluation evaluates itself. Planners formulate evaluation procedures early in the change process and make them an integral part of the change effort. They apply evaluation processes on schedule and use appropriate evaluation methodologies. Reports reach (only) appropriate people. Report authors present findings in a format useful to future planners.

Approaches to Evaluation

The following sections show how planners can approach evaluation from either a goal-based or a goal-free stance with methods that range from informal inquiry to the use of scientific quantitative or qualitative procedures.

Goal-Free and Goal-Based Evaluation

Goal-free evaluation involves standards just as much as does goal-based evaluation. The difference between the two lies in the source of standards. Goal-free evaluation uses the individual standards (values) held by participants from diverse sectors of the change scene. Planners secure these participants through snowball sampling techniques that pick the first respondents through purposive methods and then ask them who else could answer similar questions. The qualitative methodologies sometimes associated with goal-free evaluation direct planners to conduct open-ended interviews. The free-ranging nature of goal-free methods opens the change situation to fresh ideas.

Goal-based evaluation uses standards chosen or developed "officially" for use in the change episode. It compares the conduct and outcomes of the change event with general standards such as satisfaction, cost, efficiency, effectiveness, and the extent of adoption of the innovation. It looks at overall goals and objectives. It compares change procedures and outcomes with standards used as foundations for making diagnoses, developing innovations, and choosing strategies and tactics.

Scientific Methods for Evaluation

In goal-based evaluation, planners compare the actual situation with the predetermined standards employed. In making the comparison, they decide whether a quantitative approach or a qualitative approach, or both, will best suit the measurement situation. Methods include any appropriate kind of self-report, observation, projective technique, and so on. Descriptive and inferential statistical analyses and their interpretations apply to quantitative data. Planners might combine quantitative and qualitative methods in the same evaluation project.

Evaluation forms part of an inductive and deductive spiral. A loop on the spiral starts with values made explicit as standards. Next come the goals (objectives) developed in response to standards. Then planners choose indicators of "on target" (benchmark) functioning that typifies standards and determine what indicates effectiveness. For example, would absence of polio indicate the effectiveness of an immunization campaign?

In another step, planners decide what information represents the indicator they chose. Then they ask where they can obtain the necessary information (data). They need reliable and valid instruments for obtaining data. Actual data collection represents the turning point at which the evaluation heads back toward the abstract portion of the spiral. Once collected, data need aggregation and analysis, and the results of analysis require interpretation. At this point, goals (objectives) again come into view and may change as planners try to make sense of evaluation results in terms of values and the standards derived from values. After preparation of the report, planners present their findings and recommendations to appropriate parties, including future planners (who may be themselves!).

Evaluation in Planned Change Theories

The nature of a planned change theory influences evaluation in several ways. The philosophical foundation of a theory gives it a particular slant that pervades the evaluation process. What a theory does not say may be as important as what it does say. Each of the four featured theories approaches evaluation from a viewpoint that ranges from an almost total omission of discussion about evaluation to specific information about evaluation concerns.

Lewin's Microtheories

Lewin (1958) discussed evaluation only once in explanations of his microtheories. Planners evaluate as part of a planning cycle, after a round of interventions, and in preparation for further interventions. None of Lewin's microtheories gives any attention to determining whether or not interventions help adopter populations reach their own goals.

Despite the absence of instruction regarding evaluation in Lewin's microtheories, nurse planners should not dismiss them as irrelevant. Lewin's (1948, 1951) microtheories provide ideas about force field analysis that would prove very useful in a serious evaluation effort. Lewin did not provide examples of the measurement of forces; he measured results of experimental methods of changing behavior. The measurements proposed (but not illustrated) by Lewin's force field analysis microtheory would lend themselves well to goal-based evaluation if goals were stated in measurable terms. Further, planners could use ideas from his channels theory in making before-and-after depictions of channels, gates, and gatekeepers for either formative or summative evaluation.

Bennis, Benne, and Chin's Writings

Bennis, Benne, and Chin (1985) worked mostly through the words of invited authors. Their choice of ideas and materials for their edited books shows concern for evaluation. In their views, not only does evaluation judge the appropriateness of planning and actions, it also concerns the theories that guide actions. These editors themselves engaged in evaluation when they stated that they considered normative-reeducative strategies of change more suitable for today's situations than rational-empirical or power-coercive strategies. Further, Argyris and Schön (1985) furnished a section on the evaluation of theories of action. They considered the internal consistency of the espoused theory and the theory-in-use with respect to their congruence and addressed the effectiveness, value, and testability of the theory-in-use during the action phase.

Nutt (1985) wrote of the importance of evaluating innovations. Harrison (1985) discussed planners' approaches to strategy. Bermant and Warwick (1985) offered four important criteria for judging the humaneness of processes and outcomes of social interventions. The Bennis, Benne, and Chin writings lend themselves equally well to goal-based and goal-free evaluation.

The Rogers Diffusion Model

Rogers (1995) did not index the word *evaluation,* the word *goals,* or the word *objectives*; planners need to obtain guidance about the specifics of either goal-based or goal-free evaluation from other sources. But Rogers did pay a great deal of attention to evaluation on two other levels. He addressed the philosophical dimensions of diffusion and, on the practical level, provided several ideas and tools that planners could use in actual measurement.

On the philosophical level, Rogers criticized (evaluated) the pro-innovation bias and the individual-blame bias of diffusion research. At some length, he discussed the social inequality caused by diffusion of innovations and proposed ways to prevent the widening of socioeconomic gaps. He addressed adoption of innovations in terms of desirable/undesirable, direct/indirect, and anticipated/unanticipated consequences. The attention that Rogers gave to these and similar issues suggests topics and standards for the evaluation of change episodes. In addition to concepts named above, Rogers provided information related to analysis of populations, identification of social system leaders, and message tracking throughout communication networks. His time-oriented descriptions of innovation development, decision processes, and planner (change agent) roles help planners identify stages of a change episode. Such identification could assist planners in performing either a formative or a summative evaluation. Attention to characteristics of innovations would sharpen an evaluation.

Bhola's Configurations (CLER) Model

Evaluation forms an integral part of Bhola's CLER (1994) model. This model has three theoretical bases: systems theory, dialectical thinking, and constructivism. The systems theory foundation provides the outputs concept that CLER relates to goals. The dialectical formulation explains goal formation, and constructivism directs methods used in development of the innovation.

Systems theory requires an output. That output is the results of the use (adoption) of the innovation. CLER calls for goals to guide formation of the innovation so that it possesses integrity. Second, under dialectics, the formulation of goals provides input by planners (scientific knowledge) and adopters (social system knowledge) through a process of comparison and adjustment of individual and group goals. Constructivism requires comparison and contrast (evaluations according to individuals' standards) of planner and adopter viewpoints in the development of the innovation. No innovation is a completely new creation—the old and the new combine to form the "new." Evaluation forms an integral part of the successive approximations where planners {P} and adopters {A} repeatedly compare the developing innovation with objectives {O}. Thus the checks and balances that make formative evaluation an integral part of the CLER model exist under the {P} × {O} × {A} ensemble (process).

Under constructivism, the innovation (product of construction) and results of its adoption must fit within its context. In other words, the innovation (solution) was developed according to a specific pattern that planners and adopters devised together, and it has to work well in the place where adopters actually use it. Finding out if the innovation actually works calls for evaluation.

In addition to theoretical foundations, Bhola (1974, 1979, 1989, 1990, 1992) gave practical guidelines for conducting an evaluation of a change event. Bhola's emphasis on goals lends itself well to goal-based evaluation; his stress on dialectical theory suggests methods for goal-free evaluation. Both formative and summative evaluation would fit well with Bhola's CLER model.

Summary

Evaluation judges the success of a change event. Analysis precedes evaluation. Analysis identifies underlying themes and component parts of the change situation and tells planners what to evaluate. Evaluation, classified by its relationship to goals, falls into two categories. Goal-based evaluation uses "official" goals (standards) as guides for evaluating a change event. Goal-free evaluation uses the values of individuals not always officially connected with the change in judging success. Formative evaluation occurs during a change project; summative evaluation occurs after completion of a change episode.

Evaluation differs from monitoring. Monitoring looks at everyday functioning to see if everything operates "on track." Evaluation does that too, but it also looks at the major intent of the whole change plan to see if its basic assumptions fall in line with the values of planners and other involved persons.

Wise planners provide early for evaluation. The standards they use in diagnosis, goal setting, choice of innovation, and development of strategies and tactics serve them well in evaluation. They also can involve other interested groups in their plans for evaluation.

Evaluation examines the basic intent of a change episode, the four components of change (diagnosis, innovation, strategy, and evaluation), and the appropriateness of the choice and use of the planned change theory employed in the episode. Evaluative comparisons require either quantitative or qualitative scientific methods, or a combination of the two types. Planners use data collection and analysis methods appropriate to the approach they have chosen. Careful evaluation sometimes permits generalization of results to change situations in other places. A complete evaluation occupies one loop on the inductive/deductive spiral of knowledge generation.

Four major change theorists differ in their approaches to evaluation of planned change events. In spite of Lewin's lack of attention to evaluation, planners can obtain many ideas for evaluation from his force field analysis and channels microtheories.

Bennis, Benne, and Chin addressed evaluation through essays provided by a number of their invited authors. They discussed evaluation of change theories and evaluation of innovations. Two of their invited authors (Bermant & Warwick, 1985) provided a thoughtful discussion of the part that ethical issues should play in the evaluation of any change episode.

Although Rogers did not emphasize evaluation per se, he did criticize some diffusion maneuvers on the basis of their proplanner biases. He also had concern for the long-term results of innovations. In addition, the Rogers model identifies numerous dimensions along which planners could evaluate change events. Rogers supplied several instruments useful in evaluation and gave some instructions for their use.

Evaluation forms part of the theoretical foundation for Bhola's CLER model. The output (the innovation) identified by systems theory is formulated under dialectical theory (dialogue) and must fall within the realm of what planners and adopters together can develop (constructivist viewpoint) in the existing change situation. Planners and adopters work together closely throughout the entire change process to define and implement goals for the change episode. In addition, several Bhola essays provide instruction regarding summative evaluation.

References

Argyris, C., & Schön, D. A. (1985). Evaluating theories of action. In W. G. Bennis, K. D. Benne, & R. Chin (Eds.), *The planning of change* (4th ed., pp. 108-117). New York: Holt, Rinehart & Winston.

Bennis, W. G., Benne, K. D., & Chin, R. (1985). *The planning of change* (4th ed.). New York: Holt, Rinehart & Winston.

Bermant, G., & Warwick, D. P. (1985). The ethics of social intervention: Power, freedom, and accountability. In W. G. Bennis, K. D. Benne, & R. Chin (Eds.), *The planning of change* (4th ed., pp. 449-470). New York: Holt, Rinehart & Winston.

Bhola, H. S. (1974). *ETV in the Third World: A diffusionist's perspective.* Bloomington: Indiana University. (ERIC Document Reproduction Service No. ED 098 926)

Bhola, H. S. (1979). *Evaluating functional literacy.* Teheran, Iran: International Institute for Adult Literacy Methods. (ERIC Document Reproduction Service No. ED 169 498)

Bhola, H. S. (1989). Training evaluators in the Third World: Implementation of the action training model (ATM) in Kenya. *Evaluation and Program Planning, 12,* 249-258.

Bhola, H. S. (1990). *Evaluating "literacy for development": Projects, programs, and campaigns.* Hamburg, Germany: UNESCO Institute of Education. (Available from the Publications Office, UNESCO, Paris)

Bhola, H. S. (1992). A model of evaluation planning, implementation, and management: Toward a "culture of information" within organizations. *International Review of Education, 38*(2), 103-115.

Bhola, H. S. (1994). The CLER model: Thinking through change. *Nursing Management, 25*(5), 59-63.

Hamel-Craig, M. (1994). *Quality of use of planned change theory in nursing periodical literature.* Unpublished master's research project, Andrews University, Berrien Springs, MI.

Harrison, R. (1985). Strategies for a new age. In W. G. Bennis, K. D. Benne, & R. Chin (Eds.), *The planning of change* (4th ed., pp. 128-149). New York: Holt, Rinehart & Winston.

Lewin, K. (1948). *Resolving social conflicts.* New York: Harper.

Lewin, K. (1951). *Field theory in social science.* Chicago: University of Chicago Press.

Lewin, K. (1958). Group decision and social change. In T. M. Newcomb & E. L. Hartley (Eds.), *Readings in social psychology* (pp. 197-211). New York: Holt.

Nutt, P. C. (1985). The study of planning process. In W. G. Bennis, K. D. Benne, & R. Chin (Eds.), *The planning of change* (4th ed., pp. 198-215). New York: Holt, Rinehart & Winston.

Rogers, E. M. (1995). *The diffusion of innovations* (3rd ed.). New York: Free Press.

Tiffany, C. R. (1994). Analysis of planned change theories. *Nursing Management, 25*(2), 60-62.

Bridging the Gap

Altering Square Pegs
to Fit Round Holes

BOX 9.2: KEY WORDS AND PHRASES

— Adaptation
— Adaptation level
— Adaptive
— Adaptive modes
— Adaptive system modes
— Cognator subsystem
— Contextual stimuli
— Developmental approach
— Developmental category of nursing knowledge
— Discipline
— Environment
— First-level assessment
— Focal stimulus
— Goal of nursing
— Goals of human system

— Health
— Holism
— Ineffective response
— Innovator subsystem
— Interaction approach
— Interdependence adaptive mode
— Interdependence adaptive system mode
— Interpersonal adaptive system mode
— Linear
— Metaparadigm concepts
— Nursing (actions)
— Nursing diagnosis
— Nursing intervention
— Person
— Physiological adaptive system mode

— Reaction worldview
— Reciprocal interaction worldview
— Reformulation
— Regulator subsystem
— Residual stimuli
— Role adaptive system mode
— Role function adaptive mode
— Second-level assessment
— Self-concept adaptive mode
— Simultaneous action worldview
— Stabilizer subsystem
— Systems approach
— Worldview

This chapter contains two main sections. The first discusses congruence between worldviews foundational to nursing models/theories and planned change theories. The second presents a synopsis of the Roy Adaptation Model for use as a reference point in considerations of the borrowing of change theories for nursing use.

From Borrowing to Sharing

Nurses often borrow planned change theories from the social sciences and use them (generally without adaptation) for creating change in nursing situations (Tiffany, Cheatham, Doornbos, Loudermelt, & Momadi, 1994). Nurses have spent little effort in examining the congruence between planned change theories and nursing models/theories to determine if they can be shared properly. This examination is becoming increasingly necessary as more nurses use nursing models/theories as a basis for practice. Congruence between planned change theories and nursing models/theories will enable the sharing of change theories by the disciplines of social science and nursing. Shared theories will enhance the planning of change by nurses in clinical practice, administration, and education.

This part of the chapter rests on the assumption that the discipline of nursing views planned change theories as a proper subject of inquiry useful for and applicable to nursing situations. The broad level of applicability of nursing models/theories makes them ideal for use as theoretical umbrellas under which planned change theories can be examined for congruence with nursing models/theories and reformulated (translated) to plan change in nursing situations. The proper sharing of theories from other disciplines with the discipline of nursing has been discussed by several nurse theorists.

Donaldson and Crowley (1978, p. 118) stated that because of the uniqueness of each discipline's perspective and context, it is not possible simply to borrow theories from another discipline (body or branch of knowledge). Hardy (1978) stated that although nursing is free to draw upon theories developed by other disciplines, it has an obligation to alter those theories (square pegs) to fit into nursing situations (round holes). Hardy's position is consistent with that of Ellis (1968), who stated that theories used in nursing need examination in light of nursing knowledge. Whall (1980b) supported Ellis (1968) and Hardy (1978) by stating that if nursing is to develop a body of knowledge upon which to base practice, it would be counterproductive to borrow theories "as is" without first examining their consistency with nursing. Fawcett (1978) offered greater specificity by proposing that if nursing is to share a theory with another discipline, that theory first must be examined for congruence with the key concepts (metaparadigm concepts) of nursing (i.e., person, environment, health, and nursing). She further stated that reformulation (translation) of the metaparadigm concepts and the development of statements about the relationships among these key concepts are necessary before the borrowed theory can be designated as shared with nursing (Fawcett, 1993a, 1995).

> According to Schwab (1964) disciplines have both substantive and syntactical structures. The substantive structure is composed of conceptualizations [ideas] which are borrowed [for example, from change theories] or invented, but their inclusion is always based on their fit with the perspective of the discipline. (Donaldson & Crowley, 1978, p. 119)

The substantive structure in nursing reveals that the proper subject of inquiry is human beings. "Nursing studies the wholeness or health of [human beings] recognizing that [they] are in continuous interaction with their environments" (p. 119). The substantive structure in planned change theories has determined that the proper subject of inquiry is change as it relates to human beings. This book is premised on the assumption that planned change theories form a substantive knowledge base that provides a proper subject of inquiry for nursing that can be viewed from a nursing context. This assumption is supported by the fact that many nursing conceptual models/theories, such as those of Johnson, Levin, Newman, Rogers, Roy, and Parse (Fawcett, 1995), discuss change. Recently, change has been identified as a critical concern of nursing (DeFeo, 1990). The challenge for the authors is to determine the acceptability of the conceptualizations (ideas) within planned change theories with respect to their goodness of fit with nursing theory (syntactical structure).

The syntactical structure, according to Schwab (1964), is "the way in which the discipline synthesizes and examines the substantive knowledge" (Whall, 1980a, p. 60). According to Whall (1980a), nursing conceptual models/theories can be used as the syntax by which existing theories may be examined for adequacy of concepts and identification of weaknesses. The purpose of the examination is reformulation (translation) of the existing theories—in this case, planned change theories.

The following sections contain discussions of worldviews and their influence on disciplines, descriptions of several categories of nursing knowledge, and explanations of relationships between categories of nursing knowledge, holism, and linearity.

Worldviews

Worldviews, which may include beliefs about change, influence the ways people in a discipline view their knowledge base and key concepts. It is important to examine planned change theories to discover their worldviews and

TABLE 9.1 Reaction, Reciprocal Interaction, and Simultaneous Action Worldviews

The Reaction Worldview	The Reciprocal Interaction Worldview	The Simultaneous Action Worldview
Humans are bio-psycho-social-spiritual beings.	Human beings are holistic. Parts are viewed only in the context of the whole.	Unitary human beings are identified by pattern.
Human beings react to external environmental stimuli in a linear, causal manner.	Human beings are active. Interactions between human beings and their environments are reciprocal. Reality is multidimensional, context dependent, and relative.	Human beings are in mutual rhythmical interchange with their environments. Human beings change continuously and evolve as self-organized systems.
Change occurs only for survival and as a consequence of predictable and controllable antecedent conditions.	Change is a function of multiple antecedent factors. Change is probabilistic and may be continuous or may be only for survival.	Change is unidirectional and unpredictable as human beings move through stages of organization and disorganization to more complex organizations.
Only objective phenomena that can be isolated, defined, observed, and measured are studied.	Both objective and subjective phenomena are studied through quantitative and qualitative methods of inquiry. Emphasis is placed on empirical observations, methodological controls, and inferential data analytic techniques.	Phenomena of interest are personal knowledge and pattern recognition.

SOURCE: Fawcett, J. (1993). From a plethora of paradigms to parsimony in world views. *Nursing Science Quarterly, 6*(2), 58. Reprinted by permission.

to determine the congruency of these worldviews with nursing models/theories. *Worldviews* have been defined by Fawcett (1993b) as "philosophic claims about the nature of human beings and the human-environment relationship" (p. 56). Recently, Fawcett proposed one set of three worldviews. The inherent beliefs involved in these worldviews (titled *reaction, reciprocal interaction,* and *simultaneous action*) are listed in Table 9.1.

Three of the four change theories (or models, or collections of writings) discussed in this book (Lewin; Bennis, Benne, and Chin; and Rogers) demonstrate *reciprocal interaction* worldviews. This is not surprising given

TABLE 9.2 Characteristics of Three Categories of Nursing Knowledge:
Developmental, Systems, and Interaction

Characteristics of the Developmental Approach	Characteristics of the Systems Approach	Characteristics of the Interaction Approach
Growth, development, and maturation	Integration of parts	Social acts and relationships
Change	System	Perception
Direction of change	Environment	Communication
Identifiable state	Open and closed systems	Role
Form of progression	Boundary	Self-concept
Forces	Tension, stress, strain, conflict	
Potentiality	Equilibrium and steady state	
	Feedback	

SOURCE: Fawcett, J. (1995). *Analysis and evaluation of conceptual models of nursing* (3rd ed.), p. 22. Philadelphia: F. A. Davis. Reprinted by permission.

the nature of the subject matter—planned change. Bhola's writings show a worldview consistent with the characteristics of *simultaneous action.* (See Table 9.1.) These characteristics appear most often in his discussions on dialectics and constructivism.

Fawcett (1995) identified the Neuman Systems Model, the Self-Care Framework, and the Roy Adaptation Model as nursing conceptual models that hold a *reciprocal interaction* worldview. She further identified the Science of Unitary Human Beings as holding a *simultaneous action* worldview. Contemporary nursing models/theories have moved beyond a reaction worldview.

Categories of Nursing Knowledge

Philosophical claims by nursing about the nature of human beings also are reflected in broad categories of nursing knowledge. Drawing upon the disciplines of psychology, biology and physics, and sociology, Fawcett (1995) identified three categories of nursing knowledge: developmental, systems, and interaction. Characteristics of the three categories of nursing knowledge, as described by Fawcett, are listed in Table 9.2

All four of the planned change theories discussed in this book have been developed using the systems approach. This is consistent given that the targets for change most often are social units. Additionally, all have *interactionist* levels of analysis. This is expected, given that the interaction approach comes from sociology, and the theoretical knowledge base of planned change theories is the social sciences. An excellent example of an interactionist level of analysis is the identification and measurement of driving and restraining forces found in Lewin's change theories.

Among nursing conceptual models, Fawcett (1995) categorized the Self-Care Framework as an example of a *developmental* model, the Neuman Systems Model as a *systems* model, and the Roy Adaptation Model as a *systems* model with *interactionist* levels of analysis.

Holism and Linearity

Holism and *linearity* are two interrelated concepts (idea structures) that are prominent in differing worldviews and categories of nursing knowledge. In the holistic view, one must consider the total, not the parts, because the total is different than the parts. The Cartesian position that the mind and body are separate is contrary to holistic thinking. *Reductionism,* which follows the Cartesian position, holds that summing the parts equals the total, the whole. In contrast, the holistic view is that mind, body, and spirit are one and are different than the sum of the parts. The person, viewed holistically, is considered the proper subject for nursing. Moreover, from a true holistic perspective, the family, or any other social unit, would be considered a different entity than the combination of individual members (Whall, 1980b; Whall & Fawcett, 1991). Although family members contribute to and influence the family, the family differs from its members.

The health-illness continuum is a familiar example of linearity. If one believes that persons at any point in time can separate themselves from their present environment and go back in time to solve a problem in the past, this is linear thinking. Linear thinking is not consistent with holistic thinking. Given nursing's strong position that holistic persons are the proper subject for nursing, an understanding of the positions on holism and linearity taken by planned change theories is warranted.

Many linear terms and linear diagrams are found in the four planned change theories discussed in this book because their basic approach comes from systems theory. However, some of the theoretical discussions appear to be more illustrative of holistic than linear thinking. Bhola's Configurations (CLER) model appears to be the most holistic of the four.

The Science of Unitary Human Beings is a nursing conceptual model that exemplifies consistency with holistic (nonlinear) thinking. Readers will find that not all nursing models/theories are as consistent as this one.

**The Round Hole: Change From
the Roy Adaptation Model Perspective**

Many nursing conceptual models/theories are available for nurses to choose from when selecting a framework for practice. This part of the chapter discusses relationships between the planned change theories of Lewin; Bennis, Benne, and Chin; Rogers; and Bhola and the Roy Adaptation Model (RAM). The RAM was chosen because the model is used widely in practice and education and has been developed and used in an organizational context (DiIorio, 1989; Lutjens, 1992, 1994; Roy & Anway, 1989) to a greater extent than other nursing models/theories. Moreover, Roy's use of the term *adaptive* to describe individuals as well as her stated scientific assumptions (Roy, 1980) about the ability of individuals to change provide a strong, clear conceptual fit with planned change theories.

This section introduces basic concepts in the RAM that will be used as building blocks for subsequent discussions. The section includes (a) a short description of the origin and foundations of the RAM, (b) a description of the key nursing concepts and other major concepts of the RAM, and (c) a brief discussion of major modifications of the RAM applied to selected organizations. Later chapters (d) look at the four change theories featured in the book from a Roy perspective and (e) apply the combined models (the RAM and a change theory) to a nursing situation. The RAM and all change theories hold a worldview of change as inherent, natural, and continuous. Moreover, they all assume that people adapt to a changing environment—albeit to differing degrees.

Foundation and History
of the Roy Adaptation Model

Roy began work on the RAM in 1964 while she was a graduate student at the University of California, Los Angeles (Lutjens, 1991). The concept of adaptation was introduced to Roy in a psychology class. As a pediatric nurse, she had been impressed with the ability of children to bounce back from critical illness. This clinical experience struck Roy as a poignant example of adaptation and a suitable concept upon which to build a theory of nursing. This example is illustrative of Roy's reciprocal interaction worldview. In addition to her clinical observations, Roy creatively combined ideas from several other theories to develop the RAM. The most notable influences come from Bertalanffy's General Systems Theory and Helson's Adaptation-Level Theory.

The RAM was used first in 1968 as the conceptual framework for a baccalaureate nursing curriculum at Mount St. Mary's College in Los Angeles. The first publication on the RAM appeared in 1970. Since that time, the RAM continues to be used by many clinical nurses and nurse administrators, educators, and researchers in their practice settings. Many publications on the experiences of nurses working with the RAM appear in the nursing literature. The RAM is one of the most highly developed and widely used conceptual models of nursing.

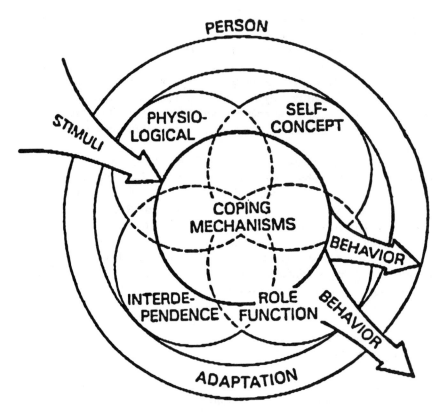

Figure 9.1. The Person as an Adaptive System

SOURCE: From "Essentials of the Roy Adaptation Model," by H. A. Andrews and C. Roy. In C. Roy & H. A. Andrews (Eds.), *The Roy Adaptation Model: The Definitive Statement*, p. 17. Copyright © 1991 by Appleton & Lange. Reprinted by permission.

Essentials of the Roy Adaptation Model

The RAM is a systems model; thus the major features of this model are the system and its environment. A system is a set of parts connected to function as a whole for some purpose. It is the interrelationship of these parts that allows the system to function as a whole. The specific and unique interrelationships of any given system differentiate that system from other systems. The cardiovascular system and the gastrointestinal system are familiar examples of human systems. The idea of system is clearly seen in Roy's description of the recipient of nursing care—the person.

Person. In all nursing models, there are four common key concepts (metaparadigm concepts) that serve as cornerstones upon which the model is built. The metaparadigm concepts are person, environment, health, and nursing (actions). Person is defined by Roy as a holistic adaptive system. According to Roy, holistic "pertains to the idea that the human system functions as a whole and is more than the mere sum of its parts" (Andrews & Roy, 1991a, p. 6). The term *adaptive* "means that the human system has the capacity to adjust effectively to changes in the environment and, in turn, affects the environment" (Andrews & Roy, 1991a, p. 7). Systems have *inputs, controls, output,* and a *feedback loop* (Andrews & Roy, 1991a). (See Figure 9.1.) Although these terms in systems theory are considered linear, the RAM appears more holistic than linear.

Environment. According to Roy, "environment includes all conditions, circumstances, and influences that surround and affect the development and behavior of the person" (Andrews & Roy, 1991a, p. 18). Environment is the world within and around the recipient of care, the person. In systems terminology, environmental stimuli are inputs. These conditions, circumstances, and influences can be categorized as focal, contextual, or residual stimuli. The focal stimulus is the stressor, that which immediately confronts and provokes the adaptive system. A disease or surgical event is an example of a focal stimulus. Contextual stimuli are those that add to the effect of the focal stimulus. These are often sociodemographic characteristics of clients. Residual stimuli are unknown or otherwise unmeasurable factors contributing to the effect of the focal stimulus on the adaptive system. These stimuli might be hunches or "gut" feelings.

The processing of environmental stimuli by an adaptive system is accomplished by regulator and cognator systems. In systems terminology, these subsystems are the controls or processors. The regulator subsystem consists of neural, chemical, endocrine, and perception/psychomotor processes. The cognator subsystem consists of apparatus and pathways for adaptive systems to perceive, process information, learn, make judgments, and display emotion. In addition to the particular stimuli, the pooled effect of the stimuli, that is, the adaptation level, also influences the person. "Adaptation level is a constantly changing point that represents a person's ability to cope with the changing environment in a positive manner" (Lutjens, 1991, p. 14).

Health. Health is defined as "a state and a process of being and becoming an integrated and whole person" (Andrews & Roy, 1991a, p. 19). A person's health is a reflection of adaptation. Thus adaptive responses that promote integrity or wholeness are outputs that represent health. Ineffective responses reflect a lack of integration or a disruption in wholeness and therefore represent a lack of health.

Adaptive responses resulting in health are observed and measured in four adaptive modes: physiological, self-concept, role function, and interdependence. The physiological mode is concerned with maintaining the physical and physiological integrity of a person. The self-concept mode is concerned with a person's perception of his or her personal self. The role function mode is concerned with the performance of a person's roles in society, such as parent, nurse, or church worker. The interdependence mode is concerned with the development and maintenance of satisfying relationships.

Nursing. The goal of nursing is to promote adaptation, thereby contributing in a positive manner to the person's health, quality of life, or dignified death (Andrews & Roy, 1991a). Nursing promotes adaptation by enhancing the interaction between the person and the environment for the purpose of attaining the goals of the human system: survival, growth, reproduction, and mastery. These goals are viewed in a broad sense. For example, growth can be psychological and/or spiritual as well as physical. Reproduction includes producing creative work in addition to producing children (Roy, 1990). The nursing process is the method that nurses use to promote adaptation and, thereby, health.

The nursing process, according to the RAM, consists of six steps—assessment of behavior, assessment of stimuli, nursing diagnosis, goal setting, intervention, and evaluation (Andrews & Roy, 1991b). First-level assessment gathers data about behavior. In second-level assessment, nurses categorize client responses to stimuli in four adaptive modes: physiological, self-concept, role function, and interdependence. A tentative judgment is made at this point regarding the effectiveness of the client's behavioral responses to internal and external environmental stimuli. The assessment process continues by identifying the stimuli influencing the client's behavioral responses. Nursing diagnosis, according to the RAM, is a statement about the person's adaptation status. It results from the judgment process (critical thinking) of the nurse. (See Figure 9.2.)

Goal setting is "the establishment of clear statements of the behavioral outcomes of nursing care for the patient" (Andrews & Roy, 1991b, p. 42). Intervention is the management of the stimuli, specifically the focal stimulus, and the adaptive level, to maintain and enhance adaptive behavior or to change ineffective behavior to adaptive behavior. Evaluation is determining "the effectiveness of the nursing intervention in relation to the person's behavior" (Andrews & Roy, 1991b, p. 46).

In summary, the RAM views the person as constantly growing and developing within a changing environment to which one must adapt. Adaptation is both a process and an end state. Adaptive responses—proactive and reactive—promote health. The nurse's role is to promote adaptation so that health may be attained and/or maintained or death with dignity may be achieved.

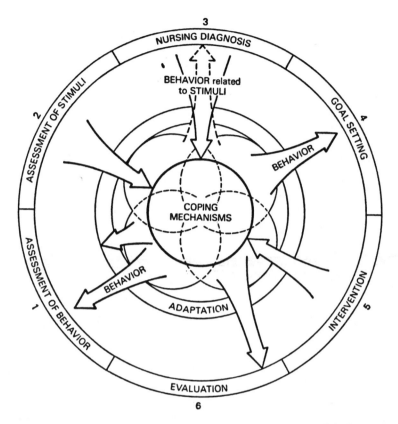

Figure 9.2. The Nursing Process as It Relates to Roy's Description of the Person
SOURCE: From "The Nursing Process According to the Roy Adaptation Model," by H. A. Andrews and C. Roy. In C. Roy & H. A. Andrews (Eds.), *The Roy Adaptation Model: The Definitive Statement,* p. 30. Copyright © 1991 by Appleton & Lange. Reprinted by permission.

The Roy Adaptation Model
Applied to Administration (RAMA)

Although the RAM is built upon the concept of an individual person, as are all nursing conceptual models and theories, the foundational concept of person can extend to families, groups, communities, and other social systems (Schultz, 1988). That is, the recipient of care can be a family, a group, a community, or an organizational unit such as the nursing staff on a clinical unit. Roy's own work includes beginning theories derived from the RAM applied to families (Roy, 1983), communities (Roy, 1984), and, most recently, organizations (Roy

& Anway, 1989). DiIorio (1989) and Lutjens (1992) also have used the RAM to derive theories for organizations. Because change theories are most often used to effect change at some level of an organization, it is important to know those modifications of the RAM that are specific to organizations as adaptive systems.

Organizational adaptive systems. Just as clients have regulator and cognator subsystems as sources of adaptation, likewise, organizations have stabilizer and innovator subsystems. The stabilizer subsystem consists of structures and processes that maintain the organization on a day-to-day basis. "Stabilizers involve the established structures, values, and daily activities whereby staff accomplish the primary purpose of the organization" (Roy & Anway, 1989, p. 79). Examples of stabilizers in nursing service would be staffing and scheduling plans, standard plans of care, unit culture, and the delivery of patient care.

The innovator subsystem consists of structures and processes that enable organizational change and growth. Examples of innovators would be new technology, like lasers, that change the ways things are done, task forces that are organized to solve problems, and educational programs presented to teach about new technologies or problem-solving methods.

Adaptive system modes. The adaptive modes also are modified for organizations and given new labels: physical, interpersonal, role, and interdependence systems (Roy & Anway, 1989). The physical system includes communication systems, technology, physical plant, organizational structure, and financial systems, to name several. The interpersonal system includes such factors as the organization's image, organizational culture, and interpersonal relationships among health care team members. The role system includes the duties and responsibilities of roles undertaken or positions assumed by people within an organization, for example, staff nurse, nurse manager, and quality assurance officer. The last adaptive system, interdependence, includes external contacts such as suppliers, vendors, government and legal regulations, and the market for the services provided by the organization. Internal contacts include liaisons with units within organizations such as other divisions, departments, offices, and agencies.

Nursing management process. Like clients, organizations are influenced by stimuli internal and external to themselves. The focal stimulus is that which demands a management focus. A diagnosis-related group (DRG) that is losing money for the hospital is an example of a focal stimulus. Certain contextual stimuli would contribute to the effect of this focal stimulus. These might include nurse practice behaviors, physician ordering practices, and sources of payment for clients' hospital stays (Lutjens, 1994). Such contextual stimuli could aggravate the problem or, in other words, exaggerate the effect of the focal stimulus. Residual stimuli include attitudes of physicians and nurses toward government

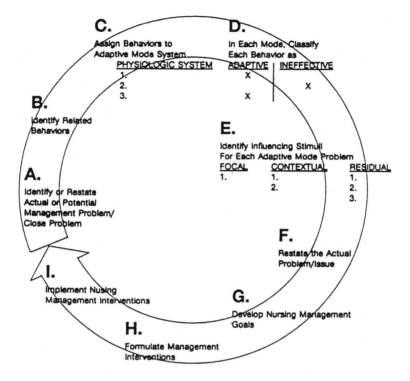

Figure 9.3. RAMA Nursing Process From Assessment Through Evaluation

SOURCE: From "Roy's Adaptation Model: Theories for Nursing Administration," by C. Roy and J. Anway. In B. Henry, C. Arndt, M. Di Vincenti, & A. Marriner-Tomey (Eds.), *Dimensions of Nursing Administration: Theory, Research, Education, Practice*, p. 84. Copyright © 1989 by Blackwell Scientific Ltd. Reprinted by permission.

intervention in their respective practices and of hospitals toward government regulatory practices in health care.

In nursing management, steps of the nursing process remain the same as in clinical care of clients but the focus is different—the organizational unit becomes the client. The "caregiver" for the organization might be the nurse manager who needs to assess the behavioral responses of the nursing unit, assign behaviors to adaptive system modes, and classify, in each mode, each behavior as adaptive or ineffective. (See Figure 9.3.) The assessment process concludes with a nursing management diagnosis, a statement about the organization's adaptive status. Goals set for the nursing unit clearly delineate the expected unit outcomes. The nurse manager formulates management interventions, often called strategies, to manage stimuli affronting the unit. Strategies are implemented and then are evaluated in relation to progress toward the established nursing management goals.

Summary

The first part of this book discussed general considerations necessary to the proper use of planned change theories. The second part presents four planned change theories and discusses relationships between them and nursing models/theories. This chapter provided an interlude between the two book parts.

This chapter presented two aspects of the borrowing of planned change theories by nursing. It started with a discussion about differences between borrowing and sharing theories. The second part of the chapter, a presentation of the Roy Adaptation Model, anticipates discussions in later chapters.

First, this chapter differentiated between theory borrowing and theory sharing. It continued with a presentation of a set of three worldviews proposed by Fawcett (1993b): reaction, reciprocal interaction, and simultaneous action. The worldviews reflected in the four change theories discussed in the book were identified and examples were given of worldviews found in selected nursing models/theories. Compatibility was evident.

Areas of nursing knowledge (developmental, systems, and interaction) categorized in nursing literature by Fawcett (1995) were presented. The four change theories were examined in light of these categories of nursing knowledge. All used a systems approach with interactionist levels of analysis.

The interrelated concepts of holism and linearity were defined, followed by a short discussion of their use in the four planned change theories. The CLER model was found to be the most holistic of the planned change theories. Among nursing conceptual models/theories, the Science of Unitary Human Beings was identified as an exemplar of holistic thinking. Chapters in the second part of the book will examine the four planned change theories for congruence with the Roy Adaptation Model (RAM) and will translate aspects of theories, as necessary, to achieve consistency with the RAM.

The second part of this chapter started with a brief description of the foundation and history of the Roy Adaptation Model. The model first appeared in 1968 as the conceptual framework for a nursing curriculum and was published in 1970. The chapter continued with a presentation of key concepts and relationships found in the Roy Adaptation Model. These concepts include the four key concepts found in any nursing model/theory (person, environment, health, and nursing). The modification of the RAM for use in nursing organizations described the stabilizer and innovator subsystems that enable organizations to adapt. The modified RAM gave new labels to adaptive system modes (physical, interpersonal, role, and interdependence systems) and provided examples for each mode. Nursing management processes deal with the focal, contextual, and residual stimuli described in the last part of the chapter. In later chapters, the RAM, with the previously discussed modifications for organizations, will be used to examine a planned change theory and to apply the translated change theory to a nursing situation.

References

Andrews, H. A., & Roy, C. (1991a). Essentials of the Roy Adaptation Model. In C. Roy & H. A. Andrews (Eds.), *The Roy Adaptation Model: The definitive statement* (pp. 3-25). East Norwalk, CT: Appleton & Lange.

Andrews, H. A., & Roy, C. (1991b). The nursing process according to the Roy Adaptation Model. In C. Roy & H. A. Andrews (Eds.), *The Roy Adaptation Model: The definitive statement* (pp. 27-54). East Norwalk, CT: Appleton & Lange.

DeFeo, D. J. (1990). Change: A central concern of nursing. *Nursing Science Quarterly, 3,* 88-94.

DiIorio, C. K. (1989). Application of the Roy model to nursing administration. In B. Henry, C. Arndt, M. Di Vincenti, & A. Marriner-Tomey (Eds.), *Dimensions of nursing administration: Theory, research, education, practice* (pp. 89-104). Boston: Blackwell Scientific.

Donaldson, S. K., & Crowley, D. M. (1978). The discipline of nursing. *Nursing Outlook, 26,* 113-120.

Ellis, R. (1968). Characteristics of significant theories. *Nursing Research, 17,* 217-222.

Fawcett, J. (1978). The what of theory development. In *What, why, and how of theory development* (Publication No. 15-798, pp. 17-33). New York: National League for Nursing.

Fawcett, J. (1993a). *Analysis and evaluation of nursing theories.* Philadelphia: F. A. Davis.

Fawcett, J. (1993b). From a plethora of paradigms to parsimony in world views. *Nursing Science Quarterly, 6,* 56-58.

Fawcett, J. (1995). *Analysis and evaluation of conceptual models of nursing* (3rd ed.). Philadelphia: F. A. Davis.

Hardy, M. E. (1978). Evaluating nursing theory. In *What, why, and how of theory development* (Publication No. 15-798, pp. 75-86). New York: National League for Nursing.

Lutjens, L. R. J. (1991). Callista Roy: An adaptation model. In C. M. McQuiston & A. A. Webb (Eds.), *Notes on nursing theories* (Vol. 3). Newbury Park, CA: Sage.

Lutjens, L. R. J. (1992). Derivation and testing of tenets of a theory of social organizations as adaptive systems. *Nursing Science Quarterly, 5,* 62-71.

Lutjens, L. R. J. (1994). Hospital payment source and length-of-stay. *Nursing Science Quarterly, 7,* 174-179.

Roy, C. (1980). The Roy Adaptation Model. In J. P. Riehl & C. Roy (Eds.), *Conceptual models for nursing practice* (pp. 179-192). New York: Appleton-Century-Crofts.

Roy, C. (1983). Roy Adaptation Model. In I. W. Clements & F. B. Roberts (Eds.), *Family health: A theoretical approach to nursing care* (pp. 298-303). New York: John Wiley.

Roy, C. (1984). The Roy Adaptation Model: Applications in community health nursing. In M. K. Assoy & C. C. Ossler (Eds.), *Conceptual models of nursing: Applications in community health nursing: Proceedings of the Eighth Annual Community Health Nursing Conference* (pp. 51-73). Chapel Hill: University of North Carolina Press.

Roy, C. (1990). Strengthening the Roy Adaptation Model through conceptual clarification-response. *Nursing Science Quarterly, 3,* 64-66.

Roy, C., & Anway, J. (1989). Roy's adaptation model: Theories for nursing administration. In B. Henry, C. Arndt, M. Di Vincenti, & A. Marriner-Tomey (Eds.), *Dimensions of nursing administration: Theory, research, education, practice* (pp. 75-88). Boston: Blackwell Scientific.

Schultz, P. R. (1988). When client means more than one: Extending the foundational concept of person. *Advances in Nursing Science, 10,* 71-86.

Schwab, J. (1964). Structure of the disciplines: Meanings and significances. In G. Ford (Ed.), *The structure of knowledge and the curriculum* (pp. 6-30). Chicago: Rand McNally.

Tiffany, C. R., Cheatham, A. B., Doornbos, D., Loudermelt, L., & Momadi, G. G. (1994). Planned change theory: Survey of nursing periodical literature. *Nursing Management, 25*(7), 54-59.

Whall, A. L. (1980a). Congruence between existing theories of family functioning and nursing theories. *Advances in Nursing Science, 3,* 59-67.

Whall, A. L. (1980b). *Family therapy theory for nursing: Four approaches.* Norwalk, CT: Appleton-Century-Crofts.

Whall, A. L., & Fawcett, J. (1991). *Family theory development in nursing: State of the science and art.* Philadelphia: F. A. Davis.

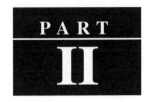

PART

II

Theory Considerations
in Planned Change

10

Lewin's Microtheories

> ## BOX 10.1: LOOKING AHEAD
>
> **Chapter 10: Lewin's Microtheories**
> **Foundations of the Theories**
> **Lewin's Contributions to Social Science**
> **Field Theory**
> **Field Theory and the Microtheories**

> ## BOX 10.2: KEY WORDS AND PHRASES
>
> — Conflict
> — Correspondence of forces
> — Driving force
> — Field
> — Field theory
> — Force
> — Force field analysis
> — Freeze
> — Gate
> — Gatekeeper
> — Gestalt
> — Gestalt psychology
> — Goal
> — Impersonal force
> — Individual-group relationships microtheory (I-G)
> — Induced force
> — Locomotion
> — Move
> — Own-needs force
> — Position
> — Restraining force
> — Unfreeze
> — Valence

In the nursing world, "everybody knows" that the words *unfreeze, move,* and *freeze* belong to Lewin. But Lewin's theories offer a great deal more than these three famous words indicate. This chapter and the next two chapters of the book explore that "something more" and offer suggestions for its use. This

117

chapter presents Lewin's theoretical work that pertains to planned change. Chapter 11 analyzes and critiques Lewin's theories. Chapter 12 coordinates Lewin's planned change theories with a nursing theory and offers suggestions for theory application in nursing situations.

The current chapter starts with an account of the background of Lewin's work. It continues with a presentation of field theory and four microtheories: (a) individual-group relationships, (b) quasi-stationary equilibria, (c) force field analysis, and (d) channels theory. Readers may wish to scan Appendix A for definitions of the glossary words in Box 10.2 before reading the chapter.

Foundations of the Theories

Kurt Lewin was born on September 9, 1890, in Mogilno, Prussia (Poland). He was educated in universities at Freiburg, Munich, and Berlin. His academic career started in Berlin in 1914 (Wessman, 1988). The Psychological Institute in Berlin provided Lewin and his students with a stimulating, supportive, and relaxed environment that nurtured creativity. Lewin's valuing of others and his tolerant stance toward them created a particularly healthful atmosphere (De Rivera, 1976). His career continued after he moved to the United States in 1933. Lewin taught at Stanford, Cornell, and Iowa universities. He founded the Research Center for Group Dynamics at the Massachusetts Institute of Technology. He died in Newtonville, Massachusetts, on February 12, 1947 (Wessman, 1988).

Lewin, a Jew, came to the United States to escape Hitler's crusade in Germany. Although he used many resources and much effort to rescue family, friends, and colleagues, his own mother died in a gas chamber (Cook, 1986). Lewin saw social science as a means for preventing, in the United States, the ills from which he had fled. As a moralist, Lewin combined values for science and for democracy in his efforts to combat the racism and anti-Semitism he saw in the United States, his beloved adopted country (Benne, 1985).

Cartwright (1951) wrote that

> [d]uring the 30 some years of Lewin's professional life, the social sciences grew from the stage of speculative system building, through a period of excessive empiricism in which facts were gathered simply for their intrinsic interest, to a more mature development in which empirical data are sought for the significance they can have for systematic theories. . . . [Lewin's] earliest work in Berlin dealt with the comparative theory of science. . . . He then proceeded throughout the rest of his life to work systematically toward establishing such a science. (p. vii)

In addition, Lewin was a major contributor to Gestalt psychology; he greatly influenced the development of modern social psychology (Wessman, 1988).

Lewin's Contributions to Social Science

Lewin's contributions fall into the two main categories of concepts and methods. Perhaps the idea of "field" best represents the concepts he developed. Lewin observed that all things happen in what he called a force field. This field consists of social, historical, situational, and physical influences surrounding individuals. Thus he emphasized relationships between individuals and forces in their environments. In his revolutionary emphasis on method, Lewin maintained that social sciences, such as psychology and sociology, are science as truly as physics and chemistry are science. He developed testable hypotheses from his theories and adapted experimentation to the problems of everyday life. He devised ways to test theory through observation of empirical data (Allport, 1948; Cartwright, 1951). His biographer called Lewin the "practical theorist" (Marrow, 1969).

Although Lewin was not interested in authorship credit, and never published a book, he provided a number of very understandable statements of his concepts and methods. In 1948, Lewin's widow, Gertrude Weiss Lewin, together with Gordon W. Allport, edited a volume of Lewin's papers that reprinted discussions of practical issues such as cultural differences and reeducation. These papers reveal Lewin's search for the laws of human behavior that later formed a unifying thread in his theoretical work. His intent was to build a bridge between social theory and social action (G. Lewin, 1948). Dorwin Cartwright edited a second Lewin volume in 1951, which presents Lewin's more theoretical papers, including those most often quoted by nurse authors. The two volumes capture the essence of Lewin's work during the 15 years that he lived in the United States. (Uppercase letters with the dates in certain Lewin citations in this chapter correspond to the reference system in Appendix C, section C.1, which was designed to help readers access Lewin's original writings.)

Field Theory

A gestalt is a configuration, an organized whole, with an emergent quality and properties more and different than the sum of its parts. Gestalt psychology considers a person's perception and behavior in light of configurational wholes. Lewin's field theory and his planned change theories clearly reflect his gestaltist viewpoints.

Lewin considered social phenomena to be as real as physical phenomena, and their recognition necessary to their scientific analysis. He believed that judging something as nonexistent puts it out of bounds for the scientist. To Lewin, the scientific analysis of social phenomena requires that both researchers and social planners have "a system of analysis which permits the representation of social forces in a group setting" ([1947A, 1947B] 1951, p. 200).

Concepts in field theory. In the course of field theory development, Lewin devised several concepts that describe social and psychological phenomena and serve as foundations for the theory. For example, he defined position as a spatial relationship of social regions. This could involve relationships such as the belongingness of an individual person to a group or to a work situation. *Position* refers to only one point, whereas *structure* is the placement of several points in relative positions in a field. *Field* is the total life space of an individual or group—the environment as it exists for the person or group. *Locomotion* is movement from one position to another; it relates to positions occupied at different times. A force is a tendency toward locomotion, an influence brought to bear on individuals or groups to motivate them to change or to remain the same. Forces can include such entities as values, peer pressures, past experiences, and the (un)availability of resources such as time, money, and influence. *Driving forces* encourage locomotion toward goals with a positive valence and away from goals with a negative valence. *Restraining forces* discourage locomotion. Locomotion occurs with a sum of forces greater than zero. A *force field* (field of forces) is the total of the influences toward change or nonchange present in the physical and social environment of an individual or group. A *goal* is a field in which all forces aim in the same direction. *Conflict* is a situation that exists when opposing forces have comparable strength and two or more force fields overlap (Lewin, [1944A] 1951).

Temporal aspects of field theory. To Allport (1948), field theory was "Lewin's system of thought" (p. ix). De Rivera (1976) described field theory as a conceptualization of behavior:

> Basically, field theory is an attempt to describe the essential here-and-now situation (field) in which a person participates. It assumes that if one fully understood a person's "situation" (in the broadest meaning of this term), one would fully understand his behavior. Hence the goal of field theory is to be able to describe fields with systematic concepts in such a precise way that a person's behavior follows logically from the relationship between the person and the dynamics and structure of his concrete situation. (p. 3)

One of the most important aspects of field theory is the idea that "any behavior or any other change in a psychological field depends only upon the psychological *field at that time*" (Lewin, [1943B] 1951, p. 45). This temporal aspect of field theory gives the theory a process orientation that holds implications for methods. The time orientation carries importance for nurse planners as they determine the characteristics of a field at a given time and choose a sequence for strategies and tactics. Strategies appropriate to one stage of the change process may not work during another stage.

Field Theory and the Microtheories

Field theory, not a usual type of theory, might better be termed "a method of *analyzing causal relations and of building scientific constructs*" (Lewin, [1943B] 1951, p. 45). Therefore, field theory is a theory for building theory. Indeed, Pepitone (1986) called field theory a metatheory. Cook (1986) named several structures "minitheories" (here called "microtheories") and placed them within field theory. Field theory thus forms a foundation for smaller theories, named here and discussed in the paragraphs that follow. One smaller theory involves relationships between individuals and groups, a concept familiar to nurses. A second microtheory deals with balances that Lewin termed "quasi-stationary equilibria." Third, at a less abstract and more practical level, Lewin advocated measurement of forces through techniques suggested by the force field analysis microtheory, which tells planners how to go about planning a change episode. Field theory also forms a foundation for channels theory, with its practical advice about the flow of ideas and materials in social systems.

Individual-Group Relationships

"Group-carried" changes work better than individual approaches. Group-carried decisions are not conscious decisions about group goals; rather, they are individual decisions made within the context of an open group discussion where participants can sense the development of a group attitude (Lewin, 1958). In this situation, nurse planners work to effect group (social) change by influencing an aggregate of individuals, as individuals. Lewin ([1944A] 1951) explained individual-group dynamics when he wrote that

> it is probably correct to say that values determine which types of activity have a positive and which have a negative valence for an individual in a given situation. In other words, values are not force fields but they "induce" force fields. That means that values are constructs which have the same psychological dimension as power fields. (p. 41)

The levels of group standards vary according to the strength of the values that form their bases. Standards act as forces that persuade group members to conform. Standards greatly influence goal setting (Lewin, 1958). "The greater the social value of a group standard the greater is the resistance of the individual group member to move away from this standard" (Lewin, [1947A, 1947B] 1951, p. 227).

Nurse planners can deal with standards with one, or both, of two approaches. First, they can work to diminish the value of a group standard against change or to increase the value of a standard for change, or both. Second, nurse planners can raise or lower the level of the standard itself.

Group approaches work better than individual approaches when planners try to change the value of group standards (Lewin, [1943B] 1951). If a person strays too far from established group standards, that person suffers sanctions that range from ridicule to ouster from the group. Lewin's (1947A, 1947B] 1951) experiences in leadership training, in changing food habits, work production, criminality, alcoholism, prejudices—all indicate that it is usually easier to change individuals formed into a group than to change any one of them separately. As long as group values are unchanged, the individual will resist change more strongly the further he or she departs from group standards. If the group standard itself is changed, the resistance that is due to the relation between the individual and the group standard is eliminated (p. 228).

Lewin mentioned approaches with deceptive appearances. They look like individual decisions made within a group but they actually are not. For example, mass media presentations place hearers in an almost private, psychologically isolated situation. Lectures operate in a similar way. One-to-one instruction also isolates the learner. In Lewin's experiments, none of these tactics worked as well as group sessions where shifts in others' sentiments became visible to participants as discussion progressed (Lewin, 1958). In group discussion, *"the individual accepts the new system of values and beliefs by accepting belongingness to a group"* (Lewin & Grabbe, [1945] 1948, p. 67).

Quasi-Stationary Equilibria

Habits resemble a river with its quasi-stationary processes. A river keeps its form as a river even while it moves. The velocity of a river reaches an equilibrium determined by such factors as the width and depth of the channel, the amount of water the river contains, and the rate of descent in a given distance. Likewise, the strength of habits results from a multitude of forces. Habits come from the interaction of the organism and its life space—the group and its setting. Nurse planners must take habits into account. The numerous political, economic, legal, psychological, physiological, and sociological factors involved in tobacco usage come to mind as an example.

Force field. A force field consists of the total of the influences toward locomotion or away from locomotion in the physical and social environment of a person or group. A force in a force field is a tendency to locomotion (Lewin, [1944A] 1951, p. 39). Forces include such factors as rainfall, climate, geography, laws, and economic conditions (Lewin, [1943C, 1947B] 1951, p. 170). Some of these forces may prevent change; the structure of life space may make certain changes impossible at a particular time. Therefore, the existence of forces toward change does not necessarily mean that change will occur. Driving forces encourage movement toward a goal with a positive valence or away from a goal with a negative valence. Restraining forces provide barriers to locomotion. Although restraining forces do not lead to change, they can neutralize driving forces and thus prevent change (Lewin, [1946B] 1951).

Correspondence of forces. Lewin described the origins of interpersonal forces. Own-needs forces correspond to the person's own needs and wishes. Induced forces relate to the wishes of another person. Impersonal forces come from the wishes of a less involved person perceived as objective and matter of fact. This third person presents a request for action in an impersonal way.

Combinations of forces. Forces combine in various ways. Each variation produces its own kind of result. Conflict situations can occur. A person may be located between two mutually exclusive positive or negative forces. Driving and restraining forces of approximately the same strength may cancel one another (Lewin, [1946B] 1951, pp. 259-269).

Two opposite forces may result in a low level of functioning or a high level of functioning. Opposing forces both may exert great strength, or they both may be very weak. Conflict characterizes a set of strong and almost equal opposing forces. A set of weak opposing forces produces a relatively unstable equilibrium because a strong force in either direction can change their balance easily (Lewin, [1946B] 1951).

The status quo is not static. Group life always exhibits change. The main difference between stable times and turbulent times is one of degree of change. Constancy can be analyzed only as compared with change. Group conduct depends upon the level at which restraining and driving forces reach an equilibrium. Both the management of change and the research into it require insight concerning the forces for and against change in group life. Force field analysis provides some of the insights necessary for nurse planners.

Force Field Analysis

In answering the question of what planned change techniques will prove effective or ineffective, Lewin recommended the field approach, in which planners ask what conditions have to be changed to produce a given result and how planners can alter these conditions with the means at their disposal (Lewin, [1943C, 1947B] 1951, pp. 171, 172). These questions lead planners to force field analysis, a careful, often measured estimation and description of the strength of influences for and against change in a particular situation. One must analyze a field before attempting to change or maintain cultural habits. "Scientific predictions or advice for methods of change should be based on an analysis of the 'field as a whole,' including both its psychological and nonpsychological aspects" (Lewin, [1943C, 1947B] 1951, p. 174). In force field analysis, nurse planners identify and analyze the forces in the environment of the individual or group to understand habits and to discover what to do to change or retain those habits. After analyses of a particular situation, planners will have some idea regarding what actions will cause change to occur. They also will get a sense regarding the appropriate sequence for those actions designed as strategies and tactics and those intended to evaluate the change event.

Sequence of strategies and tactics. To make change permanent, nurse planners must choose strategies appropriate to the stage of change involved. These stages include unfreezing, change of level, and freezing at the new level. Permanency is the objective. It is incorrect to believe that the new state becomes permanent automatically.

When the change effort first starts, planners may have to "shake up" the status quo with what Lewin called *unfreezing,* which is the process of softening toward change during which an individual or group becomes susceptible to change. Lewin suggested that this take the form of group sessions. Allport described these as a catharsis designed to remove prejudice. The unfreezing stage is a stir-up designed to "break open the shell of complacency and self-righteousness" (Lewin, [1947A, 1947B] 1951, p. 229). Group procedures promise benefits at all three stages because individuals do not change or maintain their habits in empty social space. Group work creates balances of forces that stabilize new behavior patterns. By working with groups, nurse planners avoid asking individuals to make changes that go against established custom.

Move is the action stage during which an individual or social system changes position from one point toward a different value state or condition. For this change of level, group strategies do not always work; "sometimes the value system of this face-to-face group conflicts with the values of the larger cultural setting and it is necessary to separate the group from the larger setting" (Lewin, [1947A, 1947B] 1951, pp. 231, 232) Therefore, Lewin suggested that in such situations, group sessions take place in the isolation of camps or workshops.

In the third stage, *freeze,* habits or practices become relatively fixed patterns of individual or group functioning:

Decision links motivation to action and, at the same time, seems to have a "freezing" effect which is partly due to the individual's tendency to "stick to his decision" and partly to the "commitment to a group." . . . Even decisions concerning individual achievement can be effective . . . [when] made in a group setting of persons who do not see each other again. (Lewin, [1947A, 1947B] 1951, p. 233)

Nevertheless, factors other than the freezing effects of decisions probably assume more importance than the circumstance of the decision in creating permanence. "These questions lead to problems of reconstructurization of the social field, particularly to problems of channeling social processes" (Lewin, [1947A, 1947B] 1951, p. 233). Thus nurse planners work to restructure the environment that surrounds individual decision makers.

Sequence of evaluation activities. In a cyclical replanning mode similar to the latter parts of the nursing process, Lewin likened evaluation of strategies and tactics to a reconnaissance flight. Air force personnel on such a mission quickly determine the nature and extent of a situation as accurately and objectively as they can. This reconnaissance flight has four functions: It evaluates the most recent action by comparing it with previous expectations; it serves as the basis for the next tactics; it carries implications for the overall plan; and it provides general insights regarding the strengths and weaknesses of strategies or tactics. Lewin provided what he called a circle of planning that includes planning, executing, fact finding, and possible modification of original plans. He insisted that this planning circle applies to social management (Lewin, 1958). The steps of the planning circle remind nurses of the nursing process.

Channels Theory

Lewin defined *channels* as the routes through which new ideas, practices, or products enter and travel through a social system. New ideas do not automatically enter channels; neither do new ideas move through channels by themselves. Points of entry into or critical junctures in channels are called *gates*. *Gatekeepers* are persons who have enough control of channel entry points to admit or refuse entrance to new ideas or practices. Gatekeepers speed or impede the progress of new ideas at these gates, or junctures, in the channels.

An example of channels theory. Lewin used food in a home as an example of a product that enters channels by passing the scrutiny of gatekeepers. Food moves step-by-step to reach the family table through channels such as the grocery store, the garden, a deli, or gifts from others. The psychology of gatekeepers involves (a) cognitive factors, (b) motivation, and (c) conflict. The nurse planner working with a diabetic or the mother of young children will consider all three kinds of factors. Cognitive factors, for example, may include the cultural availability of food (Does this family eat rattlesnake meat or chocolate-covered grasshoppers?), appropriateness of a particular food for various family members (real men eat meat and potatoes, not salads), meal patterns (toast and eggs for breakfast, soup for lunch), and the meaning of the eating situation (Does the diabetic diet mean loss of freedom or does it signify the opportunity to achieve better health?). Motivation includes several factors, for example, the values under several frames of reference (expense, health, taste, status), food needs (such as satiation), and obstacles (such as difficulty of preparation) to overcome before a certain food can reach the table. Under "conflict," Lewin discussed opposing forces, such as the desire to buy an attractive food balanced against an expense too great for the family food budget (Lewin, [1943C, 1947B] 1951).

Application of channels theory. Lewin stated that one can investigate the strength of food habits in a certain direction only through experimentation; questionnaires will not suffice. Appropriate interviews that explore the substitutability of essential foods help researchers plan experiments. Interviews also explore whether the basis of change of food habits results from changes in the availability of food, changes in channels (grocery store versus garden), psychological changes (alterations in the acceptability of certain foods), or changes in frames of reference such as the change from food as mere pleasure to food as a means for health as well as enjoyment.

Generality of channels theory. Lewin gave instruction regarding how channels theory could apply to situations other than the family food supply. In any situation, planners must identify channels, gates, and gatekeepers. They also must understand the psychology of the gatekeepers and must discover whether gates are guarded by impartial rules or by the individual characteristics of the gatekeepers. These kinds of information amount to the sociological analysis that "must be carried out before one knows whose psychology has to be studied or who has to be educated if a social change is to be accomplished" (Lewin, [1943C, 1947B] 1951, p. 186).

Conclusion

Nurse planners generally have used only a few concepts from Lewin's theories. In addition to these, Lewin's field theory and all of his microtheories in the area of planned change would serve nurses well. The next chapter gives an analysis and critique of Lewin's work and a later chapter provides an example of its application. Nurse readers will find many of Lewin's original English-language writings understandable and helpful. Appendix C of this book provides a chart that shows the placement, in Lewin literature, of various topics that pertain to planned change and to nursing. Appendix D lists nursing periodical articles that used Lewin literature during an 11-year time period.

Summary

This chapter started with a short biography of Kurt Lewin and a brief history of his work. Lewin's field theory relates to gestalt psychology, in which a gestalt is a configuration, an organized whole, with an emergent quality and properties more and different than the sum of its parts. Lewin founded field theory on several concepts (position, structure, locomotion, driving force, restraining force, force field, goal, conflict) related to field, which he defined as the total life space of an individual. Field theory has a temporal quality as it attempts to describe the here-and-now field in which a person participates. Along with field theory, Lewin described four microtheories: (a) individual-group relationships (this microtheory describes relationships between individual values and group standards), (b) quasi-stationary equilibria microtheory (this theory describes the ways that balances of forces exert influence toward or away from change), (c) force field analysis (a method for analyzing the forces for and against change), and (d) channels theory (which explains the social barriers and channels that new information or practices must navigate to enter a social system). These microtheories all relate to planned change.

(Note that in the Lewin references below, uppercase letters used with dates correspond to the reference system in Appendix C, section C.1.)

References

Allport, G. W. (1948). Foreword. In G. W. Lewin (Ed.), *Resolving social conflicts: Selected papers on group dynamics* (pp. vii-xiv). New York: Harper.

Benne, K. D. (1985). The process of re-education: An assessment of Kurt Lewin's views. In W. G. Bennis, K. D. Benne, & R. Chin (Eds.), *The planning of change* (4th ed., pp. 272-283). New York: Holt, Rinehart & Winston.

Cartwright, D. (1951). Foreword. In D. Cartwright (Ed.), *Field theory in social science: Selected theoretical papers* (pp. vii-xv). Chicago: University of Chicago Press.

Cook, S. (1986). An overall view. In E. Stivers & S. Wheelan (Eds.), *The Lewin legacy: Field theory in current practice* (pp. xi-xiv). New York: Springer-Verlag.

De Rivera, J. (1976). *Field theory as human science.* New York: Gardner.

Lewin, G. W. (1948). Preface. In G. W. Lewin (Ed.), *Resolving social conflicts: Selected papers on group dynamics* (pp. xv-xviii). New York: Harper.

Lewin, K. ([1943B] 1951). Defining the "field at a given time." In D. Cartwright (Ed.), *Field theory in social science: Selected theoretical papers* (pp. 43-59). Chicago: University of Chicago Press.

Lewin, K. ([1943C, 1947B] 1951). Psychological ecology. In D. Cartwright (Ed.), *Field theory in social science: Selected theoretical papers* (pp. 170-187). Chicago: University of Chicago Press.

Lewin, K. ([1944A] 1951). Constructs in field theory. In D. Cartwright (Ed.), *Field theory in social science: Selected theoretical papers* (pp. 30-42). Chicago: University of Chicago Press.

Lewin, K. ([1946B] 1951). Behavior and development as a function of the total situation. In D. Cartwright (Ed.), *Field theory in social science: Selected theoretical papers* (pp. 238-303). Chicago: University of Chicago Press.

Lewin, K. ([1947A, 1947B] 1951). Frontiers in group dynamics. In D. Cartwright (Ed.), *Field theory in social science: Selected theoretical papers* (pp. 188-237). Chicago: University of Chicago Press.

Lewin, K. (1958). Group decision and social change. In E. E. Maccoby, T. M. Newcomb, & E. L. Hartley (Eds.), *Readings in social psychology* (3rd ed., pp. 197-211). New York: Holt.

Lewin, K., & Grabbe, P. ([1945] 1948). Conduct, knowledge, and acceptance of new values. In G. W. Lewin (Ed.), *Resolving social conflicts* (pp. 56-68). New York: Harper. (Original work published 1945)

Marrow, A. J. (1969). *The practical theorist: The life and work of Kurt Lewin.* New York: Basic Books.

Pepitone, A. (1986). The creativity of field theory. In E. Stivers & S. Wheelan (Eds.), *The Lewin legacy: Field theory in current practice* (pp. xv-xvi). New York: Springer-Verlag.

Wessman, A. C. (1988). Kurt Lewin. In *Encyclopedia Americana* (Vol. 17, p. 270). Danbury, CT: Grolier.

Analysis and Critique
of Lewin's Microtheories

Although nurse authors frequently use Lewin's planned change theories, very few analyze or critique them (Tiffany, Cheatham, Doornbos, Loudermelt, & Momadi, 1994). Analysis and critique activities prove helpful to nurses; these activities enable nurse users to compare theories and make intelligent choices among them. This chapter analyzes and critiques Lewin's planned change theories.

Analysis of Lewin's Change Theories

The following analysis of Lewin's theories contains a description of Lewin's methodological stance and a general description of his theories. It continues with discussions of theory purpose, breadth, and concepts. It also describes basic and peripheral theory structures. It analyzes the use of definitions and illustrations and the sense of movement within the theories. It addresses theory assumptions.

Lewin's Methodological Stance

In the 1920s, Lewin and his students in Berlin tried to bring emotion into the laboratory. De Rivera wrote that the resultant dissertations may constitute the most brilliant experiments ever performed in psychology. Rightly termed *basic research,* these studies have relevance for those who wish to create a society responsive to human needs. De Rivera placed Lewin in the same methodological camp as Piaget and Tinbergen; Lewin employed strict experimental strategies, which he varied according to experimental conditions. De Rivera (1976) called Lewin's descriptive experiments "experimental phenomenology." He contrasted this with the "statistical experimentation" that psychologists commonly use.

General Description

Lewin's theories include field theory (a metatheory) and four microtheories. Field theory is a gestalt theory that attends to both observable and nonobservable phenomena. It does not explain any particular human behavior. Instead, field theory gives general statements about forces that induce human behavior and the ways such forces operate. Lewin called field theory a method, a theory for use in developing theory. Although field theory itself is not a change theory, it forms a foundation for change theory concepts that appear in Lewin's microtheories. Field theory explains change environments in ways that make Lewin's microtheories understandable. The microtheories include conceptual structures that describe (a) individual-group relationships, (b) quasi-stationary equilibria, (c) force field analysis, and (d) channels through which new ideas, practices, and goods enter and travel through social systems.

(Note that uppercase letters have been used with the dates in certain Lewin citations in this chapter to direct readers to Appendix C, section C.1, which was designed to help readers access Lewin's original writings.)

Theory Purposes and Breadth

Lewin ([1943B] 1951, p. 45) explicitly intended to provide a "method of *analyzing causal relations and building constructs*" when he developed field theory. Every nurse who plans change must develop his or her own conceptual models of the ways that change occurs in the world at large and in the specific change situation at hand (Lancaster, 1982). The explicit and implicit purposes of field theory serve these modeling purposes for nurse planners as well as for theorists. An implicit purpose of field theory is to contribute to the betterment of society through the application of scientific methods to solve societal problems. This implicit purpose energizes many of Lewin's general writings. Another implicit purpose of Lewin's microtheories is to explain the specifics of situational behavioral dynamics in ways that enable social planners to work effectively to cause change to occur.

Lewin's microtheories point out how change occurs at the level of the people involved in the change. The following are examples.

1. The explicit purpose of the theory of individual and group interactions is to tell readers how experiences become values, values become group standards, and standards become power fields that exert pressure toward conformity.

2. The quasi-stationary equilibria theory explains how driving forces and restraining forces form balances that cause or inhibit change.

3. Force field analysis gives lists of steps and activities for planners who assess and work with social forces in a field. The manner of presentation constitutes an "engineering theory" that explicitly tells planners what to do, how to do it, and in what order to do it. The nature of the force field analysis microtheory implies an instructional purpose.

4. The explicit purpose of channels theory is to tell and show readers how ideas, practices, and goods enter and travel in social systems.

Person, environment, and health. Lewin's change theories explicitly address person and environment; these topics form the core concerns of his theoretical work. Health issues appear but receive less emphasis than do person and environment. Attention to health usually surfaces in the more general writings rather than in Lewin's field theory or microtheories. Lewin's attention, as a psychologist, naturally centered more on mental health than on physical health.

Description, explanation, and prediction. Lewin's theories also contain extensive descriptions and explanations of phenomena and their relationships. He translated some of these into hypotheses with predictive power. Other descriptions had not yet reached the hypothesis stage of development when he died. Nevertheless, even these less developed descriptions and explanations take a form that nurses can translate into hypotheses.

Theory breadth. The Lewin theories apply to all levels of society and to any area of the workplace. They apply to individuals and groups. They consider people and environments. Field theory is a very broad theory, almost global in scope. The microtheories, with more specificity, fit within field theory. Three of these (individual-group relationships, quasi-stationary equilibria, force field analysis) lean toward narrowness; the fourth, channels theory, tends toward broadness.

Concepts

Lewin developed a large number of concepts. Many of these hold relevance for planned change theories, but not all demonstrate equal importance. This discussion centers on concepts central to planned change theories. Such concepts take the form of objects, properties, or events.

Lewin's planned change theories contain several major concepts, which Lewin called *constructs*. These include field, force, force field, position, structure, and locomotion. All but locomotion represent objects. Locomotion represents a process. All are both broad and abstract. Most minor concepts in the individual-group relationship microtheory (individual, values, group standards, goals) are narrow and abstract. These all represent objects. Minor concepts in the quasi-stationary equilibria microtheory range from narrow to medium in breadth. They range in abstractness from concrete to abstract. Several of these minor concepts relate to objects (equilibria, level of functioning, conflict, instability). Some relate to properties (psychological, nonpsychological, induced, impersonal, driving, and restraining).

Minor concepts in the force field analysis microtheory range from narrow to medium in broadness. Some of these minor concepts are quite abstract (unfreeze, move, freeze). Others tend toward concreteness (plan, find facts, intervene, monitor success). All force field analysis concepts mandate specific actions.

Minor concepts in channels microtheory (gate, gatekeeper, channel, environment) range from narrow to broad. They are quite abstract; all represent objects.

Basic Theory Structures

Cook (1986) wrote that field theory is a theory of individual psychology. He stated that in time Lewin would have formed a broad framework of field theory for his microtheories. Because Lewin died "in process," one reasonably can assume that a longer life would have given him time to complete a structure that would closely relate his four microtheories to field theory. The structures described here spring both from Lewin's writings and from what appears logical.

Cook (1986), for example, placed two of Lewin's conceptual formulations under field theory as microtheories. Actually, field theory parents four microtheories, which include conceptualization of individual-group relationships, quasi-stationary equilibria, force field analysis, and channels. (See Table 11.1.) Some relationships between field theory and the microtheories are explicit, others implicit. All these relationships are descriptive.

Individual-group relationships. The individual-group interaction structure connects several concepts. (See Figure 11.1.) Relationships in this structure are implicit, explanatory, predictive, and directional. Concepts relate in a sequenced line. All these concepts represent the targets of change; this is one of the factors that ties them together in a structure. Cognitive, affective, and motoric experiences (including reeducation) form the basis for individual values. Individuals strengthen their values within the context of group interactions. Individual values generate group standards. Standards develop into power fields that exert

TABLE 11.1 Relationships Among Lewin's Microtheories

1. Lewin's *field theory* is a theory for building theory. It takes a gestaltist view of social change situations. It attends to both observable and unobservable phenomena. This theory has a temporal quality that gives it a process orientation. Field theory is more general than the Lewin microtheories that relate to planned change; it could be described as the "parent" theory.

2. Lewin's theory of *individual-group relationships* explains how social change occurs by describing origins of forces in a field. Reeducation is an important strategy with many implications for I-G relationships.

3. Lewin's theory of *quasi-stationary equilibria* explains how social change occurs by describing kinds of balances in power fields.

4. Lewin's action theory of *force field analysis* relates the concept of force (power) to I-G theory, QSE theory, and channels theory. This action theory provides ideas about how to cause change to occur. It tells planners how to sequence strategies, tactics, and procedures for evaluation of strategies.

5. Lewin's *channels theory* explains the ways that new ideas, practices, or goods enter and travel through a social system.

---

pressure toward conformity to group standards. Individuals set goals consonant with group standards.

Quasi-stationary equilibria. All relationships in the quasi-stationary equilibria theory involve balance of driving and restraining forces. Lewin repeatedly depicted these balances by showing groups of opposing arrows that face each other across a straight line. The line represents the level of social functioning related to a particular balance of forces; the arrows show the strength and direction of the forces. (See Figures 11.2 through 11.5.) As the two sets of forces push the line toward change or away from change, the forces cluster under the specific headings of induced forces, impersonal forces, and nonpsychological forces. Characteristics of individuals fall under the psychological heading. Lewin's textual material and his graphic representations of theory combine to make relationships in this microtheory very specific. These relationships are descriptive, explanatory, predictive, and directional.

Force field analysis. Force field analysis presents a time-oriented and linear sequence of concepts; all of these mandate planner actions. It clumps change processes into two groups of stages. The first group of stages includes unfreezing (softening of position), moving (locomotion), and freezing (solidifying new behaviors) at a different level. The second group of stages includes action phases similar to those in the nursing process—plan, intervene, monitor success of interventions (strategies), and modify plans as needed. (See Table 11.2.) The force field analysis microtheory describes a working mode for planners. It tells

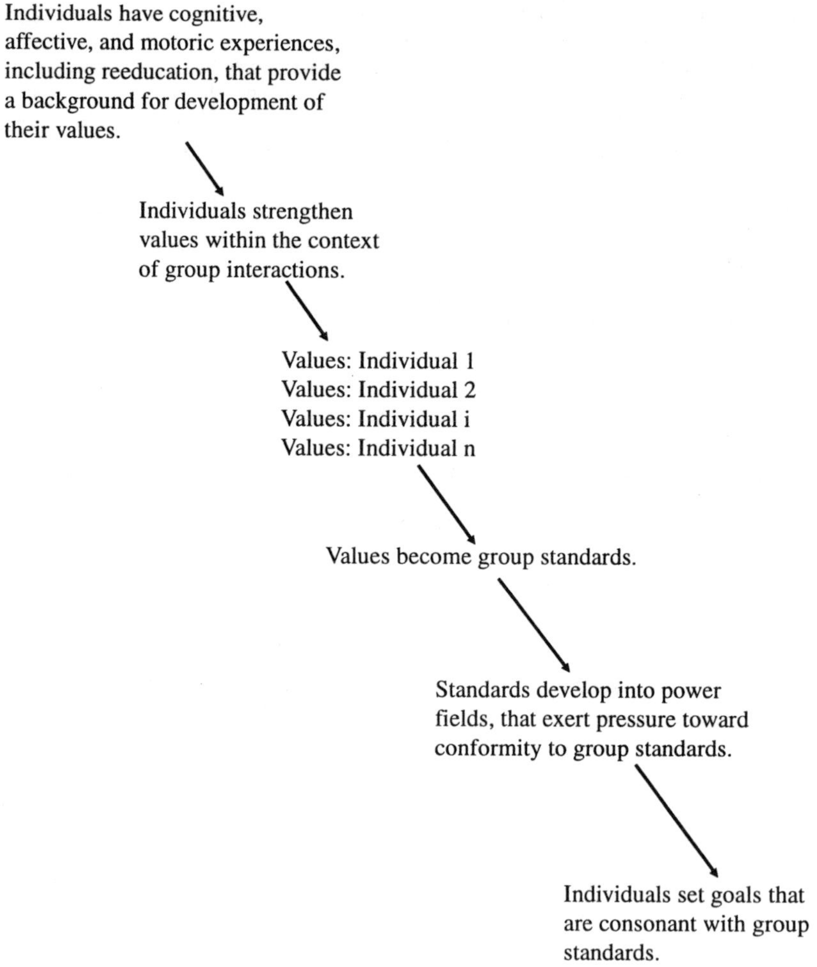

Individuals have cognitive,
affective, and motoric experiences,
including reeducation, that provide
a background for development of
their values.

Individuals strengthen
values within the context
of group interactions.

Values: Individual 1
Values: Individual 2
Values: Individual i
Values: Individual n

Values become group standards.

Standards develop into power
fields, that exert pressure toward
conformity to group standards.

Individuals set goals that
are consonant with group
standards.

Figure 11.1. Graphic Representation of Lewin's Theory of Individual-Group
Relationships

how to produce change, a stance that puts it in an engineering (planning)
category. It does not, itself, constitute an explanatory and predictive theory.

Channels theory. Lewin made relationships in the channels microtheory explicit
through verbal explanations and graphic representations. He related theory
concepts through a time-ordered sequence that describes the movement of new
ideas, practices, or goods from the environment, through channels with gates

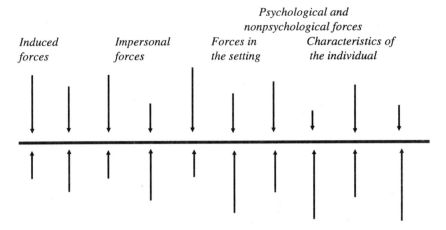

Figure 11.2. Graphic Representation of Lewin's Theory of Quasi-Stationary
Equilibria
SOURCE: Adapted from "Frontiers in Group Dynamics," by K. Lewin, 1951. In K. Lewin, *Field Theory in Social Science,* pp. 188-237. Copyright © 1951 by Harper & Row Publishers. Adapted with permission of Miriam Lewin.

Figure 11.3. Graphic Representation of Equilibria That Ensure a High Level or a
Low Level of Functioning
SOURCE: Adapted from "Frontiers in Group Dynamics," by K. Lewin, 1951. In K. Lewin, *Field Theory in Social Science,* pp. 188-237. Copyright © 1951 by Harper & Row Publishers. Adapted with permission of Miriam Lewin.

and gatekeepers, into a social system. This microtheory has explanatory, predictive, and directional relationships. (See Figure 11.6.)

Peripheral Structures

Peripheral structures flourish in Lewin's theoretical work. Any person who describes Lewin's change theories faces the question of what to include and what

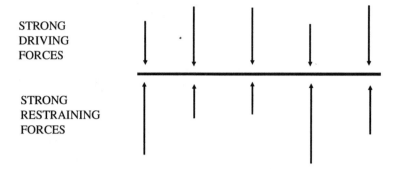

STRONG
DRIVING
FORCES

STRONG
RESTRAINING
FORCES

Figure 11.4. Graphic Representation of an Equilibrium With the Strong Driving and Restraining Forces That Foster Conflict
SOURCE: Adapted from "Frontiers in Group Dynamics," by K. Lewin, 1951. In K. Lewin, *Field Theory in Social Science*, pp. 188-237. Copyright © 1951 by Harper & Row Publishers. Adapted with permission of Miriam Lewin.

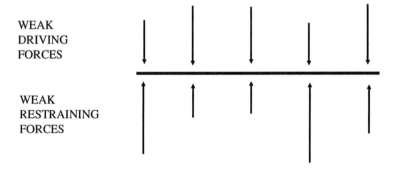

WEAK
DRIVING
FORCES

WEAK
RESTRAINING
FORCES

Figure 11.5. Graphic Representation of the Weak Driving and Restraining Forces That Foster an Unstable Equilibrium
SOURCE: Adapted from "Frontiers in Group Dynamics," by K. Lewin, 1951. In K. Lewin, Field Theory in Social Science, pp. 188-237. Copyright © 1951 by Harper & Row Publishers. Adapted with permission of Miriam Lewin.

to omit from his interesting, thoughtful, related, and voluminous writings. One way to answer this question is to look at the timing of his publications; earlier writings provide background concepts for his planned change microtheories.

Definitions and Illustrations

Lewin seemed to thrive on numerous, clear, and explicit definitions. His extended writings amplify his definitions by stating them in different words. His

TABLE 11.2 The Use of Force Field Analysis and the Deep Freeze

1. Examine data regarding nonpsychological factors (boundaries) in the change situation. These include factors such as law, climate, institutional policies, and availability of goods and services.
2. Identify psychological aspects of the change situation.
3. Identify, analyze, and measure forces named in items 1 and 2 above.
4. Diminish the value of negative group standards or increase the value of positive group standards, or both.
5. Sequence intervention strategies and tactics in three stages: unfreeze, move, freeze.
6. Sequence activities in four phases: plan, intervene, evaluate action, and modify plans as needed.

definitions and explanations do not compete; they complement one another. As they differentiate among concepts, they also reveal the consistency of Lewin's lines of thought. Over three fourths of the definitions necessary to field theory and the four microtheories discussed in this chapter are both clear and explicit, leaving the meaning of fewer than one fourth of the definitions for readers to surmise.

Conceptual representation was one of Lewin's most important tools. The sheer quantity and excellence of Lewin's figures demonstrates the significance he attached to graphic illustrations. One may look, as an example, at Lewin's

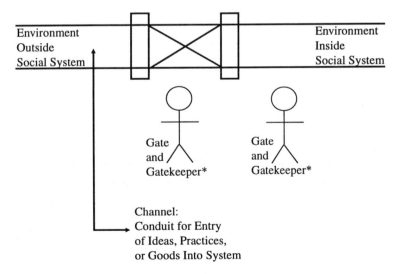

Figure 11.6. Graphic Representation of Lewin's Channels Theory
NOTE: *Forces for and against allowing entry of new ideas, goods, or practices include cognitive factors, motivation, and conflict.

chapter, "Frontiers in Group Dynamics" ([1947A, 1947B] 1951). This chapter, taken alone, includes 37 clearly understandable and relevant figures in 49 pages of text. Another chapter, "Behavior and Development as a Function of the Total Situation" ([1946B] 1951), contains 53 figures in 65 pages. Although not all of Lewin's publications display such high numbers of figures, graphic representations appear frequently. In addition, Lewin's penchant for illustration led him to provide numerous and understandable verbal examples of theoretical concepts.

Movement Within the Theory

In articles or chapters where Lewin was building a line of logic for the purpose of developing ideas, he generally moved from specific to general, from simple to complex, and from known to unknown. On the other hand, an examination of Lewin's concepts, put together in the framework of field theory and the microtheories, shows movement from broad to specific and from complex to simple. These sequences pertain not only to the structures of the theories but also to their development over time. The very general field theory took shape during the early years of Lewin's career. The channels theory, much more specific, was under construction at the time of his death.

All parts of Lewin's theories relate to one another. They show consistency among concepts and contain a fair amount of overlap. Some parts of the microtheories (i.e., individual-group relationships and force field analysis) show definite linear characteristics.

Theory Assumptions

This section addresses both the explicit and the implicit assumptions related to Lewin's field theory and his four microtheories.

Explicit assumptions. Field theory and its microtheories explicitly assume the importance of both observable and nonobservable characteristics of individuals and of their environments, over time. The theories also assume the importance of social forces and of balances among forces. They openly assume the importance of the impact of the environment upon the individual. They value the mechanics of planned change. Lewin explicitly advocated scientific, quantitative measurement and stated his assumption that scientific methods have worth in social planning. These statements require nurse planners to take an objective, scientific attitude toward planned change. Lewin's theory assumptions are consistent not only among themselves but with his philosophical outlook and more general writings.

Implicit assumptions. Although all of Lewin's theories explicitly assume that forces in their environments act upon persons who are targets of change, his work "ignores the equally valid perspective that it is the person as subject who participates in the formation of the very field that determines his behavior" (De Rivera, 1976, p. 29). This important omission in the theories implies that targets of change can do little to alter their own environmental circumstances. Such omissions show more value for planner action than for target population action in social change episodes.

Critique of Lewin's Change Theories

This critique of Lewin's change theories describes the extent to which nurse authors use Lewin theories in nursing periodical literature. It also presents affirmation for Lewin's work, addresses theory problems, and gives a nursing viewpoint. The critique ends with a discussion of the usefulness of Lewin's change theories.

The Lewin Theories in Nursing Periodical Literature

An 11-year survey (1982 through 1992) revealed a total of 155 articles that used 58 planned change theories in English-language nursing periodicals (Tiffany et al., 1994). "Theories" included planned change models or formal planned change conceptualizations such as those in the Bennis, Benne, and Chin books of readings. The Lewin microtheories took first place in terms of the number of articles that featured a particular theory, with 65 (42%) of the 155 articles appealing to the Lewin theories. The 155 articles presented 383 citations of sources of the 58 theories; the Lewin microtheories received 78 (20%) of these. Nurse authors named nine sources for their Lewin citations (they sometimes failed to name sources). Of these nine sources, *Field Theory in Social Science* (1951) received 24 citations; the Lewin chapter ([1947C]) in the 1947 edition of *Readings in Social Psychology* (T. M. Newcomb and E. L. Hartley, editors) had 13 citations.

Affirmation for Lewin's Work

Specifically, Lewin's scientific work and theories have been acknowledged in many ways. For example, De Rivera (1976) described Lewin's conceptualizations as having a systematic elegance. Cook (1986) noted that research in Lewin's institutes exerted considerable influence on the emergence of social, developmental, and organizational psychology. Additionally, Lewin's research forms the basis for group dynamics and several varieties of action research (Cook, 1986). On a more general level, Lewin's work was honored by development of the International Kurt Lewin Conferences and founding of the Society for the Advancement of Field Theory. In 1963, the Society for the Psychological Study of Social Issues voted to use money from the Kurt Lewin Memorial Fund to translate certain early Lewin papers and the dissertations of some Lewin students from the Berlin institute (De Rivera, 1976).

Bennis, Benne, and Chin (1985) credited Lewin as one of the intellectual inspirations for their volumes on planned change. They cited his many contributions to the normative-reeducative strategies that they considered appropriate for contemporary society. The frequent references that they and their invited authors made to Lewin's concepts demonstrate the strength of Lewin's influence on their thinking. In addition, the epilogue ("An Enduring Influence") in the Marrow (1969) biography of Lewin describes the influence of the Lewin legacy.

Theory Problems

Two kinds of problems appear in the Lewin planned change theories. The first, described by De Rivera, limits the scope of the theories; Lewin's theories touch only one direction of individual-group influence. The second concerns the omission of parts essential to a truly workable planned change theory.

Limited viewpoint. De Rivera wrote that when Lewin conceptualized individual behavior as a product of the structure and dynamics of an individual's field at a given time, he ignored an equally important consideration: Environmental forces do arise from valenced objects that direct a person's behavior, but this viewpoint, taken alone, neglects the fact that people participate in the formation of the fields that surround them. Lewin's viewpoint characterizes person-environment interactions as a one-way street in which behavioral activity relates to the ways that forces in the environment influence individuals; it ignores the ways that individuals influence and shape their environments. Although he called Lewin's theories elegant, De Rivera believed that individuals can and should shape their environments. Lewin's viewpoint does not rule out the possibility that humans shape their environments; it simply overlooks it. De Rivera developed the complementary perspective in his book, *Field Theory as Human Science* (1976).

Readers may wonder why the gestaltist Lewin would take a one-way view of what De Rivera saw as a two-way interaction. Several possibilities emerge. Lewin could not entirely escape his own environment. His cultural background may have given him a paternalistic bent that eroded only slowly over time. No one would call Lewin a behavioristic psychologist, but many of Lewin's contemporaries leaned in a behavioristic direction; he could not ignore their influence completely. Not long before his death, Lewin began to develop action research principles. Here, he included community leaders in planning. Given time, Lewin might have expanded his views.

Incompleteness. A complete planned change theory should contain four parts. It should have a system for diagnosing social system problems, a way of choosing or developing a solution to those problems, a method of choosing, devising, and sequencing strategies and tactics, and a means of evaluating the quality of both the innovation outcomes and the strategies in a planned change episode (Tiffany et al., 1994). Lewin's theories lack three of these parts.

First, Lewin's examples show that he accepted someone else's judgment that current practices constitute problems. The diagnostic processes he described in his writings refer to readiness of social systems to accept change. The context within which Lewin used the word *diagnosis* is one of strategy, not diagnosis of social system problems (Lewin, [1943B] 1951, pp. 48-59, 186, 231; [1946A] 1948, pp. 210, 213; 1958, pp. 200, 201). Neither Lewin's theories nor his examples show how to diagnose a social system problem through use of standards. Standards, to Lewin, referred to standards held by group members; this left little room for planner standards or objective standards from the outside. The use he made of group standards indicates that these assume importance only within the context of strategy plans. When Lewin addressed the way that individual values contribute to group standards, he was referring to the kinds of restraining or driving forces that group standards provide. He did not refer to standards as guides for diagnosing social system problems or choosing solutions to problems.

Second, in Lewin's examples, planners accepted the solutions to problems that someone else (in most cases, government) decided should become the norm. Planners did not develop solutions specifically related to goals and values important either to themselves or to target system members. Only in his descriptions of action research did Lewin deviate from this stance. Last, Lewin's theories (1958) make almost no provision for evaluation of the outcomes of the innovation. They do make room for evaluation of the success of strategies, but only in terms of planners. All the theories ignore evaluation of the extent to which strategies achieve the goals of the target population.

A careful examination of Lewin's planned change theories thus reveals that they concern strategy almost exclusively. The exception appears in his community-oriented methods for action research. Thus the theories have one of the four parts necessary for a complete planned change theory.

A Nursing Viewpoint

Lewin's planning cycle omits diagnosis of social system problems, choice of solution, and monitoring of success of solutions; cooperative planning is absent from the four microtheories. These omissions relate to De Rivera's observations about the absence of attention to influences that individuals have on their environments. Lewin's microtheories pay more attention to doing things "to people" than to doing things "with people."

Lewin's examples limit target population participation to membership in group discussion sessions where the goal is predetermined by someone other than the participants. This limitation implies that change planners should be in charge and that they do not need to solicit the actual participation of people who are targets of change. Omissions and theory examples also imply that someone in a position superior even to that of the planner has access to the most reliable knowledge about what ought to occur in a given instance. Paternalistic assumptions run directly counter to nursing values in terms of the mutuality that promotes collaboration among nurse, patient, and family.

Usefulness of Lewin's
Planned Change Theories

With careful consideration, Lewin's science-based theories prove very useful to nurse planners. Nevertheless, nurse users would do well to recognize their incompleteness. Planners might best consider them to be guides that explain some of the dynamics of the strategies and tactics they choose or devise. The Lewin microtheories fit well within the context of a more general planned change theory.

When combined with a general planned change theory, the force field analysis microtheory would help planners concerned with the selection of specific strategies and tactics to identify forces for and against change. Once they have made such determinations, they could use the individual-group relationships microtheory in planning ways to alter group values to favor change. The quasi-stationary equilibrium microtheory tells planners to manipulate balances among forces in power fields so that they strengthen some forces and lessen the activity of others. The channels microtheory offers ideas about the ways that communication strategies and tactics work in the transport of change-oriented messages into and through social systems. Planners could sequence strategies and tactics under all the microtheories through the use of the unfreeze, move, and freeze concepts that form a part of the force field analysis microtheory.

Summary

This chapter described Lewin's methodological stance and his planned change theories. It then analyzed the theories in terms of their purposes, breadth, and concepts. The chapter continued with a discussion of the ways that Lewin defined concepts and the ways he related concepts in theory structures. It highlighted Lewin's penchant for definition, graphic illustration, and textual examples and described the sense of movement that Lewin's time-oriented sequences provide. The analysis section of the chapter ended with a description of theory assumptions.

The critique of Lewin's theories reports on the use of Lewin's change theories in nursing periodical literature. It also states that, in spite of some concerns, Lewin's planned change theories remain very popular with nurses. Field theory and its attendant microtheories apply best as strategies combined with a more general change theory or with a nursing theory. The individual-group relationships microtheory suggests ways that nurse planners could influence the formation of values that either encourage or inhibit planned change. The quasi-stationary microtheory instructs planners concerning the alteration of forces in a psychological field to encourage or inhibit planned change. The force field analysis microtheory offers techniques useful to planners when they assess the dynamics of a social situation. The channels microtheory offers planners suggestions for ways to send change-oriented messages into and through a social system.

Using Lewin's theories as strategies within a planned change theory devoted to mutuality would give nurse planners access to Lewin's concepts and techniques while allowing them to keep nursing values. A later chapter provides ideas about the actual application of Lewin's planned microtheories.

(Note that in the Lewin references below, uppercase letters used with dates correspond to the reference system in Appendix C, section C.1.)

References

Bennis, W. G., Benne, K. D., & Chin, R. (1985). *The planning of change* (4th ed.). New York: Holt, Rinehart & Winston.

Cook, S. (1986). An overall view. In E. Stivers & S. Wheelan (Eds.), *The Lewin legacy: Field theory in current practice* (pp. xi-xiv). New York: Springer-Verlag.

De Rivera, J. (1976). *Field theory as human science*. New York: Gardner.

Lancaster, W. (1982). Model building and the change process. In J. Lancaster & W. Lancaster (Eds.), *Concepts for advanced nursing practice: The nurse as change agent* (pp. 229-315). St. Louis: Mosby.

Lewin, K. ([1943B] 1951). Defining the "field at a given time." In D. Cartwright (Ed.), *Field theory in social science: Selected theoretical papers* (pp. 43-59). Chicago: University of Chicago Press.

Lewin, K. ([1946A] 1948). Action research and minority problems. In G. W. Lewin (Ed.), *Resolving social conflicts* (pp. 201-216). New York: Harper.

Lewin, K. ([1946B] 1951). Behavior and development as a function of the total situation. In D. Cartwright (Ed.), *Field theory in social science: Selected theoretical papers* (pp. 238-304). Chicago: University of Chicago Press.

Lewin, K. ([1947A, 1947B] 1951). Frontiers in group dynamics. In D. Cartwright (Ed.), *Field theory in social science: Selected theoretical papers* (pp. 188-237). Chicago: University of Chicago Press.

Lewin, K. ([1947C] 1947). Group decision and social change. In T. M. Newcomb & E. L. Hartley (Eds.), *Readings in social psychology.* New York: Holt, Rinehart & Winston.

Lewin, K. (1958). Group decision and social change. In E. E. Maccoby, T. M. Newcomb, & E. L. Hartley (Eds.), *Readings in social psychology* (3rd ed.). New York: Holt.

Marrow, A. F. (1969). *The practical theorist: The life and work of Kurt Lewin.* New York: Basic Books.

Tiffany, C. R., Cheatham, A. B., Doornbos, D., Loudermelt, L., & Momadi, G. G. (1994). Planned change theory: Survey of nursing periodical literature. *Nursing Management, 25*(7), 54-59.

Altering the Lewin Square Peg

This chapter consists of three parts: a discussion of how Lewin's (KL) planned change theories fit with the Roy Adaptation Model (RAM; Roy, 1980), a combination of the RAM and Lewin's theories in a translated change process, and an application of that change process to a nursing situation.

Congruence of Lewin's Change Theories With Key Concepts in the Roy Adaptation Model (RAM)

Roy's educational background includes a doctorate in sociology; Lewin was a psychologist. Therefore, similarities in their conceptualizations of individuals and social environments offer no surprise. The works of both authors reveal reciprocal interaction worldviews. The RAM and Lewin's field theory, together with its microtheories, focus on organized wholes (the gestalt) and view individuals from a holistic perspective.

The following sections use the terms *person, environment, health,* and *nursing* to organize a discussion of the congruence that exists between the RAM and Lewin's microtheories.

Person

The RAM, initially developed for use with individuals, recognizes the client as the subject or recipient of nursing care who functions as an adaptive system. As noted earlier, clients, according to the RAM, can include groups or social systems. The person in Lewin's theories functions as a decision maker who chooses to adopt or reject a proposed change. Potential decision makers become the subjects or recipients of the "care" provided or effort expended by nurses who plan change. Decision makers, according to Lewin, include groups or social systems in addition to individuals. Lewin's theories, despite his psychology background, view change in individuals as occurring within the context of a group. Lewin viewed group standards, norms, and values as powerful environmental influences on individual decision makers. These perspectives reflect a reciprocal interaction worldview.

Environment

Both Roy and Lewin defined *environment* in broad terms and spent considerable time discussing the specifics of the environment. Roy specifies the environment as consisting of external and internal environmental stimuli that influence individuals. Similarly, Lewin used force field concepts to describe an environment as a field of forces that influences individuals to change or to remain the same. Roy's description of the environment includes external and internal stimuli, whereas Lewin discussed field (environment) from the perspective of the group and the social system in which individuals find themselves (individual-group relationships microtheory). Thus environment as conceptualized by Lewin is congruent with Roy's definition of "external stimuli." The RAM emphasizes the identification of environmental stimuli. Similarly, Lewin's quasi-stationary equilibria microtheory emphasizes the identification of driving and restraining forces.

The RAM's focal stimulus, conceptualized by the authors as congruent with a Lewin perspective, is the specific situation or event that makes the need for change evident to nurse planners. For example, this could be an administrative directive. Contextual and residual environmental stimuli consist of group standards, norms, and values that influence individual decision makers.

In Roy's model, contextual stimuli can be identified, verified, and measured. Residual stimuli include hunches, uncertainties, or unknowns. Residual stimuli discovered and verified during the change process become contextual stimuli. Those residual stimuli that remain unknown and/or unmeasurable throughout the change process may be useful during the evaluation of the change process. Lewin's quasi-stationary equilibria microtheory categorizes environmental stimuli as driving or restraining forces. Lewin strongly advocated measurement of forces (focal and contextual stimuli) through the use of force field analysis, another of his microtheories.

Health

Although Lewin did not address health specifically in his theories, his work is compatible with Roy's conceptualization of health. In the RAM, health comprises the process of moving toward integration and wholeness as the clients (decision makers) proceed through the steps of the nursing (change) process. Health exists, in the minds of planners, when clients (decision makers) adopt the desirable processes, relationships, or products designed or chosen to solve the problem. Nurse planners expect that individuals, through the change process, will understand the problem and accept the change toward health as a desirable solution.

Nursing

According to the RAM, the goal of nursing is "to enhance positive life processes and to promote adaptation" (Andrews & Roy, 1991, p. 37). Similarly, the goal in Lewin's planned change theories is to promote adaptation to a change deemed necessary to solve a social system problem.

Similarities and differences exist between the nursing process in the RAM and the change processes described by Lewin. Both cyclical problem-solving methods have overlapping steps; both involve human behavior. The RAM identifies six steps in the nursing process—assess behavior, assess stimuli, diagnose, set goals, intervene, and evaluate. Nurses follow these steps as they work with individuals in health-related situations. Lewin's theories directly address only two of these—assess stimuli and plan strategies (interventions). His theories leave two of the steps—assess behavior and diagnose (social system problems)—to the judgment of others. Most of what Lewin wrote about goals referred to formation of group standards rather than to objectives for planned change episodes. He paid a great deal of attention to strategies but his theories deal with only part of the sixth step (evaluate).

The RAM provides for assessment of behaviors; this assessment sets the tone for understanding the client's situation. Lewin covered behavioral assessment by saying that a planner who understands the environment understands behaviors. Both viewpoints value environmental assessment.

The two perspectives differ in the matter of diagnosis; Roy provided for diagnostic processes while Lewin left problem diagnosis to others. Both employ standards, but the standards are used by caregivers in the RAM to facilitate diagnosis, and by someone else, somewhere else, in the Lewin examples. In the RAM, nurse caregivers compare a situation with standards. Professional nurses draw from an extensive scientific knowledge and nursing experience base when they choose standards to determine whether or not a situation constitutes a problem. Their knowledge base includes standards from a RAM typology of indicators of positive adaptation in each of the four adaptive modes. A complementary typology indicates commonly recurring adaptation problems.

In Lewin's examples, problems that indicate a need for change were identified by outsiders or those not directly involved at local levels. This is a common situation in a government-regulated industry such as health care. The determination by the federal government that health care, especially hospital care, is too costly provides an example. Government agencies used standards in identifying this problem. Their standards took the form of information regarding percentages of national income spent for health care in various developed nations. They also had testimony from citizen consumers, from insurance company executives, and from businesses that provide health care benefits as part of a wage package.

The RAM and the Lewin theories differ in their approaches to goal setting. In the RAM, goals represent end-point behaviors. Long-term goals concern resolution of ineffective responses to problems, which frees energy to meet other goals. Short-term goals identify behaviors expected after interventions and pinpoint behaviors that indicate adaptive processes. Most of what Lewin (1958) wrote related goals to the formation of group standards. He gave minor attention to goals as objectives for planned change efforts; for him, goals were objectives that planners might not be able to describe clearly. In a series of educated trial-and-error actions, the means of reaching goals come into question but goals do not. Thus Lewin provided neither for adjustment of goals nor for decision makers' participation in goal formulation. This system differs widely from Roy's admonition that clients should participate in goal formulation whenever possible. It is important to note that toward the end of Lewin's life, his research involved projects that advocated greater participation by adopters.

Although the RAM takes the environment into account in the preparation of plans for interventions, Meleis (1991) noted a limitation of the RAM framework for understanding person-environment interactions. This is the point where the Lewin theories excel. Indeed, Lewin's theories actually amount to sophisticated strategies for achieving goals set by a higher authority. His field theory and all its accompanying microtheories offer a great deal of practical advice regarding environmental stimuli, their impact on decision makers, and the ways that various forces in the environment function and interact.

In the evaluation step, the RAM compares real and ideal behaviors, measures movement toward or away from behavior described by goals, and evaluates data to permit readjustment of goals and iinterventions designed to achieve goals. Lewin's evaluation system, on the other hand, concentrates on the quality of strategies. It does not question goals.

A RAM-KL Change Process

Nurses who base their practice on the RAM might want to use the RAM view of the nursing process as an organizing framework and to extend RAM concepts by incorporating ideas from Lewin's change theories. This section presents a reconceptualization that permits such usage. The combined Roy Adaptation Model-Kurt Lewin (RAM-KL) change process incorporates Lewinian change concepts with the RAM view of the nursing process. Lewin died at the height of his career, leaving his monumental work unfinished. Therefore, this description of a planned change process claims the creative license necessary to apply Lewinian concepts to the steps of the nursing process. The RAM-KL change process minimizes differences between the RAM and the Lewinian microtheories and, to a reasonable extent, fills resultant gaps with extrapolations from Lewin's published work. Nevertheless, it does not supply concepts completely missing in both the RAM and the Lewin microtheories.

Assess Behavior

The combined RAM and Lewin view asks planners to make an initial assessment of behaviors exhibited by individuals in a social system. Behavior depends on the field (environment) at a given time. When planners fully understand the environment, they understand behaviors that occur in the individuals and groups who inhabit that environment. Planners categorize the information on behaviors they collect in the four adaptive system modes (physical, interpersonal, role, interdependence) found in the Roy Adaptation Model Applied to Administration (RAMA). Behavioral assessment clarifies the focus of the planner-decision maker interaction and sets the tone for understanding the decision makers' situation. After this initial assessment, the nurse planner analyzes patterns of behaviors and uses descriptions of adaptive responses (standards) to identify ineffective responses. Planners employ professional judgment to make an initial determination of whether or not the situation calls for planned change. If persons in the situation need nurse planner support, then the nurse planner moves into second-level assessment.

Assess Stimuli

In second-level assessment, the nurse planner collects data regarding the focal, contextual, and residual stimuli in a social system. Focal stimuli could include stressors such as economic downturns, social inequities, epidemics, natural disasters, social pressure toward new practices, lack of resources, law, climate, or institutional policies. The contextual stimuli (e.g., sociodemographic characteristics that add to the effects of the focal stimulus) could include characteristics such as individual and group values, persons' needs to exert peer pressure, past interpersonal relationship experiences, or ethnic backgrounds. Residual stimuli (unknown or otherwise unmeasurable factors contributing to the effect of the focal stimulus on decision makers) in social situations could include such things as the many unstated and private political realities related to policies in the social system.

Field is the total life space, the environment as it exists for the person or group. Planners who operate under the RAM-KL process assess many kinds of forces in the environment. A thorough assessment of environmental stimuli helps to clarify the etiology of the problem.

Diagnose

Anyone who diagnoses a problem compares the situation under consideration with some sort of standard. This comparison may be informal and unrecognized. Just as nurses compare laboratory values with the norms for people having the test in question, so planners compare social situations with certain norms or standards. These come from sources such as government agencies, professional organizations like the American Nurses Association, science-based professional knowledge, or professional experience.

Diagnosis entails a cyclical process in which planners rule out competing explanations for the behaviors they observe. The diagnostic process may include a series of tries (successive approximations) where planners repeat portions of behavioral and environmental stimuli assessments and make comparisons with standards.

Set Goals

Planners work together with decision makers to set goals; mutuality prevails. Together, they prioritize goals as important or merely desirable. At first, goals may not be clear. As planners consider an initial idea, they collect information needed to clarify goals. They devise an overall plan and make decisions about the first action step. In change situations, goals relate to diverse problems. Planners set goals that aim for a correspondence between environmental stimuli and abilities of decision makers to cope with their environments.

Intervene

When planners devise strategies designed to meet goals, they create mental representations (mental pictures) and perhaps graphic representations (pictures on paper) of the situation and the means required to produce change in it. When using the RAM-KL change process, planners start the representation process with the assessment of behavior and of the field (total life space) that supplies environmental stimuli. Mental and graphic representations continue as planners consider additional factors in the change situation.

Channels and gatekeepers. Planners also make representations of channels through which ideas, practices, goods, or services enter and travel in the social system. What do channels contain? What is the nature of the internal and external environments of the social system? Where are the gates and who are the gatekeepers? Through what steps must the new idea or product travel? What are the rates of flow in the channels? An examination of the psychology of gatekeepers includes cognitive factors, motivation, and conflict. Planners determine whether gatekeepers are guided by rules and regulations or their own free will. The study of channels assists in the identification of forces in the change environment.

Force field analysis. Next, planners measure the strength and direction of forces in the field. These forces may include law, climate, peer pressures, values, past experiences, social system policies, and availability of resources such as personnel, money, goods, and services. The survey includes the wishes of persons close to the change scene in addition to the characteristics of persons who will experience change.

Unfreeze. Planners sequence change strategies so that they occur in three stages: unfreeze, move, and freeze. In the unfreeze stage, planners create doubt or concern about the wisdom of current behaviors or habits. Change strategies unfreeze situations. They "soften" the system by creating dissatisfaction with existing conditions and suggesting that better ways of doing things exist and might function well at local levels. Planners form mental and perhaps graphic representations of the balance between driving and restraining forces and think about strategies necessary to change that balance. A situation becomes tense as planners increase forces driving toward change and diminish restraining forces that resist change. Group sessions work well at this unfreezing stage.

Move. As planners prepare for the move stage, they either alter stimuli so that they fall within the adaptive zones of decision makers or introduce strategies designed to increase the coping abilities of the decision makers. Planners usually increase the likelihood of locomotion toward change through group work designed to alter balances of forces for and against change.

Decision making occurs in the context of group work so that individuals involved in the change do not have to change in isolation. Cognitive, affective, and what Lewin called motoric experiences form the basis for values. Individuals strengthen their values best in the context of group interactions. Individual values generate group standards, which become power fields that exert pressure toward conformity to standards. Therefore, planners employ group work, such as decision making by consensus, as a change strategy. In group work, members witness shifts in others' value positions. Thus individuals have an opportunity to accept a new value while they experience belongingness to the group. Planners avoid strategies such as mass media approaches, lectures, and one-to-one sessions between a planner and a decision maker; these counterfeit group work. Pseudo-group strategies do not include individuals in groups; in truth, pseudo-group work isolates individuals from group decision making. When the group climate so strongly opposes the new values that change has no chance, planners work with individuals to address the values that generate group standards and pressures toward conformity. They give information and supply other resources that make change as easy as possible.

Freeze. Strategies also must create permanency for the change. The freeze step solidifies the situation to create a permanent adaptation. This stabilizes the balance of forces at the new level. Planners work to increase whatever forces encourage adherence to new standards. They reward and support behavior related to the new group standards and try to reduce forces that push people away from new standards.

Nurse planners use education, coaching, facilitation, technostructural, persuasive, and data-based strategies to assist decision makers to change their behavior. With change imposed from the external environment, nurse planners do what they must to get decision makers to decide in favor of change. They use creativity when they implement strategies to optimize driving forces and minimize restraining forces that act as barriers to change. For example, the attitudes of nurse caregivers have changed from a purely clinical perspective to one that includes the economics of health care. Caring for clients from a holistic perspective now includes economic caring in addition to the traditional physiological, psychological, spiritual, and sociocultural caring.

Evaluate

In the RAM-KL change process, nurse planners compare end-point behaviors with ideal behaviors envisioned in goals. Evaluation measures movement away from or toward goals. The process permits readjustment of both goals and strategies employed to achieve goals. In the best evaluations, planners and decision makers look together at the decision makers' behavior to determine movement away from or toward goal behavior.

Planners do not wait until the end of an entire change sequence to evaluate and replan goals and strategies. As they intervene, they consider the effects of each strategy on the overall plan. Evaluation (Lewin's fact finding) has four functions. It helps planners know whether results met expectations; it provides information about how to correct plans; it guides modifications of the overall plan; and it gives insight into the quality of the strategies. Intervention and evaluation cycles continue throughout the change process. These include comparison with objective standards so that planners can judge whether the actions taken have led forward or backward. In the RAM-KL change process, evaluation entails an ongoing activity, not merely a terminal step.

In summary, the RAM-KL change process views people as systems capable of adapting to change. The environment exerts a critical influence on individual behavior. It often imposes change that persons must deal with whether they like it or not. Government health care regulations give an example of a focal stimulus over which hospitals or nurse caregivers have little control. The RAM-KL change process offers a sense of the familiar and a way to exert a degree of control through an implementation phase. It provides nurses with a planning approach to social change that does not conflict with clinical practice viewpoints. The combination of the RAM with Lewin's emphasis on strategy enlarges the RAM perspective; nurse "doers" strongly value intervention.

Application of the RAM-KL
Change Process to a Nursing Situation:
An Example

The following example applies the RAM-KL change process. It relates to a financial dilemma in a hospital. Planners could consider the problem at a national, regional or state, corporate, or institutional level. This example shows a clear progression, over time, of a change episode throughout an institution: hospital executive committee (including chief financial officer and chief nurse executive), chief nurse executive (CNE), nursing administration committee (nurse managers and nurse coordinators of staff support departments), and nurse caregivers on units. Involvement of increasing numbers of people as change

TABLE 12.1 Application of the RAM-KL Change Process

Step	Application of Step	Restraining (R) or Driving (D) Force
Assess behavior	*Physical adaptive system mode:*	
	Current skill mix	(D)
	Currently open positions	(D)
	Projected open positions	(D)
Assess stimuli	*Focal:* High RN skill mix	(D)
	Contextual: Nurse, physician, and community expectations	(R)
	Nurses educated for primary care	(R)
	Gatekeepers	(D & R)
	Residual: Past and present interrelationships	(D & R)
Diagnose	High nursing labor costs related to current skill mix	
Set goal	Lower nursing labor costs	
Intervene	*Unfreeze:* Attain consensus about need to change and of appropriateness of new skill mix	
	Move: Gain acceptance of revised strategic plan, change process implemented on target units	
	Freeze: Progress reports, recognition ceremony	
Evaluate	Analyze labor costs for division, average skill mix for division, average skill mix for individual units, quality improvement documents	

progressed toward application on the units shifted the balance of forces toward change and provided a climate of mutuality.

Repetition of a particular cycle of change activities—that is, each activity reported here but in a greater or lesser amount—occurred at each level. Activities included assessment of behaviors and stimuli related to behaviors, and diagnosis of a problem that called for change. Activities also included goal selection and prioritization. Each cycle contained plans for strategies designed to cause change. Plans and strategies included channel recognition and analysis, force field analysis, and group participation in changing standards toward new ways of functioning. Strategies softened a social system toward change, moved participants toward change, and froze behaviors in new patterns. All cycles involved some evaluation of the goal, the solution, and the strategies designed to increase the likelihood of change. (See Table 12.1.)

The Hospital Scene

The executive committee of a medium-sized rural hospital (the social setting) had been discussing the financial status of the hospital at several recent meetings. The chief financial officer, a committee member in charge of the Financial Department (a RAMA stabilizer structure), brought the matter to the committee's attention. As committee members expressed concern over current and forecasted labor costs, they began to think of ways to solve the problem. The committee, with the chief nurse executive (CNE) as a member, agreed, after much discussion, that the 80:20 skill mix ratio of registered nurses to other nursing personnel was higher than necessary. The CNE stated that she would meet with the nursing administrative committee and present a rudimentary proposal at the next meeting. Unbeknownst to the hospital executive committee, the CNE and the nursing administration committee had anticipated this move by the executive committee. Much discussion already had taken place and tentative plans had been made. This initial proposal from the CNE satisfied the executive committee as being responsible and prudent. Thus the CNE, in collaboration with the executive committee, accepted a share of responsibility for solving the problem.

The Problem and the Goal

Due to the nature and organizational level of the problem (high hospital labor costs), the CNE will function (for purposes of illustration) as nurse planner. The CNE, in the planner role, will coordinate and facilitate the change planning activities of the nursing administration committee. This nursing committee included nurse directors, nurse managers of the clinical units, and managers/coordinators of the staff support departments/offices such as continuing nursing education and quality improvement. The hospital executive committee already had selected the long-term goal of lower labor costs. The CNE and the nursing administration committee could contribute to this goal by reducing nursing labor costs through a permanent change in the skill mix of unit nursing personnel. Unlicensed personnel could be teamed with registered nurses. The nursing administration committee (a RAMA innovator structure) had already decided that special care units would retain 100% registered nurse caregivers with one unlicensed assistive person assigned to each unit for indirect care activities. Skill mixes on the other units could vary according to guidelines that she and other planners would establish later, after giving the situation more study. Reaching the long-term hospital goal of lower costs would contribute to the general survival goal of the hospital and thus would preserve employment for nurses,

including herself. Now the CNE, in concert with the nursing administration committee, must face the question of exactly how to promote adaptation to the new skill
mix in a manner acceptable to those who would have to live with the results.

Assess Behavior

The CNE, as nurse planner, delegated many of the assessment activities to
nursing administration committee members. She coordinated the first-level
assessment activities that examined behaviors (current skill mix, currently open
and projected open positions) on the units. All behaviors were assigned to the
physical adaptive system mode. The CNE and selected committee members
looked closely at unit schedules and requested additional accounting printouts
from the chief financial officer. Together, they made a tentative decision that
units with skill mixes most similar to the desired ratio and with a greater number
of open positions would serve as driving forces to facilitate the change process.

Assess Stimuli

In second-level assessment, the CNE and the committee identified environmental stimuli and specific driving and restraining forces. They also identified
gatekeepers, such as clinical nurse managers, influential physicians with many
admissions to the units, and politically correct unit personnel. Influential persons
could speed or impede the entry and internal flow of information vital to the
units. The nursing administration planning committee appraised each driving
and restraining force to determine its influence on decision makers, in this case,
the clinical nurse managers. As the committee identified the forces in the
situation, they made graphic representations of balances of driving and restraining forces on a series of worksheets. When the worksheets were completed, the
committee made educated guesses about the readiness of each unit and each unit
manager to adapt. This prioritization of the units that seemed the most likely to
change easily to the new skill mix amounted to an initial selection of units
targeted as the first to change. The focal stimulus, the high RN skill mix, was
influenced by gatekeepers; nurse, physician, and community expectations; and
large numbers of nurses educated for primary care delivery systems (contextual
stimuli). Past and present interrelationships of individuals unknown to the
committee provided many residual stimuli, some of which would become known
(contextual stimuli) during the change episode.

Diagnose

During and after second-level assessment, the CNE and the nursing administration planning committee compared the current nursing division labor costs

and skill mix with facts gathered from sources outside the hospital. The sources included descriptions of current practice from hospitals of similar size and type in the local geographic area, literature sources, and statistics from a magnet hospital of comparable size and kind in a nearby city. The facts thus gathered provided comparison standards to which the committee could relate current costs and skill mix in the nursing division as they made the diagnosis of high nursing labor costs related to the current skill mix.

Set Goals

The assessment and diagnostic information affirmed the goal of lower nursing labor costs. It also provided detailed data that nurse managers could use later when they worked with the nursing administration committee to redefine the skill mix for each unit. The nursing administration planning committee now developed a time line (Gantt chart) to set broad goals for the various nursing units to change to the new skill mix ratio. On the chart, they sequenced strategies and tactics in unfreeze, move, and freeze stages. This completed preliminary work and early plans to implement the change process.

Intervene

Unfreeze. The CNE reported on agenda items discussed at the hospital executive committee at her regularly scheduled meeting of the nursing administration committee. Therefore, the committee members knew the financial concerns of the hospital executive committee. Discussion occurred at the nursing administration committee meetings about changing the skill mix as one of several strategies to address the financial (social) problem. The group reached consensus over time that a change in unit skill mix ratios was needed and they considered the change appropriate. They had already agreed that the ratio could be changed to 65:35 (65% registered nurses and 35% unlicensed assistive personnel) and continue to maintain quality.

Move. When the CNE took the completed preliminary plan to the nursing administration committee, her strategy was to discuss it thoroughly with the committee as a whole. Committee members had been involved individually with different parts of the plan, depending on their expertise and other commitments. Members of the committee identified additional driving and restraining forces and measured the forces that they could measure. The CNE planner, as chair of the group, used strategies with a rational approach, including acknowledgment of previous committee input and contributions of individual members. When members of the nursing administration committee reached a consensus that change was imminent and that together they had developed a sound course of action, they shifted from their role as decision makers to the role of nurse planners. This shift was appropriate because the nurse managers were the ones best able to determine the readiness of the staff nurses on their individual units to make the required change.

As nurse planners, the managers repeated the change process on their units using the overall plan agreed to by the committee. Managers/coordinators of staff support departments/offices became nurse coplanners. They assisted the nurse manager planners as they implemented the change on all targeted units. The unit staff now took the role of decision makers. The planners and coplanners refined the preliminary plan to reach consensus regarding the details of the solution they would implement to achieve the goal of lower nursing labor costs. They collaborated to develop specific strategies to implement the desired change on their own units in accord with the mutually agreed upon time lines.

Freeze. The CNE arranged with the editor of the in-house newsletter to give complimentary accounts of gains of the nursing division toward established goals. When the units met the targeted skill mix ratios, the CNE reported their progress to the hospital executive committee and planned a recognition ceremony for the nursing division.

Evaluate

At an early date, nursing administration committee members decided to evaluate progress toward and maintenance of desired skill mix ratios on clinical nursing units. Several measurements taken at intervals revealed the degree of adaptation. These included labor costs for the division of nursing, the average skill mix for the division, and skill mix ratios for the individual units. They examined the findings in terms of the divisional goal of lower nursing labor costs. Additionally, they examined quality improvement documents to determine if there were indications of reduced quality. Evaluation suggested several minor adjustments of skill mix ratios as well as the Gantt time line, strategies, and specific tactics.

Summary

This chapter consisted of three parts. First, it drew parallels between the Roy Adaptation Model and Lewin's planned change theories. Both Roy's and Lewin's work stems from similar philosophical perspectives and disciplinary backgrounds—sociology and psychology. They both espouse reciprocal interaction worldviews. Both use essentially a systems approach but also have characteristics of the interaction approach. The chapter examined ways that Lewin's theories relate to the key nursing concepts as developed by Roy.

Second, the chapter provided a format for a combined RAM-KL change process. The RAM provided concepts of assessment, diagnosis, goal setting, intervention, evaluation, and mutuality. Lewin concepts include force field analysis, channels, and group work to deal with individual-group relationships. Lewin's work also supplied the techniques of mental and graphic representation of forces in planned change situations.

The chapter ended with a scenario that applied the RAM-KL change process. This scenario identified four levels of change: hospital executives, chief nurse executive, nurse administrators, and nurse caregivers. The level of change shifted as the scenario progressed. At each level, planners had a degree of control over the implementation of strategies with the survival of the hospital as the common overall goal. Decision makers at all levels contributed to this goal by deciding to adopt the change in unit skill mix as a permanent way of providing care on the units.

References

Andrews, H. A., & Roy, C. (1991). The nursing process according to the Roy Adaptation Model. In C. Roy & H. A. Andrews (Eds.), *The Roy Adaptation Model: The definitive statement* (pp. 27-54). Norwalk, CT: Appleton & Lange.

Lewin, K. L. (1958). Group decision and social change. In T. M. Newcomb & E. L. Hartley (Eds.), *Readings in social psychology* (pp. 197-211). New York: Holt.

Meleis, A. I. (1991). *Theoretical nursing: Development and progress* (2nd ed.). Philadelphia: J. B. Lippincott.

Roy, C. (1980). The Roy Adaptation Model. In J. P. Riehl & C. Roy (Eds.), *Conceptual models for nursing practice* (pp. 179-192). New York: Appleton-Century-Crofts.

Bennis, Benne, and Chin's Planned Change Writings

BOX 13.1: LOOKING AHEAD

Chapter 13: Bennis, Benne, and Chin's Planned Change Writings

Foundations and History of Bennis, Benne, and Chin's Planned Change Writings
Change Writings by Bennis, Benne, Chin, and Their Invited Authors

---

BOX 13.2: KEY WORDS AND PHRASES

— Epistemology   — Morphology
— Laboratory learning   — Positivism
— Logical positivism   — Teleological

This chapter on the writings of Bennis, Benne, and Chin and their invited authors starts with a discussion of the history and foundations of their edited books of readings and ends with a review of the 1985 edition.

Warren G. Bennis was born in 1925 in New York City and educated at Antioch College, the London School of Economics and Political Science, and the Massachusetts Institute of Technology (MIT). He taught at MIT and Boston University and was a senior research associate at the Human Relations Center in Boston (Evory, Gareffa, & Metzger, 1982).

Kenneth D. Benne, born in 1908 and the son of a Kansas farmer, received his education at the Kansas State University of Agricultural and Applied Science, the University of Michigan, and Columbia University. He began his career with rural elementary and high school teaching in Kansas. Later, he taught at the University of Illinois and Columbia University. A coinventor of the "training group" and cofounder of the National Training Laboratories, Benne also taught at Boston University (Evory, 1978).

Robert Chin, born in 1918 in New York City (now deceased), received his education at Columbia University. Chin spent many years teaching at Boston University. He also served as director of the Human Relations Center in Boston (Fadool, 1976). Thus all three editors of *The Planning of Change* spent part or all of their professional careers in the Boston area.

Prior to the time that Bennis, Benne, and Chin (BB&C) edited their first book, many persons chose either a laissez-faire or an armed-conflict solution to new-knowledge upheavals. Bennis, Benne, and Chin refused to consider either response. Instead, they advocated the application of social science knowledge to human problems. One main question they encountered was how to use such knowledge. An attempt to answer this main question forms the major thrust of all editions of their book. Their approach calls for the *"planful application of valid and appropriate knowledge in human affairs for the purpose of creating intelligent action and change"* (Bennis, Benne, & Chin, 1985, p. 4).

The BB&C emphasis on practical theory and knowledge use mandates the formation of knowledge-based social technologies and the development of responsible agents of change. Bennis, Benne, and Chin solicited essays that describe processes, conditions antecedent to change, and consequences of change. Client systems include individuals, groups, formal organizations, and cultures. Value orientations permeate these writings; collaborative processes become an ethical imperative. Last, but not least, Bennis, Benne, and Chin did more than salute their intellectual and moral ancestors. Through their attention to historical perspectives, they identified a chronology for three major philosophical positions with respect to planned change. They clarified criteria for these viewpoints and demonstrated time-oriented and philosophical relationships among them.

Foundations and History of Bennis, Benne, and Chin's Planned Change Writings

Bennis, Benne, and Chin (1961, 1969, 1985; Bennis, Benne, Chin, & Corey, 1976) cooperated in the production of four editions of *The Planning of Change*. (Corey, a geography and urban planning educator, joined BB&C for the 1976 edition.) Their volumes take second place to Lewin's work in popularity with authors of nursing periodical literature on planned change (Tiffany, Cheatham, Doornbos, Loudermelt, & Momadi, 1994).

In the first edition (1961) of *The Planning of Change,* the editors sought to define an emerging field of study. Quite long (781 pages), it emphasized the dynamics of face-to-face groups, a topic that received less emphasis in the second and shorter edition. Group dynamics, by 1969, had found adequate and previously unavailable coverage in widely circulated publications. The experience of producing the first edition helped the editors to clarify their focus and shorten the book to 627 pages in the second (1969) edition. The focus of this edition reflected developments in theory building, research, and experimentation in the applied behavioral sciences both in the United States and abroad.

Changes in readers' needs and in society at large contributed to changes in each edition of the book. For example, nine tenths of the writings in the second edition were new. The third (1976, 517-page) edition discussed the effects of the liberation movements of the 1960s, the Vietnam War, and the social turbulence of the 1960s. The fourth (1985) and shortest (487-page) edition added input on open systems. It also dealt with the interests of the less advantaged in society as planners seek change to benefit the poor. The remainder of this chapter reviews the fourth (1985) edition of the BB&C book, *The Planning of Change.*

Bennis, Benne, and Chin recognized the influence that Lewin had on the perspectives from which they viewed planned change. They claimed him as one of the intellectual forebears of their work. Lewin founded the Research Center for Group Dynamics at the Massachusetts Institute of Technology (MIT) in the mid-1940s. By 1945, he had assembled a staff. Benne, along with others, collaborated with Lewin during these formative years, so the heavy emphasis on group dynamics that appears in the first edition of the BB&C book comes as no surprise. The following quotation explains some facets of the connection between Lewin's ideas, many of which he did not live to refine and publish, and the choice of the normative-reeducative approach chosen by the Bennis, Benne, and Chin group.

> We may use the organization of the National Training Laboratories in 1947 as a milestone in the development of normative-reeducative approaches to changing in America. The first summer laboratory program grew out of earlier collaborations among Kurt Lewin, Ronald Lippitt, Leland Bradford, and Kenneth Benne. The idea behind the laboratory was that participants, staff, and students would learn about themselves and their back-home problems by collaboratively building a laboratory in which participants would become both experimenters and subjects in the study of their own developing interpersonal and group behavior within the laboratory setting. It seems evident that the five conditions of a normative-reeducative approach to changing were met in the conception of the training laboratory. Kurt Lewin died [February 11, 1947] before the 1947 session of the training laboratory opened. (Chin & Benne, 1985, p. 33)

The five conditions of the normative-reeducative approach include (a) a truly dialogic relationship between the client and the planner; (b) the notion that the client's problem might need something more than a technical approach, that is, a social-psychological approach; and (c) the necessity for collaboration between client and planner in diagnosing a social problem and in solving it. Further, (d) planners must attend to the nonconscious elements of the change situation and (e) planners and clients should learn to use behavioral science methods appropriately in solving social problems (Chin & Benne, 1985).

The 1985 edition of *The Planning of Change* names some of the theoretical roots of the normative-reeducative approach. These include the use of technologies for participative learning and self-study invented by Leland Bradford. Also, Benne had sought to resolve conflict through techniques that combine democratic and scientific values. Another influence on the training laboratory perspective involved the Tavistock Clinic work in the application of therapeutic methods in industrial settings. Roethlisberger and Dickson advocated personal counseling as an organizational change strategy. Elton Mayo's work in industrial sociology and the Carl Rogers counseling methods also had a part in the founding of the National Training Laboratories and the subsequent development of the normative-reeducative family of strategies advocated by Bennis, Benne, and Chin (Chin & Benne, 1985).

Change Writings by Bennis, Benne, Chin, and Their Invited Authors

In the fourth edition of *The Planning of Change* (1985), the editors provided four parts: (a) planned change in perspective, (b) diagnostics in social systems, (c) interventions in planned change, and (d) the place of values and goals in the planning of change. The detail included in the following summary of the Bennis, Benne, and Chin work assumes importance in the light of the advanced age or death of the editors. Additionally, their books, with their valuable contributions to the study of planned change, now have gone out of print.

Section D.2 in Appendix D lists nursing periodical articles that used Bennis, Benne, and Chin literature during an 11-year time period. Because readers will find such information in the index of the 1985 edition of the BB&C book, Appendix D does not include a chart that shows the placement of specific topics in the Bennis, Benne, and Chin literature.

Planned Change in Perspective

This first part of the (1985) book has two chapters (four essays) that address two kinds of issues. Reading 1.1 provides historical perspectives. Three other essays, taken together (1.2, 2.1, and 2.2), categorize strategies.

Planned change in America. The Benne, Bennis, and Chin (1985) reading (1.1) on planned change in America places the emerging discipline of planned change in a historical context. Between 1900 and the 1950s, behaviorally oriented social scientists entered the service of government to assist in the mapping of government change programs such as the New Deal. Later, in the 1960s, grassroots movements protested the ascendancy of technostructures (e.g., the "military-industrial complex"). These two circumstances, and possibly others, refocused attitudes toward planned change. During the first half of the century, people asked whether or not they should seek to shape their futures. Should they try to make deliberate changes? Or should they simply let things happen? Planners saw opportunities for service; natural-adjustment proponents thought social scientists should watch from the sidelines.

By 1950, laissez-faire postures had lost out to social activists in the form of professional managers in business and industry and to practitioners in the helping professions such as psychiatry, social work, nursing, and counseling. The question had shifted from whether people should plan change to how they should plan it. *Progress* took on a meaning that mandated the use of science in the service of humans and said that experts should meet peoples' needs according to the ways the experts interpreted those needs.

By the 1960s, the horror of genocide through atomic warfare had imprinted itself on the consciousness of many. Liberation movements denounced oppressive conditions of life. Protest groups included racial-minority groups, women, the poor, homosexuals, and the environmentally conservative. Protests encouraged a proactive stance. An emphasis on redistribution of social power debunked the value-neutral stance previously assumed by social scientists. New ways of thinking laid the groundwork for win-win strategies of changing.

Even though liberation movements created readiness for learning about change strategies, gaps developed between liberation leaders and social scientists. Benne, Bennis, and Chin concluded that the liberationists were wrong to isolate themselves from the help of social scientists of goodwill. They also decried the conduct of the Vietnam War and its aftereffects, saying that it demonstrated the futility of using power-coercive strategies in the face of the human power associated with belief in a cause. The war also illustrated the effects of manipulating information for the purpose of rendering the public helpless to protest a public policy. BB&C concluded that agents of planned change must accept a profound degree of ethical responsibility. They must summon the opinions of adopters on matters of values so that they can service the universal good—human survival.

General strategies for effecting change. The first part of the essay (1.2) by Chin and Benne (1985) provides descriptions of the empirical-rational, normative-reeducative, and power-coercive strategies for changing. Under empirical-rational strategies, the authors described basic research and knowledge dissemination through education, personnel selection and replacement, systems analysis, diffusion systems, utopian thinking, and clarification of language. Normative-reeducative strategies emphasize dialogue, the use of social science information in addition to technical information, collaboration between planner and client, the recognition of nonconscious elements of change, and the appropriate use of behavioral science methods. These require the problem-solving capacities, and therefore the personal growth, of system members. Descriptions of power-coercive strategies discuss nonviolence, the use of political institutions, and working with power elites.

Section 1.2 includes a chart from an earlier edition that shows placement of the various lines of thought about deliberate changing. Like the narrative that precedes it, the chart divides the theorists or other major proponents of planned change strategies into the empirical-rational, normative-reeducative, and power-coercive strategies camps. It arranges them with respect to degrees of coercion involved, with the most neutral (rational-empirical) at the left, running through the midrange interactive strategies in the center, into the power-coercive strategies at the right. The vertical dimension of the chart places the earlier change strategy developers and their forerunners at the top; the placement runs through time and puts later strategy advocates at the bottom. Vertical and horizontal lines show ideological connections among strategies. Contributors include many U.S. citizens and a few persons from other countries. (See Figure 13.1.a and 13.1.b.)

The current state of planned changing. Section 2.2 (Benne, 1985a—purposely taken out of sequence here) describes the objects of changing in terms of group size, from individuals to societies. In terms of the changing of individuals, Benne reported trends in the revolt against psychiatrists who attach labels and treat disease stereotypes rather than persons. Likewise, he criticized schools that focus on cognitive development rather than on whole persons. Benne addressed small-group interventions and reported on methodologies for use in communities. He stressed the importance of macrosystems and asserted that persons can learn about them in laboratory settings.

Strategies of consultation. The section (2.1) by Blake and Mouton (1985) combines approximations of the progressions found in sections 1.2 and 2.2 in a chart with 25 cells. The Blake and Mouton designations for the unit of change (individual, group, intergroup, organization, society) resemble the categories provided by Benne in 2.2. The neutral-coercive progression of their types of interventions (except for theories, the last type) resembles the progression toward coercion in the earlier Chin and Benne section (1.2). Blake and Mouton

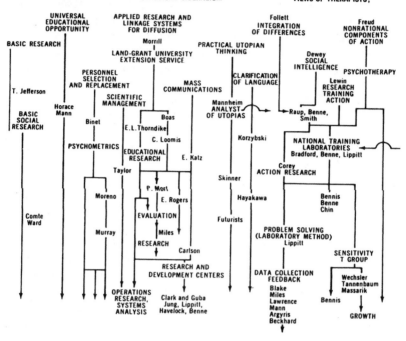

Figure 13.1.a. Strategies of Deliberate Changing

SOURCE: From "General Strategies for Effecting Changes in Human Systems," by R. Chin and K. D. Benne, 1985. In W. G. Bennis, K. D. Benne, & R. Chin (Eds.), *The Planning of Change* (4th ed.), pp. 44, 45. Copyright © 1985 by Holt, Rinehart and Winston, Inc. Reprinted by permission.

briefly described the kind of situation that would pertain in each cell in their matrix. They also included practical examples for most cells. The editors added the Benne essay to the chapter to supplement Blake and Mouton's emphasis on the development of organizations.

Diagnostics in Planned Change

The second part of the book discusses diagnostics—getting a conceptual handle on a change situation. The four chapters (nine essays) that describe the dynamics of political environments in various types of systems introduce ideas that readers can use to analyze those systems. BB&C included essays that deal with systems, knowledge use, new ideas about organizations, and the internal and external environments of organizations.

RE-EDUCATIVE   **C. POWER—COERCIVE**

TRAINERS, AND SITUATION CHANGERS

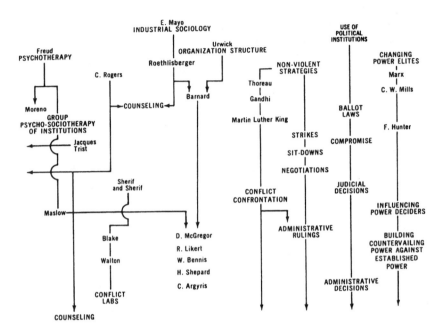

Figure 13.1.b. Strategies of Deliberate Changing

SOURCE: From "General Strategies for Effecting Changes in Human Systems," by R. Chin and K. D. Benne, 1985. In W. G. Bennis, K. D. Benne, & R. Chin (Eds.), *The Planning of Change* (4th ed.), pp. 44, 45. Copyright © 1985 by Holt, Rinehart, and Winston, Inc. Reprinted by permission.

Models of environments. Chin (1985, 3.1) described three basic approaches planners can take concerning environments in change situations. First, planners can act directly to change an environment. Second, they can work on relationships between or among systems. Third, persons internal to a system can watch and analyze important developments in the environment.

An effective change plan selects the target unit at an appropriate level (person, group, organization, community), defines system boundaries, makes an orderly analysis of the environment, takes the chosen change theory into account, and considers the professional competencies needed. It identifies causal forces and determines the direction of their flow in both the system and its environment. Chin developed a matrix that characterizes environments under two dimensions: textures and contents. He wrote that conditions in cells do not exhibit equal importance as planners learn to establish "mind-holds" on social systems and their environments.

Resistant environments. Klein (1985, 3.2) considered resistance absolutely essential to individuals and to systems because individuals and systems must maintain their integrity and ward off real threats. In modern society, persons running massive change programs accumulate vast quantities of data, analyze and manipulate those data, and use them to plan rapid and irreversible changes with far-reaching and possibly dangerous effects.

Those who resist change most vociferously often occupy the fringe of the adopter group. Their arguments appear extreme, but they may represent many who would like to voice complaints but are too inarticulate or shy to do so. The resister almost always has something of great value to communicate. His or her message could help planners avoid serious pitfalls. A proper change plan includes mechanisms for heeding defenders of the status quo. Listening to resistance at all possible stages in the change event increases the likelihood of success of the change effort.

Evaluating theories of action. In dealing with knowledge use, Argyris and Schön (1985, 4.1) wrote that planners and theory developers should look at reasons that theories-in-use (theories actually employed in change situations) achieve certain kinds of results in the "real world." Questions concern the ways planners relate theories-in-use to their espoused (formally chosen) theories. Both an espoused theory and a theory-in-use should possess internal consistency. The two should be congruent with one another. The theory-in-use should be effective and should have value in the behavioral world. It is tested through use.

Dilemmas arise because people tend to use mental mechanisms when they apply their espoused theories. For example, they may so value theories-in-use that they ignore disconfirming data. Through selective inattention, they sometimes suppress uncomfortable data or remove offending elements from the situation. They might create a self-fulfilling prophecy or change the espoused theory. When discrepancies appear between the espoused theory and the theory-in-use, they sometimes change minor details, but not the core, of the theory-in-use. The mental schemes people use to confront incongruities between an espoused theory and a theory-in-use present dangers, as when a person believes in participatory democracy but uses manipulative and roughshod tactics.

Educational field experiences. In writing about knowledge use, Benne (1985b, 4.2) described two related but different worlds—the academic world and the practice world. The academic world values educational priorities; the practice world values service priorities. Deeper differences concern epistemology (a study of the sources and limits of knowledge). Academics, isolated from practical affairs, make sharp distinctions between knowledge generation and knowledge use. Practitioners, who must make practical, on-the-spot judgments, value useful, fruitful, and illuminating knowledge; they blur distinctions between knowledge building and knowledge application. Society needs a generalized method of knowing that serves both academics and practitioners. Students need to recognize the value of the two overlapping kinds of knowledge. They should lay aside mental blocking mechanisms such as stereotyping, status differentials, and fears of inadequacy. Through collaboration, academicians and practitioners should affirm epistemological differences and further the two kinds of knowledge generation.

Strategies for a new era. Harrison (1985, 5.1) wrote that organizations need both alignment and attunement. Alignment expands the individual member's identity and sense of purpose to include the organization's identity and purpose. Attunement concerns human love, as seen in empathy, understanding, caring, nurturance, and support. Harrison likened an aligned organization to a symphony orchestra in which all members "line up" with the conductor's idea of the way the music should sound. Alignment, run amok, invites dictatorial methods by leaders. Attunement resembles a jazz combo that spontaneously provides time for each musician to express musical ideas as the group improvises around a theme. Attunement requires mutual respect and a measure of peace. Attunement, taken too far, never gets the job done. Alignment and attunement require balance.

Harrison advocated the identification of high performance patterns by organizational participants. In such identification, members think about the times when they, highly in tune with the organization, experienced conditions that enabled them to achieve extraordinarily high levels of performance. The group works to duplicate such conditions for participants. The group achieves balance between alignment and attunement by fusing conditions needed for peak performance with the mission of the organization.

Paradigm shift. Mohrman and Lawler (1985, 5.2) defined *paradigm* as a way of looking at the world. They advocated a shift toward a tentatively emerging paradigm called Quality of Work Life (QWL). QWL includes attention to human welfare and a balance between individuals and organizations. The individual has worth that modern technologies should not and need not supplant. QWL technologies attend to both the individual and the organization.

Mohrman and Lawler (1985) cited the steps that Kuhn described for a paradigm shift. During "normal" times, unusual events fuel speculation and thought. Adjustment usually occurs. Later, unusual situations pile up. A crisis ensues; if extensive enough, a large-scale paradigm destruction and a subsequent shift follow. A new normal state emerges. The authors felt that a shift toward the QWL paradigm was occurring in the United States.

Corporate culture. Snyder (1985, 6.1) wrote about corporate culture, which consists of the "system of norms, beliefs and assumptions, and values that determine how people in the organization act" (p. 164). Managers of successful organizations manage corporate culture in a series of phases. These phases provide for gaining an understanding of the culture and the influence it has on the organization. Planners assess forces that favor both the status quo and cultural change. They decide what changes, if any, should occur and what changes are possible. Then they use levers ("tools") of change.

The several methods for understanding culture include direct observation by an outside person, surveys, document review, and assessment by members. Snyder made a list of 20 essential questions. The planner uses Lewin's force field analysis to determine the strength and direction of cultural forces.

Levers of change found in organizational cultures include management style and action, human resource management, organizational structure, information and communication, strategy, and physical design and setting. Snyder discussed ways that planners can use strategies for influencing people at points of leverage toward change.

Evolution of organizational environments. Terreberry (1985, 6.2) had concern for the environments of organizations. She presented four "ideal types" of environments: (a) a placid, randomized, relatively unchanging environment, with goods and bads randomly distributed; (b) a placid, clustered environment with relatively unchanging goods and bads that appear in clusters; (c) a disturbed-reactive environment that experiences similar systems in its field; and (d) a turbulent environment where dynamic processes arise from the field itself, not merely from its constituents.

Terreberry (1985) wrote that organizational environments then were approaching a turbulent state. As evidence, she cited rapidly increased organizational interconnectedness and unpredictable change in organizational interdependence. The change from placid, randomized environments to turbulent environments exhibits an increasing ratio of externally induced change as compared with internally induced change. Terreberry offered a model as a beginning conceptual framework for viewing formal organizations and their interdependencies within environments. She asserted that one cannot assess the degree of advantage offered by any type of organizational configuration without understanding the dynamics of the environment of that organization.

Adaptability and copability. According to Motamedi (1985, 6.3), *adaptability* and *copability* refer to the ways that organizations relate to their environments. Adaptability concerns an organization's match (correspondence) with the environment; copability relates to the strength of the organization's internal identity.

Adaptability looks outward and emphasizes the future; copability looks inward and relates to the here and now. Adaptability changes the external environment; copability maintains and nurtures the internal environment. Adaptability cannot occur without an understanding of both the internal and the external environments and the ways they relate. Copability concerns the ability of the system to maintain its own identity and integrity in the face of environmental pressures. Copability requires knowledge of the internal system and its processes and the ability to take actions appropriate to preserve system integrity. Such actions include problem identification and alleviation, stalling, and problem repression.

A placid, randomized environment requires low amounts of adaptability and copability. A placid, clustered environment requires highly specialized competencies for dealing with entities in the environment, but the rate of interaction remains low. Survival in a disturbed, reactive environment involves much movement (dynamics) in a few, quite well-known (static) areas. Survival in a turbulent field environment demands a great deal of knowledge about the environment and constant, dynamic adaptability and copability. As environments become turbulent, managers need knowledge about ways of dealing with them.

Interventions for Planned Change

This third part of the BB&C book is divided into three chapters (15 essays) that give readers both theoretical and practical perspectives on the interventions they might use to cause change to occur. It provides information about planning structures and processes, education and reeducation, and organizational and political factors in planned change.

Comparing the processes of planning. Nutt (1985, 7.1) presented a morphology for comparing various kinds of change processes put forth by model makers. Scholars and practitioners often pay insufficient attention to processes used for planning change. In his morphology, Nutt divided the planning process into five stages and three steps and listed techniques that planners could use in the stages and steps.

The *formulation stage* verifies the existence and nature of the problem (performance gap) identified by the sponsor. The *concept stage* develops a model that describes the problem. *Detailing* identifies possible solutions to the problem. *Evaluation* provides for a choice among possible solutions. *Implementation* involves plans for strategies designed to gain acceptance for the preferred solution. Each stage contains three steps. *Search* gathers necessary information. *Synthesis* assembles ideas found during search. *Analysis* studies the results at each stage.

Nutt (1985) showed how to use the matrix formed by the stages and steps to draw comparisons between different planning approaches. Such comparisons show that variation typifies planning methods; they follow unique paths.

The uniqueness of planning pathways poses both threats and rewards. Planners tend to emphasize the more theoretical aspects of planning; sponsors tend to favor development and implementation of solutions. An orderly progression through all the stages and steps generally improves results, but overly long planning processes might involve excessive expense. Planners with wide theoretical exposure and field experience know how to skip or combine stages or steps in ways that preserve both fiscal and product integrity. Political processes might cause planners to skip or combine steps. Requests by sponsors for progress reporting encourage what Nutt calls cycling (planner-sponsor consultation).

In his research, Nutt (1985) described the morphology he proposed as a generic model useful in making comparisons of diverse planning methods. Previously, he had profiled 50 case studies with the morphology and had demonstrated the degrees of comprehensiveness and the sequencing of stages and steps used in their various planning processes. He stated that future research should compare the patterns he discovered with the outcomes of related change episodes.

Power and strategy. According to Mason and Mitroff (1985, 7.2), organizational power has teleological (shaped by a purpose or goal) properties; it relates to purposes of the organization, which vary from site to site. Strategies are plans for acquiring power. Persons use power for either good or evil. *Power* is "the human control of the energies necessary to achieve human purposes, whatever those purposes may be" (p. 216).

A power-oriented view of strategy centers on proactive behavior rather than reactive behavior. Proactive behavior focuses more on enabling actions than on matching actions (responsive actions). Any organization that creates enabling conditions for itself possesses the ability to find a matching niche in the environment. Enabling conditions of organizational power include the ability to change or create purposes; to obtain resources of the right kind, in the right amount, and at the right time; and to eliminate conflict among concerned stakeholders. A successful strategy requires all four of these conditions of power.

Mason and Mitroff defined stakeholders as vital entities with resources, purposes, wills, and the capacity for decision making. An organization consists of a collection of internal and external stakeholders who network together in supporting or resisting behaviors. As stakeholder relationships change, organizations gain power if more activity flows through supporting relationships than through resisting relationships. Activities that range from fighting to loving will change the stakeholders; all require power. The state of the organization at any one time relates to the total of stakeholders' behavior. Planners base every strategy they try on assumptions regarding stakeholders, stakeholder relationships, and the organization's power to effect change.

In organizations, leaders must have inspiration to create new strategies; managers must have the resources required to translate new purposes into action; and other stakeholders need the spirit, dedication, and enough commitment to perform the tasks necessary to fulfill organizational purposes.

Mason and Mitroff developed the strategic assumption surfacing and testing (SAST) technique to help organizations to identify stakeholders and determine their relative importance; not all stakeholders assume equal importance. Further, SAST helps leaders in organizations identify and test their own assumptions about stakeholders through research methods, dialogue, or monitoring. SAST guides the actual implementation of strategies. In principle, SAST could help leaders develop an action plan for each stakeholder; in practice, leaders direct their efforts toward stakeholders capable of limiting the organization.

Usable knowledge: A metatheory. Dunn (1985, 7.3) wrote about usable knowledge that concerns social policy research. He did this in response to what he saw as the tangled state of theories in the field. Dunn scrutinized previously unexamined assumptions about theories and hidden standards for theory assessment. He reasoned that these assumptions and standards had obscured an understanding of the role of policy research in social problem solving.

Dunn approached his task by developing a four-cell matrix of discovery with row stubs to name the principal phenomena that *explain* cognitive relations (imposed on users, generated by users) and column heads to name the principal cognitive relations that *define* knowledge use (objective, subjective; see Table 13.1.).

Later in the discussion, Dunn expanded the row stubs by giving each main row three subheads (users, knowledge, social systems); this addition yielded a matrix with 12 cells. The six stubs and two heads in Dunn's matrix come from very general criteria. Thus Dunn avoided the problem that emerges when one uses a particular theory as a source of standards for the evaluation of itself. A system for evaluation of theories must not use, as a standard, any theory that falls into the class under evaluation. This prevents the evaluator from siding with any one of the theories undergoing evaluation.

Prompted by the stipulations that the cells indicated, Dunn developed a series of three propositions and their related corollaries. In keeping with the row subheadings, the propositions fall under the *users, knowledge,* and *social systems* categories. The first proposition states that "knowledge use is a systematic cognitive relation structured by the ways that *users* anticipate events" (p. 238, italics added). Corollaries address such topics as user individuality, frames of reference, choice mechanisms, restriction of ranges of events, and experience.

TABLE 13.1 A Basic Typology for Classifying Theories of Knowledge Use

	The Principal Cognitive Relations *That* Define *Knowledge Use Are*	
The Principal Phenomena That Explain *Cognitive Relations Are*	*Objective* *(Interactional)*	*Subjective* *(Cultural)*
Imposed on Users (Imperative)	Interactional Imperativism	Cultural Imperativism
Generated by Users (Constructed)	Interactional Constructivism	Cultural Constructivism

SOURCE: From "Usable Knowledge: A Metatheory of Policy Research in the Social Sciences," by W. N. Dunn. In W. G. Bennis, K. D. Benne, & R. Chin (Eds.), *The Planning of Change* (4th ed.), p. 231. Copyright © 1985 by Holt, Rinehart and Winston, Inc. Reprinted by permission.

The second proposition addresses *knowledge* as a cultural artifact. Corollaries deal with such issues as adequacy, relevance, and cogency. The third proposition views *social systems* as artificial entities that are created, maintained, and changed through knowledge transactions. Corollaries center on rationality, capability, and emancipation.

Conversational planning. Schön (1985, 7.4) started his exploration of conversational planning with a discussion of the dominant view of inquiry—instrumentalism. Although instrumentalism (rational planning) requires explicit objectives, no one can formulate clear objectives without first discovering the nature of the problem (problem setting). In the "real world," problems do not emerge in a well-formed state. A difficulty arises because instrumentalism judges the quality of problem setting by the achievement of objectives. This creates a chicken-and-egg situation that encourages an arbitrary choice of objectives. Planners, under this system, assume a spectator/manipulator stance.

Schön advocated the use of a dialectical approach. The dialectical approach requires that a planner immerse him- or herself in the planning situation as what Schön called an ecologically embedded agent/experient. This stance recognizes the decision-making capacities of people in the situation; it helps planners reflect on meanings and thus diminishes miscommunication. Objectives and strategies remain open to restructuring as the change episode unfolds. Planners who employ dialectics engage in problem setting and problem solving in ways that instrumentalist views ignore.

A systems approach. Churchman (1985, 7.5) wrote that people have great difficulty in seeing the incompleteness of their own disciplinary perspectives.

Humanists cry that not everything yields itself to quantification. Systems analysts reply that they do not try to quantify everything; that's impossible. Both talk; neither listens. Feeling the ineffectiveness of his usual expository approach, Churchman told a story that illustrated the issues involved. Three men (Mr. Action, Mr. C. S. Temm, and Mr. S. R. Teez), passengers in a hijacked plane, argue interminably about various models of action. Periodically, a drunk joins them. Finally, the plane banks and the pilot announces the return to New York to dump the passengers. The debaters cry, "Why?" At which time the drunk tells them that he is one of the hijackers. His country had wanted to kidnap some high-powered talent from the United States, but after hearing their discussions, he concluded they would be worthless. All they do is talk, talk, talk. And, as everybody knows, oppressed people get liberation only through revolution! Teez replies, "Oh dear," as the hijacker disappears. The flight attendant tells Teez not to worry—the hijacker is quite drunk. "Anyway," she says, "none of you three ever included a woman's view in your arguments." Thus Churchman pointed out the fact that systems analysts often fail to include themselves in the systems they describe.

Radical planning. Grabow and Heskin (1985, 7.6) favored neither the rational-comprehensive planning mode nor completely spontaneous change. They saw the rational-comprehensive mode of planning as an unattainable ideal characterized by an objectivity that sets planners apart from the planned-for, leads to centralization, and resists change. It assumes prior knowledge of probable outcomes and follows several steps of the classical problem-solving process. A spontaneous change program also presents problems.

Grabow and Heskin argued for a communal society where *synthesis* enables members to arrive at a position superordinate to the apparently contradictory points held by various entities in the society. Under this new model, a paradigm founded in dialectics and synthesis emerges. A decentralized society would place the maximum number of decisions within the reach of as many people as possible. Cities no longer would have a purpose and people would live together for the mutual benefit of all. Both upper and lower limits on the quality of life would eliminate both the poverty and the extreme wealth that hinder individual development. Under synthesis, "plan" means facilitation rather than prediction. Individual planners strive for equal participation rather than for mastery over others. People neither seize power nor destroy power; they concentrate on what they are becoming.

Lewin on reeducation. Benne's (1985c) essay (8.1) reviews Kurt Lewin's ideas about reeducation. Lewin thought of self-patterns as sustained by the norms surrounding the persons who possess them. Therefore, he emphasized the importance of reeducation that attends to the impact of society and culture on the individual. Benne assessed 10 of Lewin's principles of reeducation 25 years after Lewin developed them.

Lewin proposed that fundamental similarities exist between the acquisition of the normal and the abnormal. This principle breaks down the conceptual barrier between education and therapy. As a practical matter, lines between pathological and growthful behavior still have usefulness, but as practical judgments rather than a pedagogical necessity.

Second, reeducation equals a change in culture—as family therapy will attest. Lewin's principle still has validity, even though some deny it. Third, firsthand experiences do not automatically confer learning. Therefore, education should include attention to the processes of inquiry.

Fourth, perception steers social action, a principle confirmed by developments since Lewin's time. Fifth, people alone, on the basis of accurate knowledge, cannot correct false perceptions. They also need a supportive emotional environment that lessens their need to justify themselves. Sixth, experiences alone do not change a person's or group's theories (prejudices, stereotypes) about the world. Benne explained this principle by using examples from the research world. Seventh, changes in cognitive structures do not always produce changes in sentiments. Superficial education may result in guilt feelings rather than behavior changes. Benne reported that the depth of educational experiences relates to the degree of reconstruction of a person's values and related actions. Without deep involvement, little change in values or actions occurs.

Lewin's eighth principle states that three expressions of the same process exist: a change in action-ideology, genuine acceptance of alternative facts and values, and new perceptions of the social world. After Benne confirmed Lewin's eighth principle, he proposed two operating stances for reeducators. Reeducators should respect resistance and should seek to find ways to help hostile resisters recognize their own ambivalence.

The ninth Lewin principle states that, as a rule, people accept new beliefs and values as a package rather than one at a time. Value systems are systems. Further, many educators avoid direct confrontation between value systems by using piecemeal approaches that might accomplish other ends, but not the adoption of a new value system. Benne agreed with Lewin's idea while noting that this area needs more research.

The last Lewin principle asserts that acceptance of group membership fosters acceptance of a new system of values and beliefs. Benne agreed with this tenth Lewin principle. Before he closed his essay, he briefly discussed an omission that Lewin recognized. Lewin chose not to conceptualize motoric action. Later, within the Lewinian training movement, trainers advocated the use of prompt feedback in motoric learning. Benne expressed a hope that others, like himself, would continue to value Lewin's work.

Process consultation. In some types of consultation, a manager must diagnose the problem correctly and ask the consultant to provide the correct service or secure the correct information. In another type, the consultant makes the diagnosis and recommends changes. Schein (1985, 8.2) described process consultation as a kind of consultation that does neither. Instead, the consultant and the manager work together to make the diagnosis. In the process, the manager acquires diagnostic skills. Then the manager participates actively with the consultant in developing a remedy. The consultant may or may not have skill in the area of the problem; his or her skill lies in helping the manager to learn the processes needed for diagnosis and generation of solutions.

Models: Helping and coping. In the essay on helping and coping, Brickman et al. (1985, 8.3) cited the need for a general theory of helping and coping to build a bridge between two bodies of literature: social psychology and clinical psychology. They saw that notions about responsibility for causing and solving problems create four different value orientations and permeate helping institutions.

The moral model, the compensatory model, the medical model, and the enlightenment model combine responsibility (or lack or responsibility) for problems in a four-cell matrix in four different ways, with four different results. (See Table 13.2.) In the moral model, people experiencing a problem are responsible for both problem and solution. The people with the problem may do all they can to keep things going well, but still receive blame for failure. In addition, they assume or are given responsibility to solve their own problems. If they are financially well off, any official help they get will be called incentives and will take the form of crop subsidies, tax breaks, and so on. Poorer folk will be punished for failure. The value of this model lies in its ability to compel people to work actively to better their situations. The deficiency comes from the fact that sometimes people truly do not cause their problems and cannot muster the resources needed to solve them.

The authors discussed the consequences of choices among the models in real-life situations. They ended their essay with a set of questions designed to stimulate further thinking and, possibly, research regarding the ways people and institutions choose among the models and put them into practice. Considerations arising from the Brickman et al. essay constitute a major portion of an earlier chapter in this book.

Informal helping groups. As Cowen (1985, 8.4) wrote about sources of help for people with personal problems, he stated that many people do not take their distressing personal problems to mental health professionals. Instead, they seek help from other sources, such as hairdressers, lawyers, work supervisors, and

TABLE 13.2 Consequences of Attribution of Responsibility in Four Models of
Helping and Coping

Attribution to self of responsibility for problem	*Attribution to self of responsibility for solution*	
	High	*Low*
High	I. Moral model	II. Enlightenment model
Perception of self	Lazy	Guilty
Actions expected of self	Striving	Submission
Others besides self who must act	Peers	Authorities
Actions expected of others	Exhortation	Discipline
Implicit view of human nature	Strong	Bad
Potential pathology	Loneliness	Fanaticism
Low	III. Compensatory model	IV. Medical model
Perception of self	Deprived	Ill
Actions expected of self	Assertion	Acceptance
Others besides self who must act	Subordinates	Experts
Actions expected of others	Mobilization	Treatment
Implicit view of human nature	Good	Weak
Potential pathology	Alienation	Dependency

SOURCE: From "Models of Helping and Coping" by P. Brickman et al. In W. G. Bennis, K. D. Benne, & R. Chin (Eds.), *The Planning of Change* (4th ed.), p. 291. Copyright © 1985 by Holt, Rinehart and Winston, Inc. Reproduced by permission.

bartenders. Further, the people who write the most about the helping relationship are the people who do not do the most helping. In fact,

> at least 95% of our current knowledge about the workings and effectiveness of helping processes is based on a special sampling of less than 5% of all interpersonal help-giving interactions, that is, socially recognized and sanctioned interactions in which the help agents are formally trained, credentialed, mental health professionals. (p. 312)

The authors conducted research designed to describe four contexts for interpersonal help. They wanted also to identify cross-group differences and to develop training programs for informal helpers. Lawyers saw the fewest and the most deeply troubled persons; people addressed serious problems to them. Bartenders averaged about 500 contacts per week, but the problems posed to them tended toward superficiality. About one third of the clients of hairdressers raised interpersonal problems; 7% of the workers under supervisors asked for help with their problems. Types of problems raised ranged from difficulties with health, marriage, children, and money, to guilt, confusion, and loneliness. Helpers responded with at least 16 different kinds of responses that ranged from "just listening" to efforts to persuade the troubled person to talk with someone else (referral). Although helpers reported some feelings of anger or puzzlement, the majority of their reactions fell on the positive side. Overall, these helpers expressed comfort with the helper role. Some saw helping as a normal and very important part of their work.

Cowen concluded by saying that people obtain help for diverse problems from numerous kinds of helpers. Further, many other unofficial helping groups exist. Indeed, official mental health helpers may see only a small fraction of persons seeking help. Persons in the four groups that the researchers studied stated that they could use some training in the area of helping. This prompted the researchers to offer information sessions for the informal helpers. They felt this necessary because, as they put it, "only a small fraction of interpersonal distress, biased toward entrenched, longstanding problems housed in fiscally solvent souls, ever enters the formal mental health system" (p. 322).

Getting things done. According to Kennedy (1985, 8.5), few of a person's thoughts ever get translated into speaking or writing, and little of what a person says ever gets into the mind of a hearer. Development of a message that gives all the details needed to convey an accurate and specific set of instructions requires vast amounts of time and energy. Most things worth doing exhibit such complexity that describing them in detail would consume enormous amounts of energy. Kennedy quoted McKinsey as saying that the main problem the manager faces is keeping folks moving roughly in the correct direction. From then on, the folks in the herd will have to find their own ways to get across the river.

Kennedy emphasized the role of trust, simplicity, repetition, and reinforcement in workplace communications. These build a common core of shared meanings so that subsequent communications need to refer only to a symbol to convey a complex message. Eight implications for organizations follow: Only people can get things done. Decentralization fosters efficient communication. People who develop organizations should provide mechanisms for their change. Good policies enable managers to make decisions that "fall between the cracks." Information systems should help real people accomplish real work. Helpful management processes convey information among people. Organizations ought to provide for some socialization. Every person needs a real job and instructions that give him or her both discretion and latitude.

Laboratory learning. Bennis, Benne, and Chin thought of educational and reeducational strategies as the heart of the normative-reeducative approach to planned change; when people change, they must learn. Learning in a laboratory setting differs from learning under "ordinary" circumstances. In ordinary situations, societal norms protect members not only from the pain of everyday occurrences but from viewing aspects of their actions that may hurt others and, perhaps, destroy themselves. Laboratory experiences differ from ordinary situations. Schein and Bennis (1985, 8.6) wrote about laboratory residential groups where the staff creates a social structure and normative culture that they impose on group members. In such groups, delegates do not have their usual support persons and routines. Lacking their previous status, they experience some loss of privacy and miss their usual back-home roles. They experience an informal status based on laboratory terms, face new values, and cope with a lack of structure.

Even though they require a reevaluation of previous ways of acting, laboratory methods offer protection. Laboratory conditions resemble a game with stakes less high than those "at home." The analytical laboratory approach provides a safe outlet for intense feelings. Authentic communication increases the safety of the setting. Protection comes from psychological theories that view all feelings as coming from understandable sources that many members share. Staff people know how to deal with strong feelings and share a commitment not to let group members suffer harm. They model open and authentic communication, and a psychiatrist or psychologist helps with personal problems that emerge.

At the outset, barriers to learning exist. Personal tensions preoccupy delegates. They set up protective screens or feel that they already know how to listen even though they may not actually value what others say, think, or feel. Reduction of external threat helps delegates move beyond such barriers. The objectivity, nonevaluation, and focus on behavior rather than people help delegates to trust and to strengthen their listening skills. Staff persons help group members build supportive group norms.

Codes for dissent. Codes direct people in social systems to respond in certain ways to recurrent problems. Katz (1985, 9.1) cited religion and politics as furnishing codes that deal with dissent. Some groups concern themselves with preserving values; others concentrate on preserving organizations. Groups preserve integrity and continuity of organizations mainly through expulsion or incorporation. Each mechanism carries consequences that cause groups to choose one or the other or to vacillate between the two options. A third code licenses certain individuals to play deviant roles, but in relative isolation. This type of code tends toward preservation of both values and organizations.

Katz used the example of early movements in the Catholic Church to typify the structural effects of incorporation and exclusion. She also discussed the case of Protestantism as a federation of churches with codes programmed toward exclusion. Two dilemmas exist: Organizations that insist on purity of belief lose their adherents; those that preserve the organization lose their distinctive beliefs. Both horns of the dilemma destroy organizations. Organizations have dealt with these dilemmas in different ways. Some license deviants in their efforts to practice both exclusion and inclusion. Katz developed a dispensation scale that shows how Jews have employed a pliable code that, over time, exercises checks and balances between incorporation and exclusion.

In conclusion, Katz suggested ways to develop awareness of codes that facilitate continuity. As a code develops through a series of actions and reactions, it contains less specific content and assumes a more general nature. The code's generalized and symbolic nature permits other individuals or groups to "borrow" it. A code that affects everyone in a society assumes a highly symbolic importance that makes it hard to transfer or relinquish. In a highly heterogeneous society, much borrowing of codes occurs, but the acceptance of codes that affect the whole occurs at a retarded rate. The Katz observations assume importance in planned change because they propose the idea that entire societies accept new values with difficulty. Further, change occurs more easily within a diverse society than in a homogeneous society.

Problem solving and social action. Sarason (1985, 9.2) wrote about three universal human problems. First, people everywhere wonder how to diminish the aloneness that each feels. Second, people wonder how to develop and sustain a sense of community. Last, they ask how to justify living in the face of the knowledge of their own impending deaths. Those who try to escape subjectivity as they hunt for answers find their search for objectivity frustrated because they have no choice but to remain biased and time-bound organisms.

Science hunts for problems that fit its own problem-solving style, so it not only ignores the three universal problems, it has no method for dealing with them. Scientists who enter the world of social action find themselves bewildered by a world resistant to their problem-solving methods. For example, just when the world saw the scientists who developed the atomic bomb as climbing the pinnacle of success, the scientists found themselves plagued with self-doubt. When scientists enter the social arena, they would do well to develop clear visions of what makes life and learning worthwhile.

War and the social sciences. Bakan (1985, 9.3) used the instance of war to illustrate the importance of qualitative thinking. He described logical positivism as an orientation that stresses fact above knowledge; denies nonfactual knowledge; maintains an "anti" stance regarding such things as theology, mysticism, and introspection; and prefers data to theory and theory to speculation. Positivism works through extrapolation, which in war creates disasters. Positivism hobbles the thinking necessary to successful military strategy. Strategists need to know the intent of the enemy, not just the numbers that represent enemy forces. Bakan created a role for the brand of social science that deals with subjective and introspective states, with mentation and vitality, and with deduction and suspicion.

Planning for freedom. Scholars have addressed the concept of freedom through efforts to unify descriptions of freedom, to list the liberties concerned, and to distinguish between two kinds of concepts, such as positive freedom and negative freedom. All these attempts have drawbacks. When Van Gigch (1985, 9.4) wrote about planning for freedom, he started by "unpacking" the assumptions underlying freedom, the system conditions necessary for it, and the opportunities or barriers freedom presents.

Planners start with assumptions about the nature of humans. Are humans basically selfish and willful? Or are they basically moral, rational, and interested in improvement? What conditions prevail in the system? Dimensions for answering this question include such characteristics as rationality, equality, experts and elites, and levels of participation. Van Gigch placed these dimensions in groups that formed four types of planning systems: the liberal model of democracy, the conservative model of democracy, the broker-rule model of democracy, and the Marxian socialist-communist model. Then he described opportunities and barriers under each of the four models. He concluded by saying that more planning does not necessarily lead to less freedom, but under each model, it leads to a distinct type of freedom. The solution to the dilemma of which model to choose lies in making a selection in line with one's values.

Values and Goals

The final part of the BB&C book contains two chapters (five essays) intended to help planners find direction in planned change and to confront value dilemmas in acceptable ways.

Images of the future. Futurism transcends the currently possible. In describing futurism, Boulding (1985, 10.1) presented four modes of imaging (picturing) the nature of reality and of humans. The first judges the world as good and humans as capable of improving it. The second considers the world as good but not amenable to human efforts to make it better. The third view perceives the world as bad but yielding to betterment through human effort. The fourth considers the world to be both bad and impossible for humans to change for the better.

Futurism is important because images of the future act as self-fulfilling prophecies that shape the future itself. How necessary, then, it is to create images that transcend a mundane or destructive present!

Schools, historically elitist, have conserved the past more faithfully than they have molded the future. Society needs future visions of intentional learning communities that create an equalitarian society, draw on the existent reservoir of human knowledge, and increase individuals' capacity for otherness.

Shared culture. Mead (1985, 10.2) described a number of types of disjunctures that exist in the world. As she stressed the need for a culture with better communication, she opted for communication that brings together specialists from many fields and people from diverse walks of life. Models for such intercommunication existed in ancient Greek cities, Victorian England, and early America.

The components of a shared culture, so urgently needed, must spring from within appropriate frameworks. This culture must exhibit suitability for all peoples in all traditions without favoring those with a longer or more extensive literary tradition. It must have a form appropriate for small children as well as adults. It must attend to folk traditions. How can such a culture be constructed rapidly, indeed, almost overnight?

Construction of a shared culture would start with an accumulation of existing knowledge that finds expression in simple terms, using many graphic devices. Mead would meet the problem of shared contribution through the development of a shared language that would begin with the development of glyphs such as those found on international road signs. Within five years, the people of the world would read and speak this artificial language as a second language without giving up their original languages. Only persons beyond early childhood would learn this second language, a prohibition that would prevent the loss of humanity's mother tongues—the languages of love and of poetry. Mead described a number of necessary corrective devices such as reviews of language divergences and mechanisms for dealing with the language of specializations. She saw her visions of the future as capable of preventing fragmentations and agglomerations such as those currently existing in the world.

The "mutable self." In writing about the role of self in social change, Zurcher (1985, 10.3) described four self-concept modes and their relationship to what he called the "mutable self." In the mutable self, a person has the capacity to change at will among four self-concept modes. The person also can accommodate to, control, or change the social situations that support the four self-concept modes.

The A mode of self-concept involves responses to the body and physical senses. The B mode relates to a person's anchorages in relatively stable social structures such as those found in the workplace, volunteer activities, societal reward systems, and family groups. The C mode operates in conjunction with unstable or unacceptable social structures or role sets. In the D mode, the person separates or detaches from social contact and turns to contemplation of the broader meanings of life. When persons experience all four modes flexibly, they move toward development of the mutable self. Denial of any one mode makes achievement of the mutable self impossible.

Power, freedom, and accountability. Bermant and Warwick (1985, 11.1) wrote about power, freedom, and accountability in planned change. Specialized knowledge, favorable personal positions, and advantageous networks confer power on planners. Planners, as agents of power, should pay special attention to matters of ethics.

Bermant and Warwick understood the ramifications of power in social change. They warned that the very act of defining a problem carries implications for the conduct and outcome of social change. Further, planners must consider whether to take a neutral or advocacy role when they confront issues related to the maintenance or the destabilization of social systems they might view as unjust. Planners will confront politically oriented yardsticks for evaluation of change programs and will have to deal with several sets of competing social interests.

Confronting the ideals of freedom causes planners to think about people's capacity to understand issues and act in their own interests. Planners should consider opportunity, or lack of opportunity, and provide safeguards that exhibit improved communication, participation, and empowerment.

As they think about accountability, planners ask to whom they owe accountability and what kind of accountability they owe. They might find their current competence to be less than that required previously by an ill-defined task. They will hunt for the fine line between protection and paternalism.

Moral dilemmas. Managers often seek technical help with services or products; seldom do they ask for assistance with moral matters. Yet managers cannot escape the moral dilemmas that they so frequently confront. Benne (1985d, 11.2) wrote that managers try to avoid facing moral dilemmas through several mechanisms. Sometimes they convert moral problems into technical ones. This puts values into the technical content of a problem. Managers also might try to smuggle values into a situation by labeling moral problems as matters, for example, of organizational health. Managers sometimes revert to law rather than ethical reasoning. They might restrict morality to narrow ranges of human experience. Attempts to escape moral dilemmas will not serve when societal conditions demand attention. Society now exhibits a high degree of interdependence locally and internationally, and technology creates changes in societal conditions. Traditions have less impact than they formerly did.

Many dilemmas exist at the management level, so managers find themselves in an ideal position to attend to them. When the manager accepts differing views as valid concerns and introduces methods for dealing with them, he or she has taken two giant steps toward the collaborative resolution of moral conflicts. Managers should remember that educational processes of conflict resolution help to multiply their efforts. Deliberative and collaborative efforts can help to establish moral community in the workplace and in the world.

Summary

This chapter contains a review of the 1985 edition of *The Planning of Change* by Bennis, Benne, and Chin. It started with a review of the foundations and history of the work of these three authors and editors, all of whom spent time teaching in Boston. The book consists of four parts divided into 11 chapters. Each chapter contains an introduction by the editors and from two to six essays usually written by others. The first part of the book provides a historical perspective and vantage points from which to view planned change. Change methods range from the least coercive (rational-empirical), through those in the middle ground (normative-reeducative), to the most coercive (power-coercive).

The second part of the BB&C book deals with diagnostic issues. It considers environments of change, the use of knowledge in planned change, and relationships of organizations to their internal and external environments. The third part contains essays on interventions (strategies). Some essays provide theoretical or philosophical viewpoints. Several present methods for comparing interventions or consider other practical aspects of planned change. The last part of the BB&C book concerns values and goals. The inclusion of a long essay on the ethics of social intervention demonstrates the fact that the editors had a lively interest in moral and ethical matters.

Appendix D, section D.2, in this book lists nursing periodical articles that used Bennis, Benne, and Chin literature during an 11-year time period. Appendix D does not provide a chart to show the placement of specific topics in the Bennis, Benne, and Chin literature because readers will find such information in the index of the 1985 edition of the BB&C book.

References

Argyris, C., & Schön, D. A. (1985). Evaluating theories of action. In W. G. Bennis, K. D. Benne, & R. Chin (Eds.), *The planning of change* (4th ed., pp. 108-117). New York: Holt, Rinehart & Winston.

Bakan, D. (1985). The interface between war and the social sciences. In W. G. Bennis, K. D. Benne, & R. Chin (Eds.), *The planning of change* (4th ed., pp. 382-392). New York: Holt, Rinehart & Winston.

Benne, K. D. (1985a). The current state of planned changing in persons, groups, communities, and societies. In W. G. Bennis, K. D. Benne, & R. Chin (Eds.), *The planning of change* (4th ed., pp. 68-82). New York: Holt, Rinehart & Winston.

Benne, K. D. (1985b). Educational field experience as the negotiation of different cognitive worlds. In W. G. Bennis, K. D. Benne, & R. Chin (Eds.), *The planning of change* (4th ed., pp. 118-124). New York: Holt, Rinehart & Winston.

Benne, K. D. (1985c). The processes of re-education: An assessment of Kurt Lewin's views. In W. G. Bennis, K. D. Benne, & R. Chin (Eds.), *The planning of change* (4th ed., pp. 272-283). New York: Holt, Rinehart & Winston.

Benne, K. D. (1985d). Moral dilemmas of managers. In W. G. Bennis, K. D. Benne, & R. Chin (Eds.), *The planning of change* (4th ed., pp. 471-479). New York: Holt, Rinehart & Winston.

Benne, K. D., Bennis, W. G., & Chin, R. (1985). Planned change in America. In W. G. Bennis, K. D. Benne, & R. Chin (Eds.), *The planning of change* (4th ed., pp. 13-21). New York: Holt, Rinehart & Winston.

Bennis, W. G., Benne, K. D., & Chin, R. (1961). *The planning of change.* New York: Holt, Rinehart & Winston.

Bennis, W. G., Benne, K. D., & Chin, R. (1969). *The planning of change* (2nd ed.). New York: Holt, Rinehart & Winston.

Bennis, W. G., Benne, K. D., & Chin, R. (1985). *The planning of change* (4th ed.). New York: Holt, Rinehart & Winston.

Bennis, W. G., Benne, K. D., Chin, R., & Corey, K. E. (1976). *The planning of change* (3rd ed.). New York: Holt, Rinehart & Winston.

Bermant, G., & Warwick, D. P. (1985). The ethics of social intervention: Power, freedom and accountability. In W. G. Bennis, K. D. Benne, & R. Chin (Eds.), *The planning of change* (4th ed., pp. 449-470). New York: Holt, Rinehart & Winston.

Blake, R. R., & Mouton, J. S. (1985). Strategies of consultation. In W. G. Bennis, K. D. Benne, & R. Chin (Eds.), *The planning of change* (4th ed., pp. 48-68). New York: Holt, Rinehart & Winston.

Boulding, E. (1985). Learning to image the future. In W. G. Bennis, K. D. Benne, & R. Chin (Eds.), *The planning of change* (4th ed., pp. 413-425). New York: Holt, Rinehart & Winston.

Brickman, P., Carulli, V., Rabinowitz, J. K., Coates, D., Cohn, E., & Kidder, L. (1985). Models of helping and coping. In W. G. Bennis, K. D. Benne, & R. Chin (Eds.), *The planning of change* (4th ed., pp. 287-311). New York: Holt, Rinehart & Winston.

Chin, R. (1985). The utility of models of the environments of systems for practitioners. In W. G. Bennis, K. D. Benne, & R. Chin (Eds.), *The planning of change* (4th ed., pp. 88-97). New York: Holt, Rinehart & Winston.

Chin, R., & Benne, K. D. (1985). General strategies for effecting changes in human systems. In W. G. Bennis, K. D. Benne, & R. Chin (Eds.), *The planning of change* (4th ed., pp. 22-45). New York: Holt, Rinehart & Winston.

Churchman, C. W. (1985). Perspectives of the systems approach. In W. G. Bennis, K. D. Benne, & R. Chin (Eds.), *The planning of change* (4th ed., pp. 253-259). New York: Holt, Rinehart & Winston.

Cowen, E. L. (1985). Help is where you find it. In W. G. Bennis, K. D. Benne, & R. Chin (Eds.), *The planning of change* (4th ed., pp. 311-324). New York: Holt, Rinehart & Winston.

Dunn, W. N. (1985). Usable knowledge: A metatheory of policy research in the social sciences. In W. G. Bennis, K. D. Benne, & R. Chin (Eds.), *The planning of change* (4th ed., pp. 223-247). New York: Holt, Rinehart & Winston.

Evory, A. (Ed.). (1978). *Contemporary authors* (Vols. 33-36). Detroit, MI: Gale Research Company.

Evory, A., Gareffa, P. M., & Metzger, L. (Eds.). (1982). *Contemporary authors: New revision series* (Vol. 5). Detroit, MI: Gale Research Company.

Fadool, C. R. (Ed.). (1976). *Contemporary authors*. Detroit, MI: Gale Research Company.

Grabow, S., & Heskin, A. (1985). Foundations for a radical concept of planning. In W. G. Bennis, K. D. Benne, & R. Chin (Eds.), *The planning of change* (4th ed., pp. 259-269). New York: Holt, Rinehart & Winston.

Harrison, R. (1985). Strategies for a new age. In W. G. Bennis, K. D. Benne, & R. Chin (Eds.), *The planning of change* (4th ed., pp. 128-149). New York: Holt, Rinehart & Winston.

Katz, R. (1985). Societal codes for responding to dissent. In W. G. Bennis, K. D. Benne, & R. Chin (Eds.), *The planning of change* (4th ed., pp. 354-367). New York: Holt, Rinehart & Winston.

Kennedy, A. A. (1985). Ruminations on change: The incredible value of human beings in getting things done. In W. G. Bennis, K. D. Benne, & R. Chin (Eds.), *The planning of change* (4th ed., pp. 325-335). New York: Holt, Rinehart & Winston.

Klein, D. (1985). Some notes on the dynamics of resistance to change: The defender role. In W. G. Bennis, K. D. Benne, & R. Chin (Eds.), *The planning of change* (4th ed., pp. 98-105). New York: Holt, Rinehart & Winston.

Mason, R. O., & Mitroff, I. I. (1985). A teleological power-oriented theory of strategy. In W. G. Bennis, K. D. Benne, & R. Chin (Eds.), *The planning of change* (4th ed., pp. 215-223). New York: Holt, Rinehart & Winston.

Mead, M. (1985). The future as a basis for establishing a shared culture. In W. G. Bennis, K. D. Benne, & R. Chin (Eds.), *The planning of change* (4th ed., pp. 426-439). New York: Holt, Rinehart & Winston.

Mohrman, A. M., & Lawler, E. E. (1985). The diffusion of QWL as a paradigm shift. In W. G. Bennis, K. D. Benne, & R. Chin (Eds.), *The planning of change* (4th ed., pp. 149-161). New York: Holt, Rinehart & Winston.

Motamedi, K. K. (1985). Adaptability and copability: A study of social systems, their environment, and survival. In W. G. Bennis, K. D. Benne, & R. Chin (Eds.), *The planning of change* (4th ed., pp. 186-194). New York: Holt, Rinehart & Winston.

Nutt, P. C. (1985). A study of planning process. In W. G. Bennis, K. D. Benne, & R. Chin (Eds.), *The planning of change* (4th ed., pp. 198-215). New York: Holt, Rinehart & Winston.

Sarason, S. B. (1985). The nature of problem solving in social action. In W. G. Bennis, K. D. Benne, & R. Chin (Eds.), *The planning of change* (4th ed., pp. 368-382). New York: Holt, Rinehart & Winston.

Schein, E. (1985). Process consultation. In W. G. Bennis, K. D. Benne, & R. Chin (Eds.), *The planning of change* (4th ed., pp. 283-287). New York: Holt, Rinehart & Winston.

Schein, E. H., & Bennis, W. G. (1985). Laboratory education and re-education. In W. G. Bennis, K. D. Benne, & R. Chin (Eds.), *The planning of change* (4th ed., pp. 335-351). New York: Holt, Rinehart & Winston.

Schön, D. A. (1985). Conversational planning. In W. G. Bennis, K. D. Benne, & R. Chin (Eds.), *The planning of change* (4th ed., pp. 247-253). New York: Holt, Rinehart & Winston.

Snyder, R. (1985). To improve innovation, manage corporate culture. In W. G. Bennis, K. D. Benne, & R. Chin (Eds.), *The planning of change* (4th ed., pp. 164-176). New York: Holt, Rinehart & Winston.

Terreberry, S. (1985). The evolution of organizational environments. In W. G. Bennis, K. D. Benne, & R. Chin (Eds.), *The planning of change* (4th ed., pp. 176-186). New York: Holt, Rinehart & Winston.

Tiffany, C. R., Cheatham, A. B., Doornbos, D., Loudermelt, L., & Momadi, G. G. (1994). Planned change theory: Survey of nursing periodical literature. *Nursing Management, 25*(7), 54-59.

Van Gigch, J. P. (1985). Planning for freedom. In W. G. Bennis, K. D. Benne, & R. Chin (Eds.), *The planning of change* (4th ed., pp. 392-405). New York: Holt, Rinehart & Winston.

Zurcher, L. A. (1985). The mutable self: A self-concept for social change. In W. G. Bennis, K. D. Benne, & R. Chin (Eds.), *The planning of change* (4th ed., pp. 439-446). New York: Holt, Rinehart & Winston.

Analysis and Critique of the Planned Change Writings of Bennis, Benne, and Chin

This chapter starts with an analysis of the writings found in the 1985 edition of *The Planning of Change* by Bennis, Benne, and Chin (BB&C). It ends with a critique of the book.

Analysis of the Planned Change Writings of Bennis, Benne, and Chin

After a general description of the writings in the Bennis et al. (1985) volume, this part of the chapter discusses their purpose and breadth. It also analyzes the definitions and illustrations supplied and identifies dominant themes. The section ends with descriptions of movement found within the writings and of the underlying assumptions of the writings.

General Description of the Writings

The *Planning of Change* is an edited book of writings that contains 34 essays; the editors wrote or cowrote eight of these and provided book and chapter introductions. Several of the writings appeared in earlier editions of the book; about one fourth were written in the 1960s, over a third came from the 1970s, and about a third from the 1980s. (The dates of origin of a few of the essays do not appear in the book.) Seven essays came from persons in the discipline of education, 14 from authors in business and management, 11 from those in the social sciences, and 2 from authors who collaborated across disciplinary lines.

Purpose of the Writings

Bennis, Benne, and Chin established definite purposes for their book. First, in light of the inevitability of change, they wanted to provide information about the employment of social science methods in the planning of change. They saw these procedures as the only viable alternatives to the nonintervention and radical-intervention techniques they considered inappropriate. Second, they wanted to give practical "how-to" information to practitioners who already have theoretical knowledge about the planning of change.

Breadth of the Writings

The academic disciplines of the essay authors influenced the breadth of the writings found in the BB&C book. The book includes themes from education, business (mainly management), and the social sciences (psychology, sociology, and anthropology).

Definitions and Illustrations

The BB&C book contains many terms that might be unfamiliar to nurse readers. Essay authors sometimes defined such terms. The editors lifted quite a number of the essays from their original contexts as single book chapters, relatively unchanged.

Essay authors made frequent use of graphic illustrations. Most of the illustrations aid readers in understanding the textual material. Authors frequently used the matrix of discovery described by Moles (1964). (See Chapter 5 in this volume for a description.)

Dominant Themes

Bennis, Benne, and Chin announced two dominant themes for their volume: practical theory and the social dynamics of using knowledge in causing change to occur.

TABLE 14.1 Themes in the Bennis, Benne, and Chin (1985) Book

Theme	Section Number
Practical Theorization	
General perspectives	1.1, 1.2, 2.1, 10.1, 10.2
Evaluation of theories	4.1, 7.1, 7.3
Academic/practical knowledge	4.2
Environments of change	3.1, 3.2, 5.2, 6.1, 6.2
Dynamics of Knowledge Use	
Inadequate worldviews	9.2, 9.3
Knowledge usage in specific interventions	7.2, 7.5, 8.1, 8.3, 8.4, 8.5, 10.3
Group functioning	2.2, 5.1, 6.3, 8.6
Morality, ethics	11.1, 11.2
Worth of human beings	7.4, 7.6, 8.2
Factors that shape models of change	9.1, 9.4

Themes related to practical theorization. One theme in the BB&C book of readings relates to general perspectives regarding the context of planned change theories, models, and concepts in terms of history, placement in society, and the world of thought. Another relates to the ways that practitioners can evaluate planned change theories and planning processes. One essay differentiates between academic and practical knowledge; five provide ways to conceptualize the environments of specific change situations. (See Table 14.1.)

Themes related to the dynamics of knowledge use. Two essays in the BB&C book describe viewpoints (e.g., positivism) that don't "cut the mustard." One theme relates to the dynamics of knowledge use in specific interventions. A subset of this theme concerns the dynamics of groups. Another theme reflects the deep concern that Bennis, Benne, and Chin shared regarding moral and ethical matters. Some essays give practical instruction regarding interventions that ensure attention to the worth of human beings. Two essays discuss factors that shape models of change.

Movement Within the Writings

The BB&C book starts with a description of the placement of planned change in the context of history, society, and thought. Then a section titled "Diagnostics" leads readers into ways of evaluating knowledge use and a subsequent exploration of the kinds of social environments planners might encounter. (Like Lewin, these editors evidently considered diagnostics to be more concerned with readiness for change than with problem setting.) Action comes next, with a section that includes information on problem setting and various methods for problem solving. The last section, which involves morality and ethics, seems disconnected from the conceptualization-to-action motion found in the remainder of the book.

Assumptions in the Writings

Explicit assumptions. The authors of the essays in the BB&C book overtly assume that the use of social science knowledge is good. They also assume that normative-reeducative methods are superior to laissez-faire or coercive methods and that collaboration is superior to both nonintervention and authoritarianism. They also presumed that group participation will increase the chances for success in planned change episodes.

Implicit assumptions. Covertly, the invited authors assumed that planned change is possible, that theory-based interventions will cause change, and that Lewin's theories demonstrate an appropriate direction for action. Essays in this collection imply that humans, as objects of change, have value; that planners should seek opinions of target persons and populations; and that change that takes target persons' opinions into account will produce viable conditions of work and life.

Critique of the Work of
Bennis, Benne, and Chin

The critique section of this chapter starts with a report on the place of the BB&C writings in nursing periodical literature. It continues with affirmations for the four editions of the book edited by Bennis, Benne, and Chin. It continues with a description of some problems in the 1985 edition, an assessment of the writings from a nursing viewpoint, and an evaluation of the usefulness of the book to nurse planners.

The Bennis, Benne, and Chin Writings
in Nursing Periodical Literature

An 11-year survey (1982 through 1992) revealed a total of 155 articles that used 58 planned change theories in English-language nursing periodicals (Tiffany, Cheatham, Doornbos, Loudermelt, & Momadi, 1994). "Theories" included planned change models or formal planned change conceptualizations such as those in the BB&C books of writings. The Bennis, Benne, and Chin books of writings took second place in terms of the number of articles that used a particular theory, with 43 (28%) of the 155 articles using the BB&C writings.

The 155 articles presented 383 citations of sources of 58 theories; the BB&C writings received 56 (15%) of these. Nurse authors named 11 sources for their BB&C citations (they did not name some sources). Of these 11 sources, *The Planning of Change* (1976) received 16 citations; the 1969 edition of the book had 10 citations. The 1985 edition had only 4 citations even though this edition appeared before the midpoint year of the survey.

Affirmation for the Writings

The placement of the BB&C writings as second in popularity among 58 theoretical formulations in a survey that covered an 11-year time span (Tiffany et al., 1994) shows their popularity with nurse authors. Further, in English-language nursing periodicals from countries outside the United States, the Bennis, Benne, and Chin writings received more reference citations than any other planned change theoretical writings. This number of citations demonstrates the confidence that nurse authors abroad have in the work of Bennis, Benne, and Chin.

Problems With the Writings

Events that have occurred since the 1985 edition of the BB&C book show that futuristic prophecies do not always come true. For example, Boulding (1985, 10.1) wished that learning based in love would develop a population with a capacity for otherness. Instead, violence wracks schools, and schools still act as servants of society rather than as shapers of society. Mead (1985, 10.2) wrote about the global connectedness of people. Communication connectedness indeed has developed, but the expense and expertise requirements of the electronic devices making the connections threaten to polarize societies and separate the rich and advantaged from the poor and disadvantaged. Grabow and Heskin (1985, 7.6) lauded communism as the great equalizer; communism ended up turning out a cadre of well-appointed despots more bent on "living high" than on "living equal." Mohrman and Lawler (1985, 5.2) felt that a shift toward a new paradigm, such as the Quality of Work Life (QWL) paradigm they described, would replace inefficient management practices with those better calculated to solve organizational effectiveness problems. Such a shift has occurred in some industries and organizations, but a shift to QWL conditions remains far from universal.

The BB&C writings come from many different authors and remain too scattered in both subject matter and levels of generality to warrant use as a theory or model. Omissions include inattention to concepts of power, to international concerns, to diagnostic processes intended to detect social problems, and to characteristics of innovations. Nevertheless, every nurse planner needs some of the information found in the Bennis, Benne, and Chin volumes.

Nurse authors should beware of attributing everything in the BB&C volumes directly to Bennis, Benne, and Chin when, in fact, multiple authors, over a 20-plus-year time span and from three different disciplinary perspectives, produced the book.

The Writings From a Nursing Viewpoint

In the preface for each book, Bennis, Benne, and Chin named nurses as one of the groups in their target audience. This relates to the fact that many of the BB&C writings demonstrate values that cohere with nursing values. No doubt, this synchrony accounts for some of the books' popularity with nurses. For example, the BB&C writings value the mutuality that nurses prize. BB&C stress the notion that dialogic action should consist of more than mere conversation; they include target populations in the development of plans, and, more than most other change authors, they attend to ethical and moral matters.

Usefulness of the Writings

The BB&C writings make a contribution by affirming Lewin's work. Not only did the editors pay tribute to Lewin's genius, they employed the tenor of his thinking in the deliberations through which they chose writings. Further, their 1961 edition filled a literature void by including the then-new topic of group dynamics, thus extending a Lewin tradition that began about 15 years earlier.

More than 10 years after its publication date, the 1985 edition of *The Planning of Change* makes a current contribution to change literature by pointing conceptually to Bhola's Configurations CLER Model. Repeatedly, the BB&C writings call attention to the dialogic action, systems thinking, and constructivist concepts that serve as CLER model foundations. The Bennis, Benne, and Chin admonitions regarding collaboration sound very much like the working of Bhola's (1994) $\{P\} \times \{O\} \times \{A\}$ ensemble. (See Chapters 6, 8, and 19 in this volume.)

Nurses, who so often must think in practical ways about pharmacology, microbiology, and anatomy, will find that BB&C concepts that depict organizations and organizational characteristics will prove valuable as they plan change. No naive reader could avoid learning to conceptualize social organizations while reading the BB&C books.

Summary

From a nursing viewpoint, this chapter analyzed and critiqued planned change writings collected from authors in three academic disciplines (education, business, behavioral science) by Bennis, Benne, and Chin. The first purpose of the BB&C writings was to provide planners with information about the use of social science methods in the planning of change. Fulfillment of the second purpose gives "how-to" information about the application of theoretical knowledge.

Some essays in the 1985 edition of the BB&C book *The Planning of Change* contain a fairly high number of obscure words. The many illustrations included in the book often illuminate the text through the use of matrices of discovery or other means.

Bennis, Benne, and Chin announced two dominant themes for their book: practical theory and the social dynamics of knowledge use. Under the first theme, they included essays about the context and evaluation of planned change theories, models, and conceptualizations. They differentiated between academic and practical knowledge and provided ways to view the environments of change situations.

In the BB&C writings, normative-reeducative strategies outweigh laissez-faire and coercive methods for producing social change. BB&C rejected positivism as inappropriate and inefficient. They wrote about the dynamics of knowledge use in practical situations and gave special attention to group dynamics. They linked collaboration to moral and ethical principles.

The writings included in the BB&C book move from conceptualization to action. Although the writings overtly assume the goodness of social science knowledge use, some authors openly expressed concern regarding the possibility of victimization and destabilization through the misuse of power in social change situations. Covertly, the editors assumed the goodness of planned change theory, the value of human beings, and the worth of ideas held by target populations.

Events since the publication of the latest (1985) BB&C book demonstrate the fallibility of futurism: The love envisioned for the educational system by Boulding did not materialize as she hoped. Mead dreamed that global communication would be an aid to social connectedness but it threatens to divide rather than connect humans. The social equalization that Grabow and Heskin envisioned for communism did not transpire.

The diverse writings included in the BB&C book do not have enough cohesion to form a theory. Nevertheless, they provide a great many conceptualizations useful to nurse planners. Many of the values these editors espoused are synchronized with nursing values for mutuality and collaboration. The writings affirm Lewin's work and point to the usefulness of Bhola's CLER model. In an 11-year time period, authors of English-language nursing periodical literature valued the BB&C writings and used them with a frequency second only to that accorded Lewin's microtheories. Nurses, who so often must think in concrete terms, will find the BB&C writings useful as they attempt to grapple with social problems that require them to act as the planners of change.

References

Bennis, W. G., Benne, K. D., & Chin, R. (Eds.). (1985). *The planning of change* (4th ed.). New York: Holt, Rinehart & Winston.

Bhola, H. S. (1994). The CLER model: Thinking through change. *Nursing Management, 25*(5), 59-63.

Boulding, E. (1985). Learning to image the future. In W. G. Bennis, K. D. Benne, & R. Chin (Eds.), *The planning of change* (4th ed., pp. 413-425). New York: Holt, Rinehart & Winston.

Grabow, S., & Heskin, A. (1985). Foundations for a radical concept of planning. In W. G. Bennis, K. D. Benne, & R. Chin (Eds.), *The planning of change* (4th ed., pp. 259-269). New York: Holt, Rinehart & Winston.

Mead, M. (1985). The future as a basis for establishing a shared culture. In W. G. Bennis, K. D. Benne, & R. Chin (Eds.), *The planning of change* (4th ed., pp. 426-439). New York: Holt, Rinehart & Winston.

Mohrman, A. M., & Lawler, E. E. (1985). The diffusion of QWL as a paradigm shift. In W. G. Bennis, K. D. Benne, & R. Chin (Eds.), *The planning of change* (4th ed., pp. 149-161). New York: Holt, Rinehart & Winston.

Moles, A. (1964). Le contenu d'une méthodologie appliquée: Un essai de recensement des méthodes [The content of an applied methodology: An attempt at reviewing methods]. In R. Caude & A. Moles, *Methodology: Toward a science of action* (pp. 45-82). Paris: Gauthier-Villars. (Selected portions of the text translated by F. Augsberger, 1976, for Tiffany)

Tiffany, C. R., Cheatham, A. B., Doornbos, D., Loudermelt, L., & Momadi, G. G. (1994). Planned change theory: Survey of nursing periodical literature. *Nursing Management, 25*(7), 54-59.

Altering the Bennis, Benne, and Chin Square Peg

BOX 16.12: LOOKING AHEAD

Chapter 15: Altering the Bennis, Benne, and Chin Square Peg

Congruence of the Bennis, Benne, and Chin Writings With Key Concepts in the Roy Adaptation Model (RAM)

A RAM-BB&C Change Process

Application of the RAM-BB&C Change Process to a Nursing Situation: An Example

This chapter consists of three parts: a discussion of how the Bennis, Benne, and Chin (BB&C) writings fit with the Roy Adaptation Model (RAM), a translation of concepts in the BB&C writings from a RAM perspective, and an application of the translated (combined) change process to a nursing situation.

Congruence of the Bennis, Benne, and Chin Writings With Key Concepts in the Roy Adaptation Model (RAM)

Of the 34 essays contained in the book *The Planning of Change* (1985) edited by BB&C, 7 come from the discipline of education and 11 come from social science. The disciplinary background of the authors of these essays parallels that of Roy, a nurse educator with a doctorate in sociology who used her knowledge to develop the RAM. Bennis, Benne, and Chin wanted to provide information about the use of social science methods in planning change. They also proposed to give useful information to practitioners of change. This second purpose finds favor with practitioners of nursing.

Both the writings of BB&C and the RAM espouse reciprocal interaction worldviews; both use a systems approach as a foundation; both have interactionist levels of analysis. Benne (1985) criticized schools that focus solely on cognitive development. Likewise, the nurse-client interaction process encourages the health-related growth of clients and the experiential growth of nurse caregivers. Thus both the BB&C and the RAM viewpoints see individuals from a holistic perspective. Nevertheless, differences exist. The BB&C writings deal specifically with planned change and give detailed information on the processes of planned change. The RAM makes no claim to deal with planned change. Further, the BB&C writings address many topics; the RAM/RAMA formulations present concise and unified models.

Adaptation, a foundational concept of the RAM, infers "that the human system has the capacity to adjust effectively to changes in the environment and, in turn, affects the environment" (Andrews & Roy, 1991a, p. 7). Just as the behavior of human systems signals the quality of a person's adaptation to his or her environment, so the behavior of social systems indicates the extent and quality of organizational adaptation to change. In fact, Motamedi (one of the BB&C [1985] invited authors) stated that adaptation concerns the match between a social system and its external environment. Thus both the RAM and the BB&C writings view systems as capable of adapting to and affecting the environment. The key concepts of person, environment, health, and nursing organize the following discussions of congruence between the RAM and the writings of BB&C and their invited authors.

Person

The RAM defines the recipients of nursing care as adaptive systems. Roy has long identified these recipients as families, other groups, organizations, communities, or other social systems (see Chapter 9). The BB&C writings see the person as the recipient of (decision maker in) the change process; the person chooses to adopt or reject the proposed change. This view assumes that if recipients so choose, they can adapt. As Roy did, Bennis, Benne, and Chin and their invited authors also emphasized groups, social systems, and cultures. The 1961 edition of *The Planning of Change* (1961) had a particularly strong emphasis on groups, an approach in keeping with the historical background of the book. The editors acknowledged Lewinian theories, which find their basis in the interplay of social forces associated with group and individual interactions, as providing the foundation for their work.

Although Lewin believed that group standards, norms, and values exert powerful environmental influences on individual decision makers, he did not concern himself with the influence of the individual on the environment (De Rivera, 1976). Nevertheless, the BB&C writings, which build upon Lewin's work (see Chapter 13), give as much evidence of the reciprocal interaction worldview as does the RAM. The group-dynamics approach used by Lewin at the National Training Laboratories (NTL) strongly influenced BB&C. In their edited books, BB&C further expanded the reciprocal-interaction view through writing and choosing essays that discuss and refine the role of values in the change process.

Environment

The RAM defines the environment in broad terms but specifies that it consists of external and internal environmental stimuli that influence individuals. Similarly, Chin (1985) discussed external and internal environments of organizations as causal forces. The 1985 BB&C book offered four essays that provide ways to conceptualize environments. These essays focus on groups and social systems composed of individuals. One author (Terreberry, 1985) provided a model that emphasizes the relationship between formal organizations and their environments. Although the RAM and the BB&C views both consider external and internal environments, their focus differs. Their diverse approaches seem appropriate given the disciplinary background of Roy (nursing), which focuses on the nurse-client relationship, and the disciplinary backgrounds of BB&C, which focus on relationships among individuals in a group.

The RAM provides detailed discussions of specific stimuli found in external and internal environments. The focal stimulus is that which provokes a response. From a BB&C view, an event or situation makes the need for change evident to planners. According to the RAM, contextual and residual environmental stimuli influence the effect of the focal stimulus. The BB&C writings hold that group standards, norms, and values influence decision makers. Snyder (1985), for example, defined *corporate culture* as a "system of norms, beliefs and assumptions, and values that determine how people in the organization act" (p. 164). The specific influences of individuals and organizations appear as contextual stimuli.

Roy's model provides for the identification, verification, and measurement of contextual stimuli. Residual stimuli consist of hunches, uncertainties, or unknowns. Residual stimuli verified during the change process become contextual stimuli. Information regarding any residual stimuli that remain unknown and/or unmeasurable throughout the change process may prove useful during the evaluation of the process itself. Model users can view group standards, norms, values, morals, and ethics as contextual or residual stimuli, depending on whether the stimuli yield to articulation and measurement. The adaptation level, a changeable point determined by the pooled effect of focal, contextual, and residual stimuli, represents an individual or group's ability to respond.

Health

A question arises concerning the compatibility of broad conceptualizations of health with planned change theories. The BB&C writings do not specifically address health. In the RAM, health is the process of moving toward integration and wholeness as clients proceed through the adaptation process. Similarly, the BB&C perspective sees health as movement toward the personal growth of system members as planners and adopters proceed through the change process.

Nursing

Bennis, Benne, and Chin's four volumes on the planning of change build on Lewin's work. Lewin's examples (with the exception of his posthumous action research) discussed change in the context of a predetermined innovation. In expanding Lewin's work, Bennis, Benne, and Chin (1985) did not revise or elaborate Lewin's views on the choice of an innovation. Likewise, the example in this chapter addresses the change process from the perspective of planning the strategies and tactics necessary to implement a predetermined innovation. BB&C chose writings that addressed many diverse, yet related, viewpoints concerned with restricted aspects of planning processes; some deal with less central (but important) issues, such as ethics. This dispersion of topics necessitated choosing one viewpoint for use in this chapter.

A BB&C-invited author, Nutt (1985), studied 50 different planning processes as he developed a morphology for the analysis of planning processes. (Readers can think of Nutt's morphology as a template or grid, a list of stages and steps, against which they can compare various planning processes—for example, the Program Planning Method or the systems approach.) Nutt's morphology furnishes a practical, concrete, and fairly complete picture of change planning processes. His essay highlights normative change processes congruent with the normative-reeducative viewpoint espoused by BB&C. Furthermore, Nutt's morphology accommodates either planner-driven or sponsor-driven planning. It allows for truncated (shortened by omission of an expected element) planning processes similar to the one seen in the example in this chapter. Such shortening (truncation) accommodates the high degree of regulation in a health care industry in which innovations often come from a higher authority (e.g., a government) and planners must develop strategies and tactics that increase the likelihood of acceptance of an innovation mandated from above. Thus the Nutt (1985) essay from the BB&C book of writings can fulfill needs for a discrete statement of a planning process in a mandated situation.

Nutt's (1985) planning morphology contains five stages (formulation, conceptualization, detailing, evaluation, implementation). Each stage contains three steps (search, synthesis, analysis). The formulation stage provides for clarification of the problem stipulation furnished by the sponsor in terms of a performance gap. The concept stage encourages reduction of the problem into components and subsequent development of a model that captures the planning problem. The detailing stage covers the invention or choice of potentially viable solutions. The evaluation stage fosters the informed selection of a solution from among alternatives. The implementation stage covers the planning of strategies designed to increase the likelihood of acceptance of the solution.

Nutt (1985) used his morphology as a template (pattern, guide) in the analysis of planning processes with a wide variety of forms and structures. One planning process, the Program Planning Method (PPM), applies the Nominal Group Technique (NGT) in groups that include users or clients, content experts, and administrators who control resources. This method skips some steps designated by the morphology and takes the morphology's stages out of sequence. With emphasis on acceptance (adoption), an innovation moves into full use only after approval by administrators who control resources.

By contrast, a systems planning process has 10 steps that unfold in an orderly way. The systems process skips some *steps* in the later stages but includes all *stages*. It employs the sequence stipulated by the morphology. The systems process emphasizes solution quality rather than its acceptance. Likewise, other planning processes that Nutt analyzed skip steps or stages, or take stages out of order. Nutt did not favor one planning process above others but he did point out some of the dangers inherent in various processes. For example, he wrote that some planners skip planning stages for useful reasons while others abandon orderliness to the detriment of a change project.

Nutt's (1985) five-stage planning morphology compares roughly with the six steps of the nursing process as described by Roy (1991b) (assess behavior, assess stimuli, make nursing diagnosis, set goals, intervene, and evaluate). Formulation, the first stage of Nutt's morphology of planning processes, provides for verification of the existence and nature of a problem; the purpose of this stage approximates the purposes of the two assessment steps of the nursing process according to Roy. The concept stage describes the problem. This stage fits well with the nursing diagnosis step of the RAM. In the RAM, goals provide guidelines for action and indicators of effective behaviors that later will supply evidence of adaptation. Nutt's (1985) morphology offers no goal-setting stage; in Nutt's process, acceptance of the solution preferred by the sponsor presumably indicates goal achievement. Implementation (RAM's "interventions") in Nutt's morphology involves plans for strategies designed to gain acceptance from the target population for the preferred solution. This stage of Nutt's process still involves planning, whereas in the RAM, implementation gives more emphasis to action.

Although Nutt's morphology provides no separate stage for an overall evaluation as the RAM does, each of the five stages includes evaluative steps.

Additionally, Nutt's analysis of both planner-driven and sponsor-driven processes shows cyclical planning processes that include recognition of problem realities in the field. This implies evaluation similar to that in the nursing process.

Each of Nutt's (1985) five stages has three steps (search, synthesis, and analysis). These steps resemble the cyclical nature of the nursing process: Search gathers information (much like assessment), synthesis puts ideas together (as in nursing diagnosis), and analysis studies the results. At all steps of the nursing process, nurse caregivers gather information and put ideas together. They study results during the intervention and evaluation steps. The RAM discusses both planning and action under the intervention step. Thus both Nutt's morphology and the nursing process have cyclical characteristics. The stages, and steps within stages, in the Nutt morphology can occur simultaneously just as nurse caregivers simultaneously can assess, intervene, and evaluate the client situation during the same nursing activity.

In summary, Bennis, Benne, and Chin based their work on Lewin's theories. They further developed the normative-reeducative family of strategies (interventions) initiated by Lewin at the National Training Laboratories. These strategies emphasize problem solving and personal growth among system members. The NTL staff studied interpersonal and group behavior throughout the development of a social structure and normative culture in a laboratory setting. The strong focus on face-to-face interaction, collaboration, and mutuality throughout the process of reeducation reflects approaches valued in a nurse-client relationship. Nurse-client interactions commonly propose to teach clients how to handle threats to health and well-being. Thus client education often revolves around change, such as teaching clients how to deal with the effects of chronic illness or how to live a healthier lifestyle. The BB&C writings express concern for moral and ethical behavior among people involved in the change process and for ensuring attention to the worth of human beings. Normative-reeducative strategies seek to promote the personal growth of system members and adaptation to change. The RAM aims "to enhance positive life processes and to promote adaptation" (Andrews & Roy, 1991b, p. 37). Clearly, the normative-reeducative approach resonates with the nursing strategies and values found in the RAM; the two systems obviously have similar goals.

A RAM-BB&C Change Process

The Roy Adaptation Model provides a suitable perspective for viewing change in nursing situations. Nurses can extend the RAM by incorporating ideas from the BB&C writings. This section presents a translation that facilitates the combining of the RAM and BB&C ideas. The RAM-BB&C change process incorporates BB&C (Nutt) change concepts into a RAM view of the nursing process. Nursing process steps, as seen in the RAM, organize the following discussion of the combined RAM-BB&C change process.

Assess Behavior

The combined RAM-BB&C perspective asks nurse planners to conduct an initial search for behaviors related to the social problem. Depending on the level of the problem, the search may include behaviors exhibited by individuals in the organization (social system) or behaviors of the organization. Nurse planners categorize (synthesize) information gathered during the search process into the four adaptive system modes (physical, interpersonal, role, interdependence) identified in the Roy Adaptation Model Applied to Administration (RAMA). The behavioral assessment proposes to verify the existence and nature of the social problem (Nutt's formulation). After the initial assessment, the nurse planner examines the behaviors in a search for patterns and uses descriptions of adaptive responses to identify ineffective responses. The descriptors may be industry standards or norms developed from organizational values. Ineffective responses in organizations beget performance gaps between organization and (industry) standards/norms. For example, dollars spent on particular laboratory tests might be higher in one hospital than in others in the region. Planners analyze the information and make an initial determination of the extent of the performance gap. If the sponsor (e.g., employing hospital) or the nurse planner needs assistance with changing behavior to more closely approximate standards/norms (i.e., close the performance gap), then the planner proceeds with second-level assessment.

Assess Stimuli

In second-level assessment, also covered by Nutt's formulation stage, the nurse planner collects data and information about environmental stimuli that may influence the behavior. All data and/or information gleaned from the search will need examination to determine the influence of stimuli, if any, on behavior. The focal stimulus is that which demands attention. It may, for example, come in the form of a diagnosis-related group (DRG) on which the hospital is losing money. Contextual stimuli that contribute to the effect of the focal stimulus might include a lack of educational opportunities for health care providers, an aging medical staff, lack of modern laboratory equipment and/or facilities, or a high incidence of a specific disease (DRG) in the hospital's service area. Residual stimuli (unknown and/or unmeasurable factors contributing to the effect of the focal stimulus) could include uncertainty among health care providers, fear of lawsuits, or fear of criticism from colleagues or clients. The pooled effect of the three types of environmental stimuli determines the position of the adaptation level. The level represents the group's or organization's ability to respond positively and effectively in a situation. A thorough assessment of the behaviors and stimuli influencing the behavior includes search, synthesis, and analysis activities by the planner to clearly formulate the performance gap (social problem).

Diagnose

An accurate description of the social problem (the RAM's diagnosis step, Nutt's concept stage) follows a quality assessment. The problem generally shows a deviation from an accepted standard or norm (a performance gap). Diagnosis, as a cyclical process, involves search, synthesis, and analysis activities. Searching, at this stage, involves the gathering of information that may offer competing explanations for the apparent problem. Synthesis involves comparing behaviors with standards to assemble ideas about performance. The final diagnosis involves analysis, a study of results at this stage.

Set Goals

Goal setting for behavioral change occurs best through face-to-face interaction. Bennis, Benne, and Chin's (1985) strong focus on face-to-face interaction, collaboration, and mutuality when using normative-reeducative methods demonstrates the value they placed on interpersonal processes. Planners and adopters (decision makers) must collaboratively develop and mutually establish change goals whenever possible. They must gather and synthesize information to clarify goals. They analyze potential goals to determine priority, attainability, and congruence with organizational mission, priorities, and values. They aim to achieve, or at least approximate, a match between the organization and its environment. According to the RAM, goal setting focuses on behavior. Goals aim to close the performance gap. The Nutt morphology has no goal-setting stage. At this point in the sequence, it has two stages that deal with the innovation. This chapter does not include these two Nutt stages because the innovation, as in the accompanying example, often is chosen and mandated by a higher authority. The RAM does not deal with the choice of an innovation in the same manner as do planned change theories. Instead (as seen below), it moves on to the selection of interventions, which encompasses strategies to promote patients' acceptance of solutions (innovations) specific to them and their problems.

Intervene

Regardless of the attractiveness of the solution to planners, decision makers must accept it before any solid movement toward change occurs. The information gathered and ideas assembled during the setting of goals enables planners to facilitate the implementation of strategies and tactics directed toward the preferred solution.

The RAM advocates the judgment method presented by McDonald and Harms (cited in Andrews & Roy, 1991b, p. 45) to select among possible approaches to manage environmental stimuli. In this judgment method, planners gather information about the consequences of changing each stimulus, identified in second-level assessment, that affects the specific behavior. Planners combine this information with the probability (high, moderate, low) of occurrence of the consequences. Then planners, together with decision makers whenever possible and appropriate, judge the value of each consequence as desirable or undesirable. The judgment method helps planners select strategies and tactics that have the highest probability of contributing to goal attainment (behavioral change). This method fits with both the fifth stage (implementation) of Nutt's (1985) morphology and the intervention step of the RAM.

Whenever possible, planners direct the strategy and tactics toward the focal stimulus. When they cannot eliminate or alter the focal stimulus, they should direct the strategy and tactics toward contextual stimuli in an effort to broaden the adaptation level. For example, planners in individual hospitals cannot eliminate a focal stimulus such as the diagnosis-related group (DRG) payment system any more than they can eliminate certain genetic diseases. In such situations, planners direct their efforts toward helping organizations or clients to decrease their risk and/or "live with the situation" (i.e., to adapt).

Normative-reeducative strategies. The philosophies of the normative-reeducative family of strategies developed by Lewin and advocated by BB&C coincide with principles underlying the RAM. This makes an examination of them at this point appropriate and timely.

The most prominent foundational idea in normative-reeducative strategies assumes that education will prompt decision makers to accept change. Through reeducation in a group setting, members align themselves with the group standards and norms that lead to acceptance of the preferred solution. Normative-reeducational strategies also aim to encourage the personal growth of group members.

Normative-reeducative strategies emphasize 10 Lewinian principles (Benne, 1985) that describe change in terms of complex interrelationships between persons' cognitive-perceptual orientations and their value orientations. The 10 principles have their foundations in Lewin's ideas about the impact of society and culture on individuals and organizations.

Education in a group setting commonly occurs as an intervention for either clients or nurses in health care organizations. The efficiency of the group setting makes it more fiscally responsible than individual instruction. Client education in groups includes interventions such as preoperative classes in hospitals, Lamaze classes, and parenting classes. Nurse education in groups occurs in the form of continuing education programs where nurses learn about new procedures or equipment.

Benne (1985) cautioned that the presentation of "mere facts" does not produce permanent change. Only a deep involvement in the educational experience brings about a true and lasting change in values and related actions. This caveat creates difficulties in today's hurried health care organization. Decision makers in diverse geographic or organizational locations (clinical units, affiliated offices or agencies, on varying shifts, and in positions where they commute between or among areas within a multilevel health care organization) find themselves in complex situations where they have little time for "extras." Planners find it difficult to provide the stable group relationships that Lewin (Benne, 1985) credited with fostering the acceptance of change. Often, nurse planners must employ normative-reeducative strategies in short sessions held at intervals over a long period of time. The hectic internal health care environment lies embedded in a turbulent external environment where the maintenance of a stable group presents a challenge to nurse planners.

The impact of worldwide events such as economic woes, politically oriented strife, and the prevalence of HIV/AIDS has produced tremendous life changes for myriad people. The massive reeducation efforts mounted in response have met with varying success. One reason may concern organizational culture.

Often, organizational culture finds expression in phrases such as "the way we do it around here," "we don't do it like that," or "this is the way it's done here." Culture includes employee perception. Many hospitals would like to change the piece of their cultures that fosters the perception that employees are entitled to lifelong employment.

With respect to implementing normative-reeducational strategies and tactics, BB&C advocated respect for resistance. They cautioned planners to develop tactics to help resisters recognize that their own ambivalence (Benne, 1985; Klein, 1985) may stem from the discomfort that accompanies a tension between the psychological comfort of familiarity and the psychological perception (or reality) of getting "left behind." "In tune with the times" and "poised for the next millennium" express current cultural values in the United States. Attending to, rather than disregarding, the rhetoric of resistance helps nurse planners construct effective educational strategies and tactics to increase acceptance of change.

Evaluate

In the RAM-BB&C change process, nurse planners compare poststrategy behaviors with ideal behaviors identified in goals. Such a comparison measures progress toward goals and permits modifications of both goals as well as strategies and tactics used to achieve goals. In the best evaluations, planners and adopters together examine adopters' behavior to determine progress toward closing the gap between actual behavior and desired behavior.

Nurse planners do not wait until the end of an entire change sequence, any more than nurse caregivers wait until discharge, to evaluate and modify goals, strategies, and tactics. Formative evaluation occurs throughout the deployment of strategies and tactics. Goal-setting, intervention, and evaluation steps cycle throughout the change process. These steps include comparison with objective or industry standards and norms so that planners can judge whether the actions taken have been effective in the achievement of goals. In the RAM-BB&C change process, as in the other combined change processes, evaluation constitutes an ongoing activity as well as a summative (terminal) step.

In summary, the RAM-BB&C change process views individuals and organizations as systems capable of adapting to change. The external environment exerts a critical influence on individual as well as organizational behavior. As evidenced by widespread changes in the health care industry since 1983, society imposes certain changes whether providers like them or not. Participation in change at the local level offers individuals control over the methods and details of implementing imposed changes. The RAM-BB&C change process offers nurse planners a familiar perspective and a method to attain a degree of control over how change is effected at a local level. The family of normative-reeducative strategies offers a sense of the familiar for nurse planners because its foundation coincides with their own emphasis on the worth of human beings and their values of face-to-face interaction, collaboration, and mutuality. Also, the moral and ethical stance of normative-reeducative strategies in change situations resonates with the education and professional socialization of nurses. Such familiar ground may account in part for the popularity of the BB&C writings with nurses.

Application of the RAM-BB&C
Change Process to a Nursing Situation:
An Example

After a description of the change situation, the organization of this section follows the steps of the nursing process.

The Change Situation

Multidisciplinary teams in hospitals often develop critical paths to direct the hospital stay of clients in specific diagnostic-related groups (DRGs). These paths usually designate the DRG-specific length-of-stay (LOS), that is, the number of hospital days for which the Health Care Financing Administration (HCFA) will prospectively pay the hospital for a particular DRG. The DRG-specific LOS constitutes an industry standard. Paths also denote critical client outcomes (e.g., ambulation) or client-related events (e.g., certain values on laboratory tests) that should occur on a specific day within the client's expected LOS. Caregivers usually must note variances from the planned path and a rationale for the variance. Many hospitals prefer the critical path method of guiding care over more traditional methods of managing care.

Nurse caregivers, among others, need education regarding the importance of the critical path—the predetermined, mandated, and thus preferred solution in this example. Paths constitute a way of thinking about patient care that differs greatly from the former or usual methods of managing and organizing care. Nurse caregivers must shift their thinking from an individualized plan to a critical path that, although allowing for individualization, finds its basis in "averages." (Caregivers accustomed to "standard" care plans will find the shift to critical paths less dramatic than will those accustomed to a completely individualized plan for each client.)

Often, a nurse designated for the path planning role in a hospital has considerable input into the creation of critical paths. Moreover, it is not uncommon today to find nurses as managers of critical path systems. The LOS constitutes the primary determinant of hospital costs. Therefore, the average LOS for a specific DRG constitutes the most critical determinant for selection of paths chosen for development. The DRGs that exceed the specified LOS, and those that lose money for the hospital in other ways, get prompt attention. A large urban hospital furnishes the setting for this example.

Assess Behavior

In a planned change situation, the gathering of LOS and other cost-related data on DRGs (search step of the formulation stage) assesses organizational behavior. Information gathered falls in the physical adaptive system mode. The data identify ineffective DRGs, that is, those that deviate from the industry standard set by HCFA (synthesis step of the formulation stage).

Assess Stimuli

The loss of dollars by the specific DRGs constitutes the focal stimulus. Contextual stimuli include the current high average LOS and the current high cost of caring for clients with the DRGs.

Diagnose

Diagnosis (Nutt's concept stage) identifies the specific DRGs that deviate from the industry standard set by HCFA. The diagnosis highlights a performance gap: The hospital could do a better job of caring for clients in the deviant DRGs.

Set Goals

The goal-setting step of the RAM-BB&C process focuses on behaviors intended to close the performance gap. This means that planners will seek to alter care providers' behaviors so that LOS statistics fall in line with industry standards.

Intervene

The planners develop interventions (Nutt's implementation stage) that foster acceptance of the solution (research-based critical paths) by decision makers. Specifically, decision makers need to accept the DRG-specific LOS mandated by the path(s) as a goal. In this example, nurse planners keep in mind their task of getting care providers to accept the solution preferred by the hospital (the use of research-based critical paths) to decrease costs of care for the targeted DRGs. They discuss and evaluate facilitative strategies such as hiring a consultant to develop critical paths, buying critical paths commercially, designing critical paths themselves, choosing multidisciplinary task forces to devise critical paths, or establishing a case management team for these particular DRGs.

As planners evaluate each more or less viable strategy, they keep the many ramifications of each in mind. They dismiss hiring a consultant because of cost and concern that care providers might not take ownership of paths developed by an "outsider." The same concerns surface with the idea of buying paths. Planners decide that the best idea would encompass multidisciplinary collaboration and getting care providers involved in the process. They choose the formation of multidisciplinary task forces composed of care providers most appropriate to the specific DRG. They recommend to administration that one person be responsible for managing the critical path system. Planners select a "problem DRG" that lends itself to formation of a multidisciplinary task force that could develop the critical path successfully. After initial task force members agree to accept the challenge, planners begin the necessary educational process.

In a RAM-BB&C change process, planners could choose from among several possible educational tactics (activities) under any one of a number of normative-reeducative strategies (interventions). The judgment method presented by McDonald and Harms (cited in Andrews & Roy, 1991b, p. 45) could help them choose educational strategies and tactics that have the highest probability of achieving acceptance of critical paths by care providers.

A normative-reeducative strategy, related to Nutt's implementation stage, could help to change care providers' attitudes and ways of directing client care. Such a strategy requires attention both to information (facts) and to attitudes (the values that undergird norms). With respect to facts, nurse planners educate care providers about changes in reimbursement to hospitals, the problems that DRGs present to hospitals, the causes of the immediate problem (LOSs that exceed, on average, the industry standard), the financial impact of the problem on the hospital, the preferred solution, and its rationale. Planners place emphasis on the concern of the public about the cost of health care and the ethical responsibility of care providers to deliver care in an efficient and financially responsible manner.

An affectively oriented intervention also relates to Nutt's implementation stage. Although necessary, the facts and figures of the rational approach constitute only the cognitive part of a normative-reeducative strategy. The normative portion assumes an importance equal to that of the rational, cognitive portion. Therefore, the nurse planner brings care providers together in a group setting where champions for the innovation surface early to set the tone for following research-based critical paths as part of the normative procedure for the hospital. In many real-life situations, planners need to "set up" champions for the preferred solution because operating on the mere hope that such champions will emerge carries too much risk. Planners and educators hear the views of resisters in a positive and respectful manner. Adroit nurse planners persuade resistant group members to accept research-based critical paths as a reasonable and prudent way to direct client care at the hospital without compromising quality. They attend to pervasive values, such as quality, in nurse and physician providers. They anticipate sources and forms of resistance. Tactics to deal with resisters, as well as the argument for paths in general, require forethought and careful planning by nurse planners before the implementation of the normative portion of the strategy.

After education, the multidisciplinary group members collaboratively (i.e., with equal power distribution) develop a research-based critical path for a problem DRG. The climate encourages group members to respect each other's views. Ideally, the group members who developed the critical path champion their project. Nurse members take the path to their unit meetings and physician members take it to their section meetings. Allied health care personnel who participate in the group effort share the path with their discipline(s). A start date set by the group for implementing the path allows sufficient time for obtaining institutional approval and communication to appropriate disciplines, staff, and departments. Ideally, the personal and professional growth of group members occurs through the collaborative multidisciplinary effort. Respect for each discipline's contribution to the health care team provides a positive outcome for group members.

Evaluate

The nurse planner or a designee conducts an evaluation of the effect of implementation of the path and then, in a "final" tactic, communicates results first to group members and later to the hospital at large, as appropriate. Organizational organs herald the achievement of industry standard LOSs and the concomitant decrease in hospital costs for the problem DRG. These adaptive responses signal a victory for the use of research-based critical paths and a significant contribution to the health of the hospital. The good news facilitates acceptance of other critical paths by other groups in the hospital. Success breeds success.

Summary

This chapter contains discussions on the congruence of concepts in the Bennis, Benne, and Chin (BB&C) writings with key concepts in the Roy Adaptation Model (RAM), presents a translated change process (RAM-BB&C), and provides an application of a translated normative-reeducative change strategy to a nursing situation.

Both the BB&C writings and the RAM hold reciprocal interaction worldviews. Both have foundations in a systems approach that exemplifies interactionist levels of analysis. Adaptation, from their viewpoints, concerns a correspondence between an individual or a social system and its environment. They conceptualize the key concept of person as a holistic adaptive system that acts as a recipient of or a participant in the change process. External and internal environments of the system act as forces prompting a need to change. Health for the system means the process of moving toward the personal growth of system members as planners and adopters move through the change process. The problem-solving process in the BB&C writings, especially emphasized in normative-reeducative strategies, resembles the clinical problem solving that defines the nursing process; both envision the growth of system members and appropriate adaptation to environments.

The translated BB&C change process presented in this chapter uses an adaptation of the planning morphology devised by Nutt (1985), a BB&C invited author to represent the BB&C collection of writings. The combined change process asks nurse planners to assess behaviors related to a problem and exhibited by members of an organization (social system) or by an organization itself. The identification of behaviors as adaptive or ineffective depends upon the degree of their correspondence with professional/industry standards and values. Planners identify and categorize, according to their effect on behaviors, the external and internal stimuli relevant to ineffective behaviors. Assessment of behaviors and of environmental stimuli together constitute Nutt's formulation stage.

After thorough assessment, planners make a diagnosis that accurately and succinctly summarizes a deviation from a standard. Diagnosis constitutes Nutt's conceptualization stage. Nurse planners work with adopters, whenever possible and appropriate, to collaboratively develop and mutually establish change goals consistent with the chosen solution. Together, they set goals that focus on behaviors. Intervention concerns management of environmental stimuli. Intervention in the translated process encompasses three of Nutt's adapted process stages (detailing, evaluation, and implementation). Strategies and tactics eliminate stimuli, alter stimuli, and/or increase the ability of the individual or social system to respond positively and effectively to stimuli.

Normative-reeducative strategies, appropriate for nursing and health care situations, resonate with traditional nursing values. Within the group context, resisters receive attention and respect; wise nurse planners thoughtfully consider resisters' perspectives. Evaluation measures progress toward goal attainment and gives consideration to strategies and tactics throughout the change process, which makes timely modifications possible. Keeping the process on course increases the likelihood of adaptive responses and helps to ensure goal attainment.

The third part of the chapter presents an example of the use of the combined RAM-BB&C change process. This example includes a normative-reeducative change strategy to teach care providers to adopt the concept of research-based critical paths and then to develop, use, and value critical paths as a way to direct nursing care. In the example, the assessment of organizational behavior in a hospital determined an inadequate degree of correspondence with the health care industry standard set by HCFA between LOSs and costs of care for clients with a particular DRG in a hospital. Planners used data identifying deviant DRGs to categorize them in the physical adaptive system mode. Loss of money by specific DRGs provided the focal stimulus. The current high average LOSs and the current high costs of caring for clients in the DRGs constituted the contextual stimuli. Diagnosis (Nutt's problem formulation) summarized the specific problem DRGs with regard to LOS and costs. Goals were related to behaviors that would indicate adaptation to the preferred solution—research-based critical paths. Related to the detailing, evaluation, and implementation stages of an adaptation of Nutt's planning processes, planners described alternative strategies and tactics and evaluated their potential viability and possible ramifications. The McDonald and Harms judgment method helped planners select the strategies and tactics with the highest probability of achieving acceptance of the preferred solution.

As planners intervened, they used a normative-reeducative strategy to bring care providers together in a group setting. When they introduced and explained the preferred solution (research-based critical paths), they employed the reeducational aspects of the normative reeducative family of strategies to give care providers information about current environmental stimuli affecting the fiscal position of the hospital. They employed the normative aspects of the family of strategies by using the group process and by guiding the resolution of resistance issues. These tactics helped participants move from the roles of decision maker to adopter. After the multidisciplinary care provider team developed a prototype research-based critical path for a problem DRG, the team promulgated the path to appropriate groups and determined a start date for implementation. Planners recognized the fact that they could use the search, synthesis, and analysis steps of the Nutt planning process to evaluate the effectiveness of the critical path with regard to LOS and costs. Such evaluation reveals either an adaptive or an ineffective response. They could measure the effectiveness of the normative-reeducative strategy by the attainment of the organizational behavior goals of the change process.

References

Andrews, H. A., & Roy, C. (1991a). Essentials of the Roy Adaptation Model. In C. Roy & H. A. Andrews (Eds.), *The Roy Adaptation Model: The definitive statement* (pp. 3-25). Norwalk, CT: Appleton & Lange.

Andrews, H. A., & Roy, C. (1991b). The nursing process according to the Roy Adaptation Model. In C. Roy & H. A. Andrews (Eds.), *The Roy Adaptation Model: The definitive statement* (pp. 27-54). Norwalk, CT: Appleton & Lange.

Benne, K. D. (1985). The process of re-education: An assessment of Kurt Lewin's views. In W. G. Bennis, K. D. Benne, & R. Chin (Eds.), *The planning of change* (4th ed., pp. 272-283). New York: Holt, Rinehart & Winston.

Bennis, W. G., Benne, K. D., & Chin, R. (Eds.). (1961). *The planning of change* (1st ed.). New York: Holt, Rinehart & Winston.

Bennis, W. G., Benne, K. D., & Chin, R. (Eds.). (1985). *The planning of change* (4th ed.). New York: Holt, Rinehart & Winston.

Chin, R. (1985). The utility of models of the environments of systems for practitioners. In W. G. Bennis, K. D. Benne, & R. Chin (Eds.), *The planning of change* (4th ed., pp. 88-97). New York: Holt, Rinehart & Winston.

De Rivera, J. (1976). *Field theory as human science.* New York: Gardner.

Klein, D. (1985). Some notes on the dynamics of resistance to change: The defender role. In W. G. Bennis, K. D. Benne, & R. Chin (Eds.), *The planning of change* (4th ed., pp. 98-105). New York: Holt, Rinehart & Winston.

Motamedi, K. K. (1985). Adaptability and copability: A study of social systems, their environment, and survival. In W. G. Bennis, K. D. Benne, & R. Chin (Eds.), *The planning of change* (4th ed., pp. 186-195). New York: Holt, Rinehart & Winston.

Nutt, P. C. (1985). The study of planning processes. In W. G. Bennis, K. D. Benne, & R. Chin (Eds.), *The planning of change* (4th ed., pp. 198-215). New York: Holt, Rinehart & Winston.

Snyder, R. (1985). To improve innovation, manage corporate culture. In W. G. Bennis, K. D. Benne, & R. Chin (Eds.), *The planning of change* (4th ed., pp. 164-176). New York: Holt, Rinehart & Winston.

Terreberry, S. (1985). The evolution of organizational environments. In W. G. Bennis, K. D. Benne, & R. Chin (Eds.), *The planning of change* (4th ed., pp. 176-186). New York: Holt, Rinehart & Winston.

The Rogers Diffusion Model

BOX 16.2: KEY WORDS AND PHRASES

— Adoption
— Adoption curve
— Centralization
— Competence credibility
— Confirmation stage
— Formalization

— Heterophily
— Homophily
— Innovativeness
— Network
— Persuasion stage
— Safety credibility

The study of diffusion has value for the nursing profession and the consuming public. The Rogers diffusion model, one of the most popular of the change writings used by nurses, relates to planned change by providing many insightful and research-based implications for planning the diffusion of innovations. Additionally, the diffusion approach provides "a natural framework in which to evaluate the impact of development programs in agriculture, family planning, public health, and nutrition" in developing (and developed) nations, clearly an asset in today's "global village" (Rogers, 1995, p. xvi).

This chapter starts with a short history of the Rogers diffusion model, continues with a presentation of the model, and ends with a review of the Rogers (1995) chapter on innovation in organizations. Appendix D, section D.3, lists nursing periodical articles that used the Rogers diffusion model during an 11-year time period. Readers will find information on the placement of specific topics in the Rogers literature in the index of the 1995 (or 1983) edition of *Diffusion of Innovations.*

Foundations and History of
the Rogers Diffusion Model

According to Everett M. Rogers (1983), the "curve of adoption frequency" emerged as early as 1903 in the work of a sociologist named Tarde and resurfaced later in the work of another sociologist, Bowers. It appeared again in the research of two rural sociologists, Bryce Ryan and Neal Gross (1943), at Iowa State University. Rogers cited the Ryan and Gross study as one of the most influential diffusion studies of all time. In writing about the "invisible college" of rural sociologists who made contributions to the study of diffusion, he stated that Ryan and Gross introduced "fifteen out of the eighteen most widely used intellectual innovations in the rural sociology diffusion research tradition" (Rogers, 1995, p. 35).

A pivotal year for the study of diffusion processes, 1960 saw the merging of propositions that would mold ideas from several disciplines into a relatively integrated body of generalizations. Disciplinary boundaries eased, diffusion research proliferated, internationalization occurred, and studies of knowledge, attitudes, and practices showed shortcomings in existing models and encouraged field experimental designs (Rogers, 1976). In 1961, Rogers, with Havens, presented an early paper on the topic of diffusion at a meeting of the Rural Sociological Society held at the Ohio State University (Rogers, 1962, pp. 300-316). In this paper, Rogers assembled the elements that set the direction for the formulation of a general theory of the diffusion and adoption of innovations.

During the late 1950s and early 1960s, Rogers made a comprehensive review of research literature that demonstrated the fruitfulness of interdisciplinary study. In his book *Diffusion of Innovations,* Rogers (1962) ordered findings from 405 European and U.S. studies to formulate a theoretical framework and establish generalizations (Rogers, 1995), an early and major accomplishment. As Rogers attempted to base a theory on research findings, he pinpointed various challenges inherent in diffusion research and furnished ideas for future diffusion studies (Havelock, 1973; Rogers, 1962).

According to Havelock (1973), Rogers

limited his content area to "diffusion," generally meaning the diffusion of products or specific practices. In so doing, he has excluded two major blocks of research. . . . The first is the very extensive set of general and experimental research findings in social psychology having to do with influence process, attitude change, group behavior, and organizational behavior. The second set of studies which tends to be excluded is that dealing with major personal and social change where a particular "innovation" is not clearly identifiable. Thus, we do not find in Rogers' bibliographies many of the major efforts to apply *social science* findings to organizations, work groups, classrooms, and so forth. (chap. 1, p. 3)

As a result of Rogers's decision to limit the scope of his model, many of the generalizations of the model deal with causal elements, such as characteristics of the decision-making unit and characteristics of the innovation, that do not yield readily to manipulation. Thus the emphasis of the theoretical framework of necessity centers on diffusion as it proceeds through a social system rather than on attention to variables that cause diffusion to occur.

By 1983, the Rogers diffusion model, originally published for use in agricultural diffusion, had undergone several revisions. Throughout, the model remained linear, unidirectional, and time oriented, with several stages and few feedback loops, and with its major elements intact. Although the figures depicting the model in the third (1983) and fourth (1995) editions of *Diffusion of Innovations* remain unchanged, Rogers (1995) stated that the fourth edition of the book furnishes a revised theoretical framework with additional research support (p. xv). He wrote that the linear models of communication used in most previous diffusion studies accurately describe only certain types of diffusion; a convergence model of communication, where participants create and share information, more accurately relates to other types of diffusion. Changes in chapter eight in his book reflect the broader view of communication (p. xvi), thus giving a more accurate description of diffusion. Attention to a convergence model of communication enhances the astute watching of diffusion.

The Rogers Diffusion Model

After Rogers, an "Iowa farm boy," came under the influence of Ryan and Gross, he used four findings from the Ryan and Gross study as basic elements (an innovation, communication, time, a social system) in his diffusion model. With these elements, *diffusion* is "the process by which an *innovation* is *communicated* through certain *channels* over *time* among the members of a *social system*" (Rogers, 1995, p. 10). Rogers (1995) portrayed the diffusion process as having five stages. Under conditions prior to the diffusion stages, the model addresses previous practice in a social system, looks at felt needs and problems, determines the degree of innovativeness present in a social system, and examines norms in that system. The model assumes a linear, unidirectional pattern where all arrows point toward culmination of the diffusion process in either continued adoption or final rejection.

The idea of communication channels forms an overarching concept in the Rogers diffusion model. The second (Rogers & Shoemaker, 1971) edition of Rogers's book on the diffusion of innovations carried the word *communication* in its title. Rogers repeatedly emphasized the role that communication plays in planners' (Rogers calls them "change agents") activities and discussed at length the ways that planners can minimize the widening of the rich-poor economic gap through selective communication. Communication, one of the four main elements Rogers named for the diffusion of innovations, forms one of the pivotal concepts in the Rogers diffusion model. (See Figure 16.1.)

Model Stages

The 1995 version of the Rogers model lists the five stages in the diffusion process as knowledge, persuasion, decision, implementation, and confirmation (p. 163). As potential adopters pass through this series of stages, their understanding of the innovation in question undergoes modification until they make a decision to adopt it or reject it. Rogers (1995) wrote that under certain cultural circumstances, the knowledge-persuasion-decision sequence may become the knowledge-decision-persuasion sequence. These circumstances usually pertain in societies that do not have Western notions of individual freedom (p. 172) but, instead, a strong sense of hierarchical leadership and responsibility. The discussions that describe the stages of the Rogers diffusion model follow in the order given them by the model.

Knowledge stage. The knowledge stage of the diffusion process is the time period during which persons develop awareness of the existence of an innovation and obtain some understanding of its meaning and function. Some scholars claim that the gaining of initial awareness is a process in which the person is passive; others cite selective attention to and seeking out of messages that interest the individual. These others claim that a need must exist before an innovation will obtain an onlooker's conscious attention. This raises the question of the deliberate creation of needs by planners. Further, needs and wants may not coincide; persons may want things they do not need (high-calorie sweets) and they may need things they do not want (fiber and vitamins). Rogers differentiated between awareness knowledge (finding out that an innovation exists), how-to knowledge (information about how to use an innovation properly), and principles knowledge (information that explains the reasons the

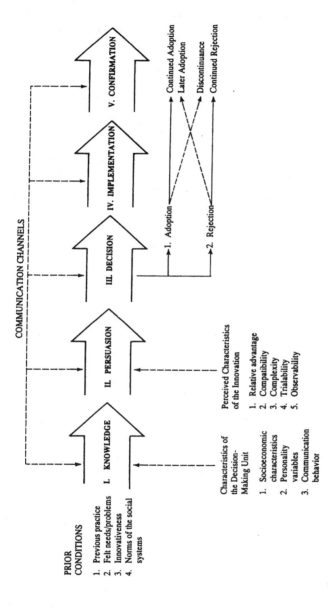

Figure 16.1. A Model of Stages in the Innovation-Decision Process

SOURCE: Reprinted with the permission of the Free Press, a division of Simon & Schuster from *Diffusion of Innovations*, Fourth Edition, by Everett M. Rogers. Copyright © by Everett M. Rogers. Copyright © 1962, 1971, 1983 by The Free Press.

NOTE: The innovation-decision process is the process through which an individual (or other decision-maikng unit) passes from first knowledge of an innovation, to fomring an attitude toward the innovation, to a decision to adopt or reject, to implementation of the new idea, and to confirmation of this decision.

innovation works as it does). Successful adoption requires all three kinds of knowledge.

Even though potential adopters gain awareness of an innovation, they do not adopt unless they perceive the innovation as important to them. Therefore, the model calls for examination of the characteristics of decision makers as associated with the nature of their perceptions of innovations and with the timing and quality of adoption.

The innovativeness dimension resulted from Rogers's association of adopters' socioeconomic characteristics, personality traits, and communication behaviors with the bell or cumulative frequency curve that results from plotting adoption frequencies over time. Although Rogers used standard statistical practices when he developed the bell curve that depicts adopter categories based on innovativeness, he made a reasoned choice to digress from the usual bell curve symmetry when he created divisions among categories. Rogers (1995, pp. 252-280) supported his generalizations regarding adopter categories with research findings. He recognized that a fair amount of empirical evidence exists to show that some deviation occurs in the linear relationship between socioeconomic status and innovativeness. The following descriptions of adopter categories present adopters as "ideal types" that do not exist in pure form in the "real world."

Innovators differ from early adopters. Innovators want to try out something new even before anyone else has sensed its value or harmfulness. Innovators have the means to try the risky, and almost always experience some losses. Not fully integrated members of the social system, these persons remain on the fringe and find their peers among like-minded persons, sometimes at quite a geographic distance from themselves. Rogers called them "cosmopolites." The innovator plays an important gatekeeper role in finding out about new things and introducing them to the local social system.

Early adopters, as localites, are fairly integrated members of their social systems. These well-respected people lead opinion in their groups. Their judicious selection and early use of an innovation enables them to give what others consider reasoned judgments about the characteristics of the innovation. Planners often seek out these responsible early adopters as an advance guard to advertise an innovation. Early adopters, well connected in the interpersonal network, have the means to adopt an innovation at an early time but they also place a high value on prudence. With their known prudence, higher than average economic status, and education, early adopters exert a great deal of opinion leadership.

Persons in the *early majority* adopt new ideas deliberately; they wait to see how things go with those who adopt earlier. Although they are great communicators, they seldom lead opinion. People in the early majority have many links in important communication networks. Early majority individuals, who adopt just before the average member, constitute about one third of the adopter group.

Persons in the skeptical *late majority* adopt innovations just after the average social system member in response to some kind of economic or social pressure. Such skeptical persons need a lot of evidence to convince them of the desirability and safety of adopting the innovation.

Laggards make their adoption decisions last. The most localite, even isolated, of all the adopter categories, laggards refer to the past more than to the future or the present. Their precarious economic position requires their deliberation; they must make certain that the innovation will succeed before they invest their resources. Rogers meant no harm when he used the term *laggard.* He wrote that any name applied to the last group to adopt soon would earn a pejorative reputation. He mentioned that the plight of laggards stems not so much from their own characteristics as from social system characteristics that deny them opportunity. Rogers also conceded that some persons never adopt; the adoption curve remains open at both ends.

Persuasion stage. The persuasion stage is the phase of the diffusion process in which potential adopters form relatively enduring attitudes (beliefs) that predispose them to adopt or reject the innovation. Persuasion, in this model, does not mean attempts by planners to secure adoption; instead, it relates to the mental and emotional processes that occur within adopters.

Whereas potential adopters gained cognitive knowledge about the innovation in the knowledge stage, they form attitudes (develop feelings) about it in the persuasion stage. Now the potential adopter actively seeks knowledge about the innovation. The source of information, the kind of information, and the interpretation of the information assume importance. The potential adopter makes a mental rehearsal of innovation usage and talks with peers to see if his or her own thinking about it is "on the right track." The main outcome of this stage is a favorable or unfavorable attitude about the innovation. The attitude develops as a result of evaluation of several characteristics of innovations that Rogers called attributes.

Adoption concerns the decision to use an innovation. Rogers (1995, pp. 205-208) linked a complex of five variables to the rate of adoption of an innovation. These include the kinds of communication channels present, the nature of the social system, and the extent and type of planners' promotion efforts. Variables also include perceived attributes of innovations (relative advantage, compatibility, complexity, trialability, observability) and type of innovation-decision process (optional, collective, or authority). Rogers stated that little research has been done to show the relative importance of the various factors that determine the rate of adoption. The following descriptions present characteristics possessed by innovations.

Relative advantage is the degree of perceived superiority of a new idea, product, or process over an old one. The idea of relative advantage compares an innovation with what it replaces or the void it fills in terms of such considerations as economic advantage, prestige or social status, efficiency, comfort, or convenience. Not all potential adopters use the same criteria when evaluating innovations; what one interprets as advantage, another considers a disadvantage. The relative advantages of a preventive innovation (i.e., insurance, immunizations, family planning methods) do not appear immediately and thus may not foster adoption of the innovation.

"*Compatibility* is the degree to which an innovation is perceived as consistent with the existing values, past experiences, and needs of potential adopters" (Rogers, 1995, p. 224). Potential adopters have no choice but to judge compatibility in terms of their values and beliefs, previously held ideas, and needs. Compatibility does not mean complete similarity; an innovation is not an innovation if it is too similar to previous practice. Technology clusters tie related innovations together in bundles and might call for package adoption deals. Schemes that artificially connect unrelated items might fail, whereas functionally related innovations might do well as a package.

"*Complexity* is the degree to which an innovation is perceived as relatively difficult to understand and use" (Rogers, 1995, p. 242). Rogers cited research that suggests that the higher the degree of perceived complexity an innovation possesses, the lower its rate of adoption.

"*Trialability* is the degree to which an innovation may be experimented with on a limited basis" (Rogers, 1995, p. 243). Adopters like trialability because it reduces uncertainty about the impact of the innovation. A new idea that permits testing on a pilot basis carries less risk and more likelihood of adoption than an innovation with no possibility of a test run. As expected, trialability appeals more to early adopters than to later adopters, to whom peers already have demonstrated positive innovation characteristics.

Observability is the degree to which others can see the results of an innovation. For example, hardware components of innovations generally have observability; software components do not. The more clearly others can view results of an innovation, the more readily the idea will be adopted—if observations reveal the innovation's advantages.

Rogers (1995) also discussed the matter of consequences of innovations. "Consequences are the changes that occur to an individual or to a social system as a result of the adoption or rejection of an innovation" (p. 405). Although they should do so, planners seldom predict the advantages and disadvantages of innovations (Rogers, 1995, p. 405). Perhaps the reason for this lack is the fact that sponsors of diffusion research overemphasize adoption and assume positive results. They also might use research methods incapable of measuring consequences.

Consequences of innovations fall into a number of categories. All innovations have both desirable and undesirable consequences, which seldom can be separated. Each innovation carries direct consequences and, later, indirect consequences. Rogers (1995) stated that "undesirable, indirect, and unanticipated consequences of an innovation usually go together, as do the desirable, direct, and anticipated consequences" (p. 421).

Decision stage. The decision stage of the diffusion process is a segment of time during which potential adopters accept or reject an innovation. If adoption occurs piecemeal with small-scale trials preceding full adoption, the decision may take shape over time.

Rogers (1995, pp. 71, 169-171) noted what he called a KAP-gap, in which potential adopters have both knowledge about and favorable attitudes toward an innovation but fail to adopt it. He cited several reasons for this gap, including undesirable side effects of innovations, the necessity for overt behaviors beyond the control of adopters, lack of connection with communication networks, and adopters' lack of feeling in control of their lives. In addition, preventive innovations provide weak adoption incentives because threatened events might never occur.

Decisions might not be permanent, but during the decision stage, the adopter either develops the intent to use the innovation or plans not to get involved with it. In active rejection, potential adopters think about using the innovation but make a considered decision against adoption. In passive rejection, adopters do not actually consider adoption; they reject by default.

Implementation stage. The implementation stage of the diffusion process is a period of time in which adopters end mental rehearsals and start behavioral use of an innovation. The start of implementation often requires active information-seeking behavior because mental trials do not answer all questions necessary to usage. Adopters need answers to such questions as where to obtain products, how to store supplies, how to maintain equipment, and how to use the innovation correctly. In an organization, the decision makers might not be the users. Uncertainty about the consequences of the innovation still exist in adopters' minds and perhaps in planners' minds as well.

Implementation ceases when use of an innovation becomes standard, familiar practice. But before that occurs, reinvention might take place. In reinvention, users, and perhaps planners, modify the innovation or the manner of using it. Inventors of innovations usually think of reinvention in negative terms; adopters consider reinvention in a favorable light. Reinvention often occurs when an innovation appears complex or in the face of inadequate knowledge about it. An innovation with multiple applications or one that can solve a wide variety of problems invites reinvention. Reinvention often occurs when planners encourage it.

Confirmation stage. The confirmation stage is the phase of the diffusion process in which adopters make "permanent" decisions about adoption or rejection of an innovation. Adopters move into the confirmation stage when they either solidify or change their earlier adoption or rejection decisions. The four options are as follows: Adopters continue or discontinue adoption; rejecters continue their rejection or now choose to adopt. In this stage, adopters may experience mental dissonance. Adopters, and also those who decided not to adopt, might hear either positive (adoption-confirming) or negative (adoption-disconfirming) messages or have positive or negative innovation usage experiences. Discontinuance (the decision to reject after adoption has occurred) has several faces. Replacement discontinuance may develop in a rapidly changing field such as computers. Disenchantment discontinuance results from displeasure with the way an innovation operates or with its secondary effects. Sometimes outside influences force adopters to discontinue, as happened when the U.S. government banned DDT.

Implications for Planners

In keeping with what Rogers called prior conditions, the nurse who uses the Rogers model to plan diffusion in a particular organization should learn a great deal about the social system in question. Planners make a real effort to see the situation from the perspective of potential adopters and to tailor efforts to the needs of the local situation. Information gathered from a thorough investigation of local circumstances forms the basis for "packaging" the information that nurse planners disperse during the diffusion episode. Social system information regarding what Rogers called "prior conditions" helps planners throughout the remainder of the diffusion process.

According to Rogers (1995), innovations have a potential for widening economic gaps in social systems. Planners who are involved with issues concerning social justice take deliberate measures to maintain justice as they diffuse innovations. They think not only of the form and function of an innovation but also consider its meaning for potential adopters. Such consideration enables planners who diffuse innovations to evaluate the equilibrium of the social system and to work toward creating a dynamic equilibrium, rather than a disequilibrium, within the system.

The Rogers diffusion model presents many implications for planners. The following discussions of those implications include descriptions of the characteristics of successful planners and the roles that planners might take throughout a diffusion process.

Characteristics of successful planners. Rogers described success in planning as related to the amount of effort planners exert. Further, successful planners develop programs in keeping with adopters' needs; they empathize with adopters. Strong research support exists for the contention that the adopters most similar to planners (i.e., with higher social status, greater social participation, more education, cosmopolite) respond most often to diffusion messages. This creates what Rogers (1995, p. 347) called a cozy circle of relationships where planners give the most help to those with the least need. He asserted that many planners do not take measures to counteract the disinclination of the lower status and least innovative adopters to respond to planner communications.

Rogers named two kinds of planner credibility: (a) competence credibility and (b) safety credibility. *Heterophilous* planners (those unlike adopters), if seen as technical experts, possess competence credibility. *Homophilous* planners (those similar to adopters), who perhaps have used the innovation beforehand, possess safety credibility. Ideally, a planner or planning team should have both kinds of credibility.

Because adopters tend to respond most readily to planners like themselves, Rogers suggested the use of paraprofessional aides to establish safety credibility. Nurses who work with paraprofessional aides will instruct these aides concerning the diffusion-oriented reasons that they should not assume an inauthentic professionalism through the inappropriate use of symbols. Aides also need competence credibility, but not at the expense of the similarity that will give them safety credibility in adopters' eyes.

Planner roles. Rogers (1995) identified and sequenced seven roles for planners. These roles, described in the following paragraphs, relate broadly to the stages Rogers proposed for the diffusion process.

The *needs identifier/creator, gatekeeper* develops the need for change:

> In order to initiate the change process, the change agent points out new alternatives to existing problems, dramatizes the importance of these problems, and may convince clients that they are capable of confronting these problems. The change agent assesses client's [sic] needs at this stage, and also may help to create needs. (Rogers, 1995, p. 337)

Because innovations cause problems as well as solve them, this role raises a moral/ethical question regarding the responsibility of planners to exert "quality control" over the nature of the innovations they introduce, the rate of the innovations' adoption, and the appropriateness of their subsequent use.

The *rapport-builder* role pertains to the establishment of an information-exchange relationship in which planners establish a camaraderie with potential adopters. Planners increase the credibility of their own competence, trustworthiness, and empathy as a step in obtaining acceptance for the innovation. They might work alongside potential adopters. They can show empathy toward adopters by both verbal and nonverbal communication that demonstrates an understanding of the adopter situation. The rapport-builder role offers nurse planners the temptation to work for their own benefit to an unwarranted extent. In response, planners can target their communications and other diffusion efforts carefully to offer equal opportunities to the poor as well as to the rich to prevent widening the gap between rich and poor. They will remember that all gap-narrowing activities come with a cost; they require a much larger number of planners and development workers than do the more divisive methods.

Nurse planners will find themselves familiar with the *diagnostician role* in which planners determine why existing practices do not meet needs. They make every effort to see the lack of appropriate practices through adopters' eyes; empathy enables the planner to assess needs accurately.

Planners fulfill the *motivator role* during the persuasion stage when they create the intent to change. They develop potential adopters' interest in the innovation through client-centered avenues of action such as the prediction of the advantages and disadvantages of the innovation in terms of the users' culture. They actively distribute information designed to picture an "ideal state" and to create dissonance between the status quo and the "ideal state." The planner also provides information regarding the ways that the proposed innovation works, how to use it, and probable short- and long-term consequences. When they choose people to convey diffusion-oriented messages, planners try to select persons who exhibit both heterophily (for the sake of competence credibility) and homophily (to confer safety credibility on an innovation). Opinion leaders, frequently heterophilous, usually come from a higher socioeconomic status than the majority of adopters. These people bring competence credibility to diffusion-oriented messages.

In the *activator role,* planners work with adopters to translate adopter intent into action (adoption). During the decision stage, the planners stand by, ready to give information, perhaps indirectly through opinion leaders and peer networks. They support adopters by showing empathy for their situation as they experience dissonance. Nurse planners heed what Rogers (1995) called indigenous knowledge systems:

> For example, Juan Flavier, a family planning official in the rural Philippines, found that villagers understood that when chicken hens ate the brown-colored seeds of the iping-iping tree, they stopped laying eggs. So Flavier explained to villagers that oral contraceptive pills for humans acted in a way similar to iping-iping seeds. (p. 240)

In the *stabilizer role,* planners solidify adoption and prevent discontinuance. During the implementation stage, they appear "everywhere" to help, guide, give reinforcing messages, and support adopters. They might offer incentives and opportunities for trial use. They work with opinion leaders. A pilot project with practice sessions allows adopters to experiment and report their results to others. The planner helps adopters use the system to the best advantage, neither overadopting nor underadopting. Planners also provide logistical support for individual adopters who want to try the innovation in other circumstances. They assist users in reinvention of the innovation whenever necessary from either a practical or a political standpoint.

In the *ability-developer role,* planners send messages to reinforce adoption decisions. They make themselves available to any laggards who still may wish to consider adoption. As the adoption sequence ends, the planner "should seek to put him or herself out of business by developing the clients' ability to be their own change agents" (Rogers, 1995, p. 337). This means that the planner works to develop self-reliance in the adopting population. Principles knowledge fits extremely well here, if not at an earlier stage in the diffusion process. At the end, the planner terminates his or her relationship with adopters.

Innovation in Organizations

Although the Rogers diffusion model applies to individuals, Rogers (1995) dedicated a chapter in his book to a discussion of innovation in organizations. This section presents highlights from that chapter.

Most early diffusion research centered on diffusion among individuals. Diffusion researchers recognized that diffusion in organizations differs from diffusion among individuals when they saw that not every individual has the social position necessary for adoption decisions. For example, individuals in organizations often cannot make optional innovation decisions to adopt or reject an innovation independently of a group. Some circumstances demand collective innovation decisions (where a group reaches a consensus regarding adoption) or authority innovation decisions (where a few persons in power make adoption decisions). Contingent innovation decisions made by individuals can occur only after an organization has made the initial adoption decision. Thus frameworks appropriate to individual adoption decisions usually do not work well for research involving innovativeness in organizations.

Rogers (1995) cited Rogers and Agarwala-Rogers, who defined an organization as "a stable system of individuals who work together to achieve common goals through a hierarchy of ranks and a division of labor" (p. 375). Five characteristics help organizations achieve stability: predetermined goals, prescribed roles, an authority structure, rules and regulations, and informal social relationship patterns.

When researchers studied innovation in organizations before the mid-1960s, they centered on characteristics of organizations related to innovativeness. They conducted a great many such studies, some with very large sample sizes. These studies used the entire organization as the unit of analysis and often collected data from a single individual, such as the chief executive officer. Researchers failed to realize that a lone individual could not depict a complex process that involved numerous persons in many parts of the organization. Their cross-sectional research designs further hampered research efforts by obliterating the effects of time from studies of a time-oriented process.

Despite shortcomings, studies of characteristics of organizations yielded important information by the late 1960s and early 1970s. Researchers found, for example, that large organizations generally exhibit more innovativeness than small ones. Perhaps size serves as a surrogate variable for such dimensions as total resources, slack resources, and the technical expertise of employees. The attitude of individual administrators toward diffusion affects the degree of organizational innovativeness, as do internal organizational characteristics (centralization, complexity, formalization, interconnectedness, organizational slack, size). System openness also helps to determine innovativeness.

The Innovation Process in Organizations

During the 1970s and 1980s, as researchers saw that organizations behave differently than do aggregates of individual organizational members, they moved research about innovation in organizations toward the study of the innovation process. Studies by Van de Ven, Rogers, and others (see Rogers, 1995, pp. 389-391 and pp. 497-498 for a discussion and listing of studies of the innovation process) on the innovation process in organizations revealed a sequence of five stages: agenda setting, matching, redefining/restructuring, clarifying, and routinizing. Agenda setting and matching constitute the initiation phase of the innovation process; the last three stages constitute the implementation phase. The names of these stages organize the sequence of the discussions that describe them.

Initiation phase. Agenda setting is a stage in the organizational innovation process in which organizational participants define a general organizational problem that creates a perceived need for an innovation. Agenda setting, which occurs constantly and might take years, has several functions. It identifies and prioritizes problems and searches for appropriate innovations within the organizational environment. Although a performance gap (a discrepancy between expectations and performance) sometimes triggers the innovation process, the sequence reverses when people who possess knowledge of an innovation hunt for a problem to solve.

In the *matching stage,* organizational members make mental rehearsals of the use of the innovation. They engage in reality testing as they think about potential problems and benefits of adoption. If they anticipate a gross mismatch, they reject the innovation, and the process stops. An adoption decision forms the watershed point between initiation and implementation in the innovation process.

Implementation phase. Redefining and restructuring are the means that organizational participants almost always use to alter the innovation to fit the organization and/or modify the structure of the organization to fit the innovation. This part of the innovation process must occur quickly, before routine sets the innovation "in stone." If the innovation was developed within the organization, redefining and restructuring might occur more quickly than they would if the innovation came from outside. Certain innovations, especially radical ones, create uncertainty. Technical uncertainty arises when an innovation requires a great deal of learning or when the possibility of rapid obsolescence appears. Financial uncertainty accompanies innovations that might not yield monetary rewards. Social uncertainty attends the possibility of labor unrest or other social problems. At this stage, an individual can act as a champion for the innovation.

Clarifying is the part of the innovation process in which the meaning and function of the innovation become clearer in the minds of organization members. Although clarification requires a fair amount of actual innovation usage by organization members, forcing premature usage invites disaster. At this stage, problems need corrective action and uncertainties require attention as users gain experience with the innovation.

When organization members no longer think of the innovation as new, *routinization* has occurred. The organization has completely absorbed the innovation.

Summary

This chapter started with a history of the Rogers (1995) diffusion model. After it presented the model, the chapter ended with a short review of Rogers's views on innovation in organizations.

Rogers developed an interest in diffusion of innovations when he came in contact with pioneer diffusion researchers Ryan and Gross at Iowa State University. In the early 1940s, Ryan and Gross had conducted an extremely influential study of the diffusion of hybrid corn seed among Iowa farmers. Rogers credited them with introducing over 80% of the most widely used scholarly innovations found in rural sociology diffusion research. By the late 1950s, Rogers had used elements from the work of Ryan and Gross and from over 400 other studies to assemble the earliest version of his diffusion model. This linear, unidirectional, and time-oriented model still retains many of its early features. The model provides useful insights into the diffusion process that have implications for nurse planners.

With model elements, diffusion constitutes a process with several important components. In diffusion, an innovation (solution to a problem) is communicated to social system members over a certain span of time. The Rogers diffusion model has five stages linked together by the concept of communication. Nurse planners who use the model need to know about the social system where they plan to cause diffusion to occur. They will attend to previous practice, the felt needs of the adopters, the degree of innovativeness present, and existing norms.

During the knowledge stage, potential adopters develop some awareness of an innovation and a degree of understanding of its meaning and function. Planners impart awareness knowledge, how-to knowledge that explains how to use the innovation, and principles knowledge that tells why the innovation works the way it does. As they prepare communications, planners consider adopter characteristics. *Innovators,* the venturesome risk takers, adopt first. Localites constitute the *early adopter* group. Not only do these respected and well-connected persons lead opinion, they have the knowledge and other resources necessary for early trial usage of the innovation. People in the deliberate *early majority* wait to see how things go with the early adopters before they try the innovation. They have a great many links in the social system and compose the bulk of those who adopt the innovation before the midpoint of diffusion.

The skeptical *late majority* adopts next. Somewhat more traditional than the early majority, they have fewer free resources to "waste" if the innovation does not perform well. *Laggards* adopt last because they must. They have so few of the resources necessary for adoption that they cannot afford to adopt unless they feel absolutely certain that the innovation will work for them. Finally, some people never adopt.

The persuasion stage of the Rogers diffusion model is the time when potential adopters form relatively enduring attitudes and feelings that predispose them to adopt the innovation. (In this model, persuasion does not mean attempts by planners to secure adoption decisions.) Adopters seek information and make mental rehearsals of innovation use. They talk with peers about the meaning of the innovation. Innovation characteristics assume importance now. An innovation might have a *relative advantage* over alternate solutions to a problem. It might or might not demonstrate *compatibility* with adopters' values, former experiences, and needs. It possesses more or less *complexity.* Some innovations lend themselves to trial usage *(trialability)* while others do not. Other persons can easily *observe* some innovations but not others. And, last, all innovations have both positive and negative consequences, not all of which appear before adoption.

In the decision stage, potential users develop an intention to adopt or reject the innovation. When they implement the innovation, adopters move from mental rehearsals to behavioral use of the innovation. Much uncertainty still exists; adopters often need help in using the innovation as standard practice. Adopters solidify or change their previous adoption decisions during the confirmation stage.

Rogers described roles that have implications for nurse planners. In addition to learning about the social system and adopters, planners *identify or create needs* and act as *gatekeepers* for the entrance of innovations into the social system. In the *rapport-builder* role, planners establish a rapport with potential adopters so that they can give them information about the innovation. Careful targeting of messages helps prevent the widening of economic gaps between rich and poor. In the *diagnostician* role, planners assess needs accurately and with empathy. They devise or select innovations and take care to name them appropriately.

As *motivators,* planners use various strategies to create the intent to change. They take into account the innovation's characteristics and existing communication networks as they develop messages for potential adopters. In the *activator* role, planners employ indigenous knowledge systems to augment their technical information messages. They furnish cues that suggest action when appropriate. As *stabilizers,* planners help, guide, and support adopters. They plan pilot projects and work with opinion leaders. In the final role, planners try to put themselves out of business by *developing the ability* of adopters to manage use of the innovation without outside help. At this point, planners provide knowledge of principles.

Recent research findings led Rogers to describe the process of innovation in organizations. This process consists of five stages occurring in two phases (initiation and implementation). In the *agenda-setting stage* of the initiation phase, organization members define a general organizational problem and search the organizational environment for a suitable innovation. During the *matching stage,* they mentally rehearse the fit between the problem and the innovation. In the *redefining/restructuring stage* of the implementation phase, organization members alter the innovation to fit the organization or modify the organization to fit the innovation, or both. In the *clarifying stage,* members increase their understanding of the meaning and function of the innovation as they start to use it. The process ends with *routinization* of the innovation; no longer do organization members think of the innovation as new.

References

Havelock, R. G. (1973). *Planning for innovation through dissemination and utilization of knowledge.* Ann Arbor, MI: Center for Research on Utilization of Scientific Knowledge.

Rogers, E. M. (1962). *Diffusion of innovations.* New York: Free Press.

Rogers, E. M. (1976). Where are we in understanding the diffusion of innovations? In W. Schramm & D. Lerner (Eds.), *Communication and change: The last ten years: And the next* (pp. 205-222). Honolulu: University Press of Hawaii.

Rogers, E. M. (1983). *Diffusion of innovations* (3rd ed.). New York: Free Press.

Rogers, E. M. (1995). *Diffusion of innovations* (4th ed.). New York: Free Press.

Rogers, E. M., & Shoemaker, F. F. (1971). *Communication of innovations: A cross-cultural approach* (2nd ed.). New York: Free Press.

Ryan, B., & Gross, N. C. (1943). The diffusion of hybrid seed corn in two Iowa communities. *Rural Sociology, 8,* 15-24.

Analysis and Critique of the Rogers Diffusion Model

BOX 17.1: LOOKING AHEAD

Chapter 17: Analysis and Critique of the Rogers Diffusion Model

Analysis of the Rogers Diffusion Model
Critique of the Rogers Diffusion Model

This chapter contains two main sections: analysis of the Rogers diffusion model and critique of the model.

Analysis of the Rogers Diffusion Model

After a general description of the model, analysis proceeds with an examination of the purposes of the model and the ways the model deals with ideas about person, environment, and health. The analysis depicts the ways the model manages the tasks of description, explanation, and prediction. It addresses the breadth of the model, explores model concepts, and examines their relationships. It gives attention to model definitions, illustrations, and movement within the model. The analysis ends with attention to the assumptions underlying the model.

Description

The Rogers diffusion model is a time-oriented, linear mental formulation that describes the spread of an innovation (solution to a social problem) through

233

communication channels over time in a social system. As a diffusion model, the Rogers model differs from an engineering theory that is designed to cause change to occur. In the Rogers model, examination of prior conditions precedes model stages. Model sequences progress from early times to later times through five irreversible stages with no feedback loops. The first stage highlights characteristics of decision-making units; the second highlights characteristics of innovations. Adopters make decisions in the third stage. Implementation occurs in the fourth stage; adopters confirm or disconfirm their decisions in the fifth stage.

The 1995 (fourth) edition of *Diffusion of Innovations* best describes the Rogers diffusion model. This edition very nearly parallels the 1983 (third) edition; the figure (1995, p. 163) that pictures the model remains unchanged from that in the former edition. A dual view is useful in any serious analysis and critique of the Rogers (1995) diffusion model. First, one considers the essence of the model as shown in the figure that illustrates it. (See Figure 16.1.) Four chapters (5-8) of the Rogers book *Diffusion of Innovations* (1983, 1995) amplify this figure. The material in the four chapters carefully follows the outline provided by the figure. The figure and the four pivotal chapters discuss, in detail, the four main elements of the diffusion process (innovation, communication through channels, time, social system) listed by Rogers (1995, p. 10).

Second, the more general chapters (2-4, 9-11) deal with issues less central to the model, such as history, research, planners, and innovation in organizations; chapter 1 in the book provides an introduction to the field of diffusion. This analysis and critique of the Rogers diffusion model does not ignore the peripheral book chapters but it does give more weight to the model figure and discussions in the four central chapters than to the material in the more general chapters.

Purposes

The purpose of the Rogers (1995) diffusion model is to describe the diffusion process that occurs over time (pp. xvi, 162). Rogers also wished to broaden scholars' understanding of the diffusion of innovations (p. xvii). He accomplished both purposes.

The Rogers diffusion model constitutes a midrange theory. Chinn and Kramer (1991) defined *midrange theory* as "theory that deals with a relatively broad scope of phenomena but does not cover the full range of phenomena that are of concern within a discipline" (p. 200). The phenomenon of diffusion is one of several of concern to planners of change but it does not treat the whole of the field of planned change.

Havelock (1973) noted that Rogers consciously chose to restrict his view of social change by eliminating two major blocks of research. First, he excluded research concerned with influence processes (attitude change, group behavior, organizational behavior); second, he excluded research related to change where no clearly identifiable innovation exists (chap. 1, p. 3). Examination of the four editions (1962, 1983, 1995; Rogers & Shoemaker, 1971) of the Rogers book on the diffusion of innovations shows that the central statement (chaps. 5-8) of the model, during the years since its inception, has retained these essential characteristics. Rogers has not claimed that his revisions have moved his diffusion model into a planned change camp. He did state that inclusion of the convergence model of communication seen in chapter 8 of the 1995 edition of *Diffusion of Innovations* helps the model do a better job of describing diffusion (p. xvi).

Person, Environment, Health

The Rogers diffusion model includes specific attention to persons as adopters by focusing on the relationship between characteristics of persons and their adoption of innovations. With several model concepts (diffusion, communication channels, social systems) that pertain to the travel of ideas among groups, the orientation of the model would enable a nurse planner to apply many model concepts to individual persons. Although the model does not mention environment, Rogers furnished numerous illustrations that show the importance of culture as the environment of the diffusion process. These include stories such as those of water boiling in a Peruvian village and the distribution of steel axes among Stone Age aborigines. Further, the model's major emphasis on communication channels shows that the model attends to the environment of diffusion. The model applies to the diffusion of health practices as well as to diffusion in any other aspect of life.

Description, Explanation, Prediction

Description typifies the Rogers diffusion model. Model clarity and its understandable definitions enable model users to describe what they see. The model's clear descriptions furnish a first step toward explanation and prediction.

Breadth and Concepts

The scope of the model remains restricted almost entirely to diffusion. Except for the treatment of change in organizations, it does not attend to aspects of planned change such as interactions among groups, social power, processes of in-depth dialogue, or feedback in social systems.

Rogers (1995) called his major model concepts the "main elements in the diffusion of innovations." These appear in his description of *"diffusion* as the process by which an *innovation* is *communicated* through certain *channels* over *time* among the members of a *social system"* (p. 10).

Relationships Among Concepts

Time, a broad concept, relates to innovativeness, model stages, indirect effects of innovations, and bell- and S-shaped curves that depict rates and completeness of adoption. The pervasiveness of the concept of time demonstrates its importance. Time relates to all five stages of the model (knowledge, persuasion, decision, implementation, confirmation).

This model has three other major concepts (communication channels, characteristics of social system members, and innovation). Rogers depicted communication channels as an overarching concept that relates to all five stages of the model. The concept of characteristics of social system members has several dimensions (socioeconomic characteristics, personality variables, communication behavior) that describe decision makers. The concept of the innovation (solution to a problem) has five dimensions (relative advantage, compatibility, complexity, trialability, observability) that characterize innovation attributes.

Several factors precede the stages of the model. Prior conditions include previous practices, felt needs and problems, innovativeness, and norms of the system. At the end of the model's time-oriented continuum, adoption and rejection decisions are divided into continued adoption, later adoption, discontinuance, and continued rejection.

Several topics and concerns not featured in the central portion of the model emerge in the less central chapters (2-4, 9-11) of the Rogers book. These topics include a focus on research concerns (history of diffusion studies, diffusion research, research methodologies) and a focus on organizations (innovation processes in organizations, planners as linkers, centralization versus decentralization). Discussions also attend to ethical concerns associated with the consequences of innovations.

Definitions, Illustrations, Movement

Most concepts in the Rogers model merited clear, explicit definitions, often followed by illuminating discussion and interesting examples. Definitions in this model consistently and clearly describe and distinguish among concepts. Clear and understandable graphic illustrations explain many model concepts. Interesting and illuminating story illustrations characterize the Rogers book.

The Rogers diffusion model, as found in chapters 5 through 8, moves in a linear fashion from earlier time to later time with infrequent side trips and the introduction of a few ideas that do not fit into the predetermined sequence. Statements in the model move between general and specific. Connections between discrete parts do not show undue overlap and the model demonstrates consistency. Feedback loops emerge in descriptions of the convergence model of communication in chapter 8. Chapter 11 of his book, which is not directly tied to the figure that depicts the model, provides an important feedback loop to innovations with its attention to innovation consequences.

Assumptions

Explicit assumptions. The Rogers diffusion model states an explicit value for efficiency in watching the progress of diffusion in a social system. Such description could lead to explanation and prediction in areas covered by the model.

Implicit assumptions. Rogers (1976, 1995) criticized the proinnovation bias that pervades diffusion research and leads to ignorance about many important aspects of diffusion. Yet his chapter on the innovation-decision process (1995, pp. 161-203) describes awareness knowledge, how-to knowledge, and principles knowledge being provided without any assistance from a planner in terms of an in-depth exploration of the meaning of the innovation for the adopter. Although chapter 8 advocates use of the convergence model of communication, with open sharing of ideas among participants, it does more to help planners describe communication networks than to explain how to formulate networks that increase participation. Nowhere does the model openly advocate planner assistance in the exploration of alternative options that adopters might consider. This omission does not prompt observers of diffusion to look for instances of adopter input or tell planners how to solicit it.

Chapter 4 of the Rogers (1995) book provides a discussion of innovation development that parallels and often describes the problem recognition and innovation development processes used in commercial industries. Here, research and development follow need identification by someone who wishes to diffuse (sell) something. The discussion and examples in the chapter cited relate more closely to industrial production than to grassroots community development or cooperative development projects such as those undertaken by Peace Corps workers. Although other parts of the book deal with certain aspects of aid and development, implicit assumptions underlying the model generally fall in line with manufacturing, advertising, and sales.

Critique of the Rogers Diffusion Model

The critique part of this chapter starts with a report of the place the Rogers diffusion model has found in nursing periodical literature. It proceeds with a discussion of affirmations of the model and problems with the model. The section also describes and critiques the ways that the Rogers diffusion model deals with each of the four components of the change planning process, and ends with suggestions regarding the usefulness of the model to nurses.

The Model in Nursing Periodical Literature

An 11-year survey (1982 through 1992) revealed a total of 155 articles that used 58 planned change theories in English-language nursing periodicals (Tiffany, Cheatham, Doornbos, Loudermelt, & Momadi, 1994). The Rogers diffusion model took third place in terms of the number of articles that featured a particular theory or model, with 27 (17%) of the 155 articles using the model in some way. The 155 articles presented 383 citations of sources of the 58 theories; the Rogers diffusion model received 42 (11%) of these. Of these sources, *The Communication of Innovations: A Cross-Cultural Approach* (Rogers & Shoemaker, 1971) received 14 citations; the 1983 edition of *Diffusion of Innovations* had 11 citations. Almost all of the nurse authors who referred to the work of Rogers used or cited the "classical" Rogers diffusion model in their articles; only three (Barker, 1990; Crane, 1985; Horsley & Crane, 1986) used or alluded to the Rogers writings on innovativeness in organizations.

Affirmation for the Model

Researchers and scholars in many disciplines investigated the matter of diffusion years before Rogers developed his diffusion model. Their efforts remained largely isolated from one another until Rogers combined the concepts they addressed. His vision in sensing the coherence among their ideas constitutes one of his greatest contributions to the field of diffusion research. Havelock (1973) commended Rogers for his review and listing of enormous numbers of diverse research reports. Together, these form the strong empirical basis for the generalizations found in the Rogers diffusion model. Havelock cited Rogers's work as a major source of information about knowledge dissemination and use (chap. 1, p. 3). The Rogers publications number well over 100. The wide acceptance of his diffusion and development writings and their translation into many languages attests to their usefulness.

Possible Problems With the Model

When Havelock described the work of Rogers in 1973, he evidently viewed the Rogers writings from a qualitative or combined quantitative-qualitative standpoint. Support for this observation stems partly from Havelock's remarks that Rogers reviewed only empirical research and ignored anecdotes and case studies. These remarks could be either negative or positive, depending upon one's opinions about qualitative versus quantitative research. Havelock wrote that Rogers directed his work toward social scientists rather than to practitioners or policymakers. Havelock also commented that Rogers excluded important research concerned with general and experimental studies on influence processes, attitude change, organizational behavior, and major personal and social change that occurs without an identifiable innovation. (These topics relate more to planned change than to diffusion.) He stated that Rogers consciously chose to limit his work to diffusion (chap. 1, pp. 2, 3), a limitation that ignores the broader field of planned change. In response to Havelock's (1973) opinions, readers might remember that the Rogers stance, although limited, then was (and still is) consistent with his emphasis on diffusion rather than on planned change.

The Rogers model started with a positivist, linear stance that has changed but little over the years. The 1995 statement of the model demonstrates the same general perspective shown in 1983. Bakan (1985) remarked that a positivist viewpoint denies mentation and vitality (mind and life), preferring logic and mathematics. This stance omits exploration of intention, purpose, design, or goal direction and, according to Greer (1977), important political aspects of decision making. In answer to Bakan and Greer's opinions, one might remember that material in the less central chapters in the Rogers book widens the model's scope.

Change Planning Processes

For purposes of consistency across chapters, this section compares a diffusion model with criteria for an engineering theory (planned change theory/model). Such a comparison serves a useful purpose because it reminds readers that the Rogers formulation is a diffusion model, geared more to watching change than to planning it, and is of premiere importance in its own sphere.

The diagnostic process. The Rogers diffusion model provides for the recognition of a problem or need as the initial phase of the innovation-development process. A scientist might foresee a need, an activist might cite a problem, or basic and applied researchers could create an innovation to fulfill the need of a firm to sell a product. Rogers did not explore ways of developing collaboration between planners and adopters, although he did very briefly state that he would like to see adopters take a more active part in problem diagnosis—the foundational activity of planned change. Thus the model covertly assumes that planners make correct diagnoses. It does not prompt observers to look for collaboration or ask planners to provide it.

The innovation-development process. One of the less central chapters in the Rogers book addresses the innovation-development process. The examples provided describe the process in terms of the research, development, and dissemination mode that features the originator, the developer, the manufacturer, and the salesperson. In others of the less central chapters, Rogers amply demonstrated his expectation that planners will develop and produce an innovation in ways that meet needs and that do not cause harm. He attended to ethical matters by expecting observers to note both the beneficial and the harmful results of the innovations they develop or choose. He did not provide for planner-adopter collaboration in the innovation-development process.

Strategy choices. Two chapters (5, 8) central to the Rogers diffusion model attend to communication strategies and tactics (i.e., provide certain kinds of information about innovations, name and position innovations appropriately, use appropriate communication networks). The model gives more attention to innovation and adopter characteristics that cause resistance and less attention to observation of organizational dynamics and interpersonal relationships that relate to resistance. In the less central chapters, Rogers addressed the planning of communication strategies and tactics in ways that avoid the widening of socioeconomic gaps. The model does not provide a system for evaluating and choosing approaches other than communication strategies.

Evaluation. Although the Rogers diffusion model does not contain specific procedures for making outcome measurements, it does provide multiple methods for tracing and measuring the diffusion of an innovation as an evaluation procedure. Its attention to the possibility of unanticipated and negative consequences of innovations gives observers a basis for the evaluation of innovation outcomes. The model omits considerations of social power and politics in the processes of diffusion; this paves the way for model users to ignore the evaluation of political strategies.

Usefulness to Nurses

The Rogers model serves well as an introduction to the diffusion dimension of social change. Further, it offers multiple concepts and intellectual tools helpful to persons tracking diffusion. Planners as well as researchers will find the Rogers chapter on communication networks particularly helpful. The attention Rogers paid to the characteristics of decision makers and innovations increases the value of his model; few other sources furnish useful descriptions of this type.

Nurse readers will appreciate the attention that Rogers paid to moral and ethical aspects of social change. For example, he discussed ways to avoid widening gaps between the "Ups" and the "Downs." He showed concern about unintended negative consequences of innovations. The broad scope of his literature reviews and professional connections enabled him to provide many interesting and illustrative scenarios that spice the writing and enlighten readers.

Additionally, his clear and interesting model definitions and illustrations make diffusion concepts understandable.

Nurses can increase the usefulness of the Rogers diffusion model in at least five ways. First, model users need an in-depth understanding of the intent of the model and of what it says and does not say; this is a diffusion model, not a planned change model. Second, nurse users should remember the nursing values of mutuality and collaboration as they employ the model. Third, nurse researchers who use the Rogers diffusion model as a basic guide in diffusion research will augment its strength if they add a means for observation of social power and power transactions. When researchers trace diffusion developed under a planned change theory, they can add measurements that reflect the concepts (such as collaboration) of that specific planned change theory.

Fourth, if nurse users employ the Rogers diffusion model for the planning of change, they should understand the central tenets of the model. This means that they will recognize the differences between the pivotal central chapters and the less central chapters in the book (*Diffusion of Innovations,* 1983, 1995) that presents the model. They will bear in mind the important practical and ethical implications for planners found in the less central chapters. They also will remember nursing values and how these relate to the model and will attend to matters of power and the political implications of placement in social systems. Last, but not least, they will recognize and consider the employment of a number of change strategies, such as facilitation, reeducation, and data-based strategies, in addition to communication strategies. They will employ outcome measures in addition to adoption statistics for the measurement of the success of plans for change.

Summary

The main sections of this chapter include an analysis and critique of the Rogers diffusion model. The Rogers model is a time-oriented, linear, unidirectional model that depicts the diffusion of an innovation through communication channels over time in a social system. Conditions that precede diffusion involve the social setting of the diffusion event. The model describes adopter characteristics that are relevant to adoption, addresses environment, and emphasizes communication channels. It applies to health just as it applies to other concerns.

Readers can take a dual view of the Rogers (1995) model. Four chapters (5-8) amplify and discuss the essence of the model as found in the figure (1995, p. 163) that illustrates it. Other chapters deal with issues less central to the model.

The Rogers diffusion model confronts person, environment, and health through implication. The model contains considerable description that facilitates explanation and prediction. Rogers restricted the scope of his model to processes of diffusion rather than broadening it to include the planning of change.

The concept of time pervades almost every aspect of this model. Other important concepts include communication channels, characteristics of social system members, and innovation. The concept of communication channels relates to all five stages of the model. The concept of characteristics of social system members has several dimensions, as does the concept of innovation. Prior conditions precede model stages.

Rogers provided many clear definitions, illuminating discussions, and interesting examples in his book. The model assumes the goodness of tracing diffusion in a social system. It also assumes that planners will display both goodwill and competency. The choice or development of innovations has a research and development flavor.

The Rogers diffusion model has found favor with nurse authors, with its popularity exceeded only by the writings by Lewin and by Bennis, Benne, and Chin. Havelock commended Rogers for the scope and importance of his work but seemed disappointed that Rogers had limited his prodigious efforts to a quantitative view of diffusion rather that to the broader field of planned change.

As a diffusion model, the Rogers model does not openly advocate collaboration between planners and adopters in any of the four processes of planned change. Nurses who use the model for tracking diffusion will find that the model provides many useful ideas but also will discover that the addition of certain other concepts will increase the usefulness of the model. The same comment holds even more true for nurses who use the Rogers diffusion model for the planning of change. All users of this interesting and insightful model would do well to gain an in-depth understanding of what the model does and does not say and of how it relates to planned change before they attempt to use it in planning either diffusion research or social change.

References

Bakan, D. (1985). The interface between war and the social sciences. In W. G. Bennis, K. D. Benne, & R. Chin (Eds.), *The planning of change* (4th ed., pp. 382-392). New York: Holt, Rinehart & Winston.

Barker, E. R. (1990). Use of diffusion of innovation model for agency consultation. *Clinical Nurse Specialist, 4,* 163-166.

Chinn, P. L., & Kramer, M. K. (1991). *Theory and nursing: A systematic approach.* St. Louis: C. V. Mosby.

Crane, J. (1985). Research utilization: Theoretical perspectives. *Western Journal of Nursing Research, 7,* 261-268.

Greer, A. L. (1977). Advances in the study of innovation in health care organizations. *Milbank Memorial Fund Quarterly, 55,* 505-532.

Havelock, R. G. (1973). *Planning for innovation through dissemination and utilization of knowledge.* Ann Arbor, MI: Center for Research on Utilization of Scientific Knowledge.

Horsley, J. A., & Crane, J. (1986). Factors associated with innovation in nursing practice. *Family and Community Health, 9*(1), 1-11.

Rogers, E. M. (1962). *Diffusion of innovations.* New York: Free Press.

Rogers, E. M. (1976). Where are we in understanding the diffusion of innovations? In W. Schramm & D. Lerner (Eds.), *Communication and change: The last ten years: And the next* (pp. 204-222). Honolulu: University Press of Hawaii.

Rogers, E. M. (1983). *Diffusion of innovations* (3rd ed.). New York: Free Press.

Rogers, E. M. (1995). *Diffusion of innovations* (4th ed.). New York: Free Press.

Rogers, E. M., & Shoemaker, F. F. (1971). *Communication of innovations: A cross cultural approach* (2nd ed.). New York: Free Press.

Tiffany, C. R., Cheatham, A. B., Doornbos, D., Loudermelt, L., & Momadi, G. G. (1994). Planned change theory: Survey of nursing periodical literature. *Nursing Management, 25*(7), 54-59.

Altering the Diffusion
Model Square Peg

BOX 18.1: LOOKING AHEAD

Chapter 18: Altering the Diffusion Model Square Peg

**Congruence of the Rogers Diffusion Model (RDM) With Key
Concepts in the Roy Adaptation Model (RAM)**
A RAM-RDM Change Process
**Application of the RAM-RDM Change Process to a Nursing
Situation: An Example**

BOX 18.2: KEY WORDS AND PHRASES

— Change agent
— Clinical protocol
— Diffuser
— Incentive
— Innovation in nursing

— Need
— Opinion leader
— Practice innovation
— Research base

The diffusion process holds special interest for nurses. In a regulated health care industry, organizations have little or nothing to say about many changes. The government, insurance companies, and consumers exert enormous pressure toward cost containment. Health care organizations often designate nurses as planners (change agents). Perhaps these assignments fall to nurses because nurses have a great deal of power in the use of patient care resources that ultimately affect the financial status of the organization.

Additionally, the effective and efficient dissemination of appropriate research-based interventions throughout a health care organization forms an important goal for nursing because research utilization leads directly to the research-based nursing practice that benefits clients, nurses, and health care organizations. (Physicians call their clinical applications of research "evidence-based medicine.")

This chapter addresses the use of a diffusion model in health care situations. It consists of three parts: a discussion of the fit between the (Everett M.) Rogers Diffusion Model (RDM) and the Roy Adaptation Model (RAM), a translation (reformulation) of the Rogers model into a RAM perspective for the diffusion of innovations in nursing, and an application of the diffusion model to a nursing research utilization project.

Congruence of the Rogers Diffusion Model (RDM) With Key Concepts in the Roy Adaptation Model (RAM)

Neither the Rogers Diffusion Model nor the Roy Adaptation Model, taken alone, provides sufficient guidance for nurses who want to plan diffusion of an innovation. The diffusion model lacks a nursing orientation; the nursing model lacks detailed information on diffusion processes. The RDM deals specifically with the diffusion of innovations. It addresses the historical and social environment of diffusion, knowledge characteristics and transmission, adopter categories, attributes of innovations, decision processes, implementation of innovations, and confirmation of adoption decisions. The RAM limits its attention to the concerns of nursing. It pertains to the wholeness of the individual in conjunction with the environment and features the nursing process as seen in the light of nursing's metaparadigm concepts (person, environment, health, nursing).

Both Everett M. Rogers and Sister Callista Roy have disciplinary backgrounds, at the doctoral level, in sociology. They apply their knowledge of sociology to specific occupational areas—Rogers to rural sociology, Roy to nursing. Rogers views his work as applicable to a wide area of social programs. He made a major contribution to knowledge through his integration of research findings from multiple disciplines in the United States and Europe; he used these to construct the Rogers diffusion model. Diffusion includes "both the planned and the spontaneous spread of new ideas" (Rogers, 1995, p. 7). Rogers described the innovation-decision process as an information-seeking/processing activity that motivates individuals to reduce their uncertainty about an innovation.

The diffusion of innovations interests many nurses, thus accounting in part for the popularity of the Rogers diffusion model in nursing literature. Nurses have used the Rogers model in a number of ways, including conducting studies similar to those that Rogers calls "diffusion research." They also have used the Rogers model for planning research utilization projects where the model facilitated the diffusion (dissemination) of nursing innovations throughout health care organizations.

The RDM takes a social-interaction approach (Crane, 1985a, 1985b; Havelock, 1973); the RAM has a systems foundation. The models share a reciprocal interaction worldview. One element of this worldview asserts that diffusion has multiple antecedent factors. This assertion aligns with the RAM's assessment steps and the RDM's prediffusion phase that calls for the identification of prior (organizational) conditions that may affect diffusion.

The concept of communication relates closely to interaction. *Interaction,* in the RDM, means communication of an innovation to social system members via communication channels in that social system. In the RAM, interaction means communication between nurse and client, which includes the patient and family/significant others. In the Roy Adaptation Model Applied to Administration (RAMA), interaction occurs between organizational units or between nurse administrator/manager and staff.

The Rogers diffusion model offers a linear, unidirectional diagram, with few feedback loops, to vivify stages in the diffusion of an innovation. In her 1984 book, Roy offered linear, unidirectional, schematic diagrams to illustrate processes within the RAM. With publication of the Andrews and Roy (1986) book, the schematic diagrams took a circular, rather than linear, form. The following sections compare the characteristics of the diffusion model with key concepts of the nursing model.

Person

The RAM identifies the recipients of nursing care as adaptive systems (individuals, members of a social system such as a health care organization, or the organization itself). Both the RAM and the RAMA identify individuals as patients, nursing staff, or organizations. The RDM identifies the recipients of the diffusion process as decision-making units. Such identification helps nurse planners to tailor the diffusion process for its recipients. Rogers categorized decision-making units, according to their time of adoption, as innovators, early adopters, early majority, late majority, or laggards.

Environment

The RAMA, like the RAM, specifies the environment through identification and categorization of external and internal environmental stimuli that influence the behavior of organizations and individuals. The RDM views the social system as the environment. The social system is influenced by external and internal factors that, in turn, change conditions in the social system.

The RDM uses the term *prior conditions* to define conditions in the social system that planners must take into account before initiating the diffusion of an innovation. The notion of prior conditions, in the RDM, parallels behaviors and environmental stimuli in the RAM/RAMA. Both influence their respective processes, that is, diffusion and nursing. Information gleaned from assessing prior conditions familiarizes nurse planners with the organizational environment. Planners can use such information to develop strategies and tactics in a manner specific to the social system, a notion similar to the individualization of client care.

The RAM/RAMA specifies external and internal environmental stimuli as focal, contextual, and residual stimuli. The RDM provides no such specification but a planner could categorize a prior condition in the environment according to the degree of influence the planner believes it would have on the likelihood of diffusion and/or the effectiveness of the diffusion process. One could categorize a condition as very influential, similar to the focal stimulus, as defined by the RAM/RAMA. Then one could consider other (contextual) conditions as contributing to the most influential (focal) condition. Many planners using the Rogers model acknowledge the existence of less understood environmental conditions in a social system. These fit the definition of residual stimuli, as used in the RAM/RAMA, to categorize hunches and uncertainties.

The RAM/RAMA defines the *adaptation level* as a changeable point determined by the pooled effect of the environmental stimuli. In a sense, this term acknowledges the cumulative effect of the prior conditions in the environment that represent the ability of the social system to respond positively to the diffusion process (i.e., to adopt the innovation).

In the RAMA, a stabilizer subsystem consists of structures and processes that maintain an organization, and an innovator subsystem consists of structures and processes designed to promote growth and change within an organization. The RAMA uses the adaptive system modes classification (physical, role, interpersonal, interdependence) to categorize organizational behavior. In the RAMA, these modes represent ways of coping that reveal the activity of the stabilizer and innovator adaptive subsystems. The modes, adapted for the RAMA from the RAM, also could serve as classifications for prior conditions in the environment.

Health

In the RAM, health is a process and a product state. It involves the process of "being and becoming an integrated and whole person" (Roy & Anway, 1989, p. 78). The product is a healthy (whole and integrated) person. "Health, defined as integration, implies a continuous process of change throughout life" (p. 78). Like planned change theories, the RDM does not discuss health. The model considers communication channels integral with and critical to effective diffusion of the innovation. The goal of diffusion states that members of a social system will adopt an innovation and work together as an integrated whole to "institutionalize" the innovation. Healthy organizations adapt to societal demands by embracing efficient and effective new solutions to old and new problems.

Nursing

The key (metaparadigm) concept, nursing, relates to steps in the process of nursing. The RAM delineates six steps (assess behavior, assess stimuli, diagnose, set goals, intervene, evaluate) in the nursing process, long defined as clinical problem solving. Nurse investigators change the stages of the Rogers diffusion process into a problem-solving process applied to a social system when they use the Rogers model as a framework in research that pictures the amount or path of diffusion as it proceeds through a social system. They likewise turn the model into a problem-solving process when they use it to plan diffusion in a social system. (Table 18.1 shows the congruence or divergence of the stages of the Rogers diffusion model with the steps of the nursing process.)

A RAM-RDM Change Process

The Roy Adaptation Model (RAM), with its emphasis on adaptation to change, provides a suitable perspective for nurse planners who desire to follow or facilitate the diffusion of innovations in health care organizations. The Rogers model, specific to diffusion, amplifies the RAM perspective. The RAMA vivifies and demonstrates the suitability and applicability of the RAM for organizations. The nursing process (according to the RAM) and concepts and ideas specific to organizations combine in the following translation (reformulation) of the Rogers model of the innovation-decision process into a nursing perspective. Labels for nursing process steps and diffusion model stages organize descriptions of the translation.

Assess Behavior

A combined RAM-RDM change process begins with assessing prior conditions in the health care organization. Prior conditions may consist of behaviors of organizational members and/or environmental stimuli. The planner initiates the needs-identifier/creator role and the rapport-builder role during the assess-

TABLE 18.1 Congruence Between the Stages of the Rogers Diffusion Model and the Steps of the Nursing Process

RAM's Nursing Process Steps	*RDM Stages*
Assess behavior, client needs, and problems; obtain information about the client's current lifestyle. Assess environmental (focal, contextual, residual) stimuli that influence behavior. Diagnose via a statement conveying the person's adaptation status. Set goals relative to behaviors that will promote adaptation.	Prior conditions • Previous practice • Felt needs/problems • Innovativeness • Norms of the social system
Intervene:	
Manage stimuli influencing behavior. Individualize intervention (strategies, tactics) according to characteristics of the client.	Knowledge stage • Characteristics of the decision-making unit • Socioeconomic characteristics • Personality variables • Communication behavior
Educate client regarding the benefit and value of the intervention.	Persuasion stage • Perceived characteristics of the innovation • Relative advantage • Compatibility • Complexity • Trialability • Observability
	Decision stage • Adoption • Rejection
Evaluate: Determine the effectiveness of the intervention (strategies, tactics) in relation to the client's behavior.	Implementation stage
Determine behaviors that are adaptive and those that are ineffective. Reassess ineffective behaviors.	Confirmation stage • Continued adoption • Later adoption • Discontinuance • Continued rejection

ment of prior conditions. While assessing, she or he also lays the groundwork for the diagnostician role and starts to think of ways to fulfill the motivator role. (See Table 18.2 for short statements describing the roles nurse planners assume during the diffusion process. Chapter 16 discusses these roles. See also Table 18.3.)

TABLE 18.2 Planner Roles in the Rogers Diffusion Model

1. The *needs identifier/creator, gatekeeper* develops the need for change.
2. The *rapport-builder* role pertains to the establishment of an information-exchange relationship in which planners establish a camaraderie with potential adopters.
3. Nurse planners will find themselves familiar with the *diagnostician* role in which planners determine why existing practices do not meet needs.
4. Planners fulfill the *motivator* role during the persuasion stage when they create the intent to change.
5. In the *activator* role, planners work with adopters to translate adopter intent into action (adoption).
6. In the *stabilizer* role, planners solidify adoption and prevent discontinuance.
7. In the *ability-developer* role, planners work to develop self-reliance in the adopting population.

The nurse planner, as a needs identifier, first assesses organizational and system member behaviors relevant to or influential in the rate or extent of diffusion of the innovation. These behaviors include previous and current practices in the organization, felt needs and problems identified in the organization, the historical and current ability of the organization to cope with environmental demands, and organizational culture. Nurse planners make tentative judgments regarding whether behaviors exemplify an adaptive or ineffective response to the demands of the environment.

Assess Stimuli

Nurse planners next assess stimuli that influence the behavior of the health care organization. For example, environmental stimuli such as changes in payment structures and processes by the federal government and insurance companies may influence a budget deficit problem.

In a combined RAM-RDM change process, some prior conditions function as environmental stimuli that planners classify as focal, contextual, or residual. The focal stimulus has the greatest influence on organizational behavior. Contextual stimuli, such as media coverage, contribute to the influence of the focal stimulus. Residual stimuli are factors that the nurse planner cannot classify with certainty, unknowns that may manifest themselves during the diffusion process. The three types of stimuli pooled together constitute the adaptation level of the organization and reflect the multicausal nature of the organizational practice, problem, or unfilled need that calls for resolution.

The stabilizer and innovator organizational coping subsystems, as described in RAMA, manifest themselves in the adaptive system modes. For example, the

TABLE 18.3 Timing of Role Activation in the RAM-RDM Process

		Planner Roles						
RAM Step	*RDM Stage*	*Needs Creator*	*Rapport Builder*	*Diagnostician*	*Motivator*	*Activator*	*Stabilizer*	*Ability Developer*
Assess behavior	Prior conditions	M	x	x	x			
Assess stimuli	Prior conditions	M	x	x	x			
Diagnose		x	M	x				
Set goals		x		x				
Intervene	Prior conditions	x	M		M			
	Knowledge	x	M		M			
	Persuasion				M			
	Decision					M		
Evaluate	Implementation						M	
	Confirmation							x	M

NOTE: An "x" designates role activation. An "M" designates major emphasis on the role at this step/stage.

stabilizer subsystem would include computer systems. Computers, necessary tools for many departments, help to maintain the health care organization by enabling it to cope with the demands of the environment. Outmoded, inefficient computers that experience frequent system problems provide signs of stabilizer ineffectiveness as manifested in the physical adaptive system mode. An inefficient computer may affect the ability of the organization to cope with budget deficit problems.

Ineffectiveness in an innovator subsystem in the organization may surface in the interdependence adaptive system mode in the form of poor judgment calls relative to changes in the environment. It also could appear as faulty processing of information coming into the organization from the environment.

Diagnose

Nurse planners, acting in the diagnostic role, determine why the existing practices and behaviors of the organization and/or its members do not meet the organization's needs. The diagnosis is a summary statement that reflects the adaptive status of the health care organization. The diagnosis should relate to the purpose of the assessment, for example, facilitating the diffusion of an innovation deemed necessary by the organization.

Set Goals

The RAM-RDM change process presumes that the adoption of the innovation by members of the social system is a goal. Nurse planners develop short-term goals to identify system member behaviors that promote adaptation, that is, adoption of the innovation. Long- and short-term goals focus on turning ineffective behaviors into adaptive behaviors and maintaining and enhancing adaptive behaviors. The diagnosis should relate to the purpose of the assessment, for example, facilitating the diffusion of an innovation deemed necessary by the organization.

Intervene

Intervention requires the introduction and use of strategies and tactics at every remaining stage of the diffusion process. Nurse planners can enhance their wise selection of strategies through the McDonald and Harms (cited in Andrews & Roy, 1991) nursing judgment method.

Strategies (interventions) that relate to *prior conditions* focus on environmental stimuli, principally the focal stimulus. Nurse planners eliminate or modify stimuli that might retard the diffusion of the desired innovation. Further, they aim to maintain, enhance, or promote stimuli that facilitate the diffusion process. If nurse planners cannot change prior conditions that impede diffusion, they aim to raise the adaptation level of the health care organization by increasing members' abilities to cope with environmental demands.

In the *knowledge stage,* planners try to ensure effective communication by learning as much as possible about system members who ultimately will make the decision to adopt or reject the innovation. They obtain needed information about potential adopters' professional characteristics and communication behaviors that relate to the innovation in question. Nurse planners impart three kinds of knowledge about the innovation (awareness knowledge, how-to knowledge, principles knowledge). Rapport deepens as planners and potential adopters exchange information.

According to Rogers (1995), the *persuasion stage* does not relate to anything done by planners but, instead, relates to the mental and emotional processes that occur in potential adopters. As they talk with peers and near-peers, potential adopters mentally rehearse the application of the innovation to the present or anticipated future situation. They evaluate the innovation on the basis of innovation characteristics, think about what adoption would mean to themselves, and consider its latent consequences. Planners now strengthen the motivator role by taking care to present information about the innovation in a way that piques interest and prompts potential adopters to consider innovation characteristics (relative advantage, compatibility, and so on) thoughtfully.

In the *decision stage,* decision makers either adopt or reject the innovation. To some degree, the crucial decision stage reflects the success of the planners' efforts to this point. Peers and near-peers who evaluate the innovation positively contribute to adoption decisions. "Satisfied customers" sell the innovation. Rogers identified planners' actions in this stage as those of the activator role, in which planners work with opinion leaders to activate peer and near-peer communication networks to move potential adopters from intent to action.

Evaluate

In the *implementation stage,* decision makers become adopters (demonstrate an adaptive behavioral response) if all has gone well in the decision stage. Rejecters of the innovation have made an ineffective (from the planner's viewpoint) behavioral response. As serious innovation use begins, the planners, in the stabilizer role, select and use strategies and tactics that support and reinforce adoption decisions. Because planners recognize the uncertainty that adopters still feel, they make themselves available to answer questions and provide technical assistance. During this stage, the planners and adopters may decide to reinvent ("tweak") the innovation. Rejecters of the innovation and decision makers "on the fence" now can see the positive results of the innovation; the enthusiasm of adopters and planners may entice them to "get on the bandwagon." The implementation stage ends with institutionalization of the innovation as standard practice (an adaptive response). This is the time when clients see the innovation as part of their practice pattern; they "just do it."

The Rogers model does not specify an evaluation stage in the innovation-decision process. Nevertheless, the idea of evaluation occurs in the implementation and confirmation stages of the model. Institutionalization of an innovation represents success. In the *confirmation stage,* continued adoption of the innovation constitutes an adaptive response (from the planner's viewpoint). Adopter behaviors that reflect the long-term adoption of and adaptation to the innovation reflect a successful adoption process. Evaluation can relate to adoption-related behaviors of social system members over the long term.

Adopters may sustain their adaptive response by continued adoption, or they may "backslide" by discontinuing innovation usage, which is an ineffective response. Rejecters may retain their ineffective response or they may decide to respond adaptively by embracing the innovation. Discontinuing adoption of an innovation does not always constitute an ineffective response; innovations may become obsolete for any variety of reasons. During confirmation, planners assume the ability-developer role to help adopters by giving them additional principles knowledge, assisting adopters' movement toward self-reliance, and teaching adopters how to plan needed changes.

In summary, the RAM-RDM change process views members of a social system as capable of adapting to change by adopting an innovation. The guidance offered by the Rogers model for the diffusion process makes the model appealing to nurses; the medical, health education, and public health examples strike a familiar chord with nurses. Nurses could use the RAM-RDM diffusion process with individual clients and in working with groups.

Application of the RAM-RDM Change Process
to a Nursing Situation: An Example

"Innovations in nursing imply changes in practice that are new to those using them and that are intended to benefit clients" (Horsley, Crane, Crabtree, & Wood, 1983, p. 120). The Rogers model provides a useful tool in research utilization studies that facilitate the adoption of innovations (especially if users amplify the model, as advocated in Chapter 17, by the addition of a means of planning and observing social power transactions). Nursing process steps and diffusion model stages organize the following application of the RAM-RDM model. Although this application presents a scenario with nurses as adopters, the RAM-RDM process also could apply to individual patients, families, or communities.

The Innovation

Studies conducted during the past two decades have identified major variations in the way health care providers treat and care for people with specific health problems (Agency for Health Care Policy and Research [AHCPR], 1994). In 1989, the U.S. Congress established the Agency for Health Care Policy and Research (AHCPR, 1992). The agency has a mandate to improve the quality, appropriateness, and effectiveness of health care in the United States. As part of its mandate, the AHCPR facilitated the development of clinical practice guidelines by commissioning experts to study selected health care problems. These problem-specific guidelines have three parts: (a) a patient guide, (b) a quick reference document for clinicians, and (c) a clinical practice guideline with recommendations throughout. Clinical practice guidelines include summary statements that offer recommendations to providers and health care organizations on ways to diagnose, treat, and manage clinical conditions. Agency personnel believe that the use of clinical practice guidelines will improve the quality of health care. Moreover, they believe that the overall cost of health care in the United States may decrease through reductions in health care use and the elimination or reduction of unnecessary and/or ineffective clinical practices of health care providers, including nurses.

Before the recent restructuring of the AHCPR guideline program (AHCPR, 1996a, 1996b) described in Chapter 21, members of the AHCPR's expert panels searched computer databases to discover literature and/or studies on the health care problems assigned to them. Then they synthesized findings from the literature to form a database on each specific health problem. They transformed pertinent knowledge derived from the database into summary recommendations (protocols) for providers and organizations. The AHCPR makes each guideline available to health care providers upon request, free of charge. Providers and organizations transform recommendations (protocols) into specific actions or behaviors (innovations) for clinical use in their organizations. They need to conduct clinical evaluation of the new practice behaviors to determine if the innovation produced the desired result. Despite the widespread dissemination of clinical practice guidelines, their effects on patient outcomes remain unclear. Moreover, the factors that contribute to the adoption and sustained use of the guidelines in clinical practice remain unknown.

Nurse planners interested in moving nursing to a research-based practice could conduct research utilization projects to disseminate AHCPR guidelines in organizations. They also could measure the degree and rate of adoption of the guidelines over time. The example below relates to the dissemination of the summary recommendations of the AHCPR guidelines for the management of cancer pain in one health care organization. The AHCPR guideline titled *Management of Cancer Pain* was published in 1994. It has recommendations throughout and ends with nine summary recommendations.

In the example, the nurse administrator taking the role of nurse planner knew of the existence of the AHCPR guidelines. Recently, some staff nurses had expressed concern about what they considered inadequate relief of pain under the current system of pain management. Additionally, she had heard a report of the successful use of the recommendations for management of cancer pain in an outpatient clinic connected with another hospital.

Assess Behavior

A nurse planner, operating in the needs-identifier/creator role, wished to assess practice patterns in her hospital to discover how nurse caregivers were managing cancer pain. She called together a small planning committee consisting of the clinical nurse specialist and the staff educator (heterophilous members who furnished competence credibility) and two caregivers from the inpatient oncology unit (homophilous members who furnished safety credibility). The planner partly fulfilled the rapport-builder role by this establishment of competence and safety credibility. When the committee first met, they discussed the tendency of the hospital to cope adaptively with environmental stimuli that call for change. The culture of the organization showed both a sensitivity to the need for acceptance of helpful innovations and a sense of caution regarding large monetary expenditures for untried practices.

In an effort to determine the nature of previous nurse behaviors *(prior conditions)* in the management of cancer pain, the planning committee developed an assessment form to collect data from nursing documentation on patient charts. Items on the form detailed the innovation derived from the summary recommendations (protocol) in the guideline for cancer pain management. The planning committee did a "walk-through" with the data collection form to determine suitability to the clinical situation, ease of use, and length of time to gather the information needed. Following a successful trial of the form, the nurse planner made a proposal to the quality improvement committee based on the oncology unit. She recruited volunteers to conduct an interrater reliability study. After the planner trained the volunteers, she determined interrater reliability, which stood at .90.

Assess Stimuli

In this example, the development and promulgation of the AHCPR clinical practice guidelines provided the focal stimulus. Contextual stimuli that contributed to the effect of the guidelines included the publicity that the guidelines had received in consumer literature (e.g., *Redbook, Wall Street Journal, USA Today*), health care provider literature, and other media. Information about practices in another hospital also provided contextual stimuli. Residual stimuli included the uncertainty felt by health care providers and the skepticism of professional and consumer groups concerned about the federal government's "intrusion" (via the AHCPR) into health care.

Diagnose and Set Goals

In the diagnostician role, the planning committee used summary recommendations from the AHCPR clinical practice guideline on managing cancer pain as the standard for diagnosis of a social system problem. The diagnosis (inconsistent use of the recommendations for managing cancer pain related to lack of knowledge about the guideline) rested on the assumption that healthy organizations respond to environmental demands by adopting efficient and effective innovations for solving old or new problems. The diagnosis summarized the ineffective behavioral responses identified by the nurse planner and the planning committee during their assessment of current nurse practice patterns. For example, one assessment finding concerned inconsistency in documentation on evaluation of relief obtained from pain intervention, as measured on a 0-10 numeric pain intensity scale. The committee set the goal of consistent and sustained use of the recommendations from the guideline on managing cancer pain.

Intervene

Prior conditions. To achieve the goals they had set, the nurse planner and committee members focused on prior conditions, especially the focal stimulus. They believed that in their situation, they could increase the ability of organization members to change ineffective responses to adaptive ones.

Knowledge stage. In the knowledge stage, planners continued in the needs-identifier/creator and rapport-builder roles as they established relationships with potential adopters. They tried to see the innovation from the viewpoint of nurse caregivers.

Planners performed some motivator role functions when they determined the level of innovativeness of the nurse caregivers (adopter population) and identified relevant professional characteristics. These included years as an oncology nurse, certification status, subscription to oncology journals, and membership in the Oncology Nursing Society (ONS). Planners saw the stability of the registered nurse population and the trust they placed in ONS publications as factors that favored adoption of the innovation. Caregivers acknowledged hearing about the guideline through an ONS journal and considered pain management very important to quality care. Planners mapped formal and informal staff communication networks because they considered them very important in the transmission of messages to staff.

The nurse planners and planning committee used the information they had collected about the nurse caregivers to develop a customized educational program directed toward reversing ineffective nurse behaviors. They presented information that provided awareness knowledge, how-to knowledge, and principles knowledge. Their teaching methods decreased anxiety among caregivers.

Persuasion stage. During the persuasion stage, caregivers evaluated the new nurse practice behaviors (innovation). These behaviors were listed as items on the assessment form that planners developed from the summary recommendations (protocol) in the AHCPR guideline. The developers' detailing of the items on the form ensured that its wording and format were specific to the institution.

In the educational program, the planning committee focused on the relative advantages of practicing according to the guideline. These included consistency for cancer pain management according to a nationally recognized standard, improved quality of care, and increased patient comfort and satisfaction. An adopter incentive, the promise of future publication of the experience, increased the degree of relative advantage to the caregivers.

As planners taught, they assumed the motivator role when they cited references, in ONS literature and other professional journals, to the guideline under consideration. Such attributions to the ONS decreased uncertainty and increased credibility for the guideline's content. Caregivers evaluated the innovation on the basis of its compatibility with professional values and previous practice. The positive tone and credibility of the educational program encouraged nurse caregivers to adopt the summary recommendations of the guideline as standards of practice.

Planners confronted the complexity issue when they presented knowledge about the nature and functioning of the protocol and chose a straightforward and simple manner of presentation. They used familiar terms and a comfortable format on the forms required by the protocol. For example, they used the more familiar terms *prn dose* and *prn dose for breakthrough pain* rather than the less familiar *rescue dose.*

With respect to trialability, planners proposed a pilot program (for the decision stage) for care of inpatients on the oncology unit. Later, protocol use could progress to the outpatient clinic or the hospice program administered by the hospital. An added incentive, publication of the pilot program experience in the hospital organ, increased the observability of the innovation.

Decision stage. The small-scale pilot project on the oncology inpatient unit influenced decision making by allowing potential adopters to make small-scale or vicarious trials. Planners fulfilled the activator role by supportive measures to help adopters translate intent into action. These measures included answering questions, giving demonstrations, and listening to adopters' concerns.

Evaluate

Implementation stage. During the implementation stage, caregivers began to use the innovation on a regular basis. Most nurse caregivers progressed from the role of decision-making units to that of adopters of the clinical practice guideline on managing cancer pain. Some remained lukewarm about the innovation. Planners soon identified an adaptive response—a practice pattern congruent with the summary recommendations (protocol) of the guideline. A pain intensity rating not greater than 4 (on a 0-10 numeric pain intensity scale) indicated a specific positive patient outcome for the pilot program. Committee members acknowledged that other outcomes of interest might emerge later when the use of the guideline would expand to the outpatient clinic and the hospice program. These outcomes could include measurement of help-seeking behaviors such as inpatient admissions and visits to care providers for purposes of pain control. The planners and adopters continued to "sell" the rejecters on the superiority of guideline use over existing practice. Planners continued to give collegial support to potential adopters during this period. The planners and caregivers sought more information about the innovation as they implemented the designated nurse practice behaviors developed from the summary recommendations of the guideline. Planners fulfilled the stabilizer role by guiding, giving reinforcing messages, supporting adopters, and providing logistical support. In other words, planners were helping "everywhere." They worked to develop caregiver abilities by on-the-spot assistance with the details of adoption and help for laggards with problems.

The nurse planner also formed a new committee composed of two current members and nurses in similar roles from the oncology clinic and the hospice program. As they planned to further disseminate the guideline to these areas, the degree of acceptance of the innovation moved toward institutionalization.

Confirmation stage. Evaluation of the continuation of an adaptive response occurs on an ongoing basis. Planners evaluated their diffusion efforts by determining the rates of new nurse practice behavior (innovation) usage six months after its introduction. They found that 87% of the oncology staff had adopted and continued to practice according to the guideline for management of cancer pain; 3% continued rejection of the innovation; 6% adopted the innovation after initial rejection; and 3% discontinued innovation use after initial adoption. Planners fulfilled the ability-developer role by reinforcing adoption decisions. They gave reports of pain relief as measured on the numeric pain intensity scale. They assisted laggards with the difficulties they experienced in attempting adoption, and offered additional principles knowledge in the form of updates of information on pharmacology and physiology for all staff. They encouraged self-reliance by teaching opinion leaders to function as planners in the introduction of guideline usage in the outpatient clinic as well as the hospice administered by the hospital. They considered their job done when unit caregivers continued to manage cancer pain according to the innovation developed from the summary recommendations (protocol) in the AHCPR guideline for the management of cancer pain.

Summary

This chapter discussed congruence of concepts in the Rogers diffusion model (RDM) with key (metaparadigm) concepts in the Roy Adaptation Model (RAM). It also presented a translated (reformulated) change process (RAM-RDM) and applied the process to a research utilization project in a hospital.

The RAM and the RDM both hold reciprocal interaction worldviews. Systems theory forms a foundation for each model. Both models display interactionist levels of analysis; both focus on adaptation to environmental demands. Individuals can adapt. Environmental stimuli, emanating either from outside or from inside the social system, influence individuals to respond. Prior conditions include behaviors and stimuli that influence the diffusion process. An integrated social system is a healthy system; integration implies a continuous process of change. The innovation-decision process (prior conditions, knowledge, persuasion, decision, implementation, confirmation) uses communication channels to integrate the innovation into the fabric of the social system. This process roughly parallels the nursing process and has a goal of adaptation (successful adoption of the innovation).

The RAM-RDM process requires assessment of behaviors and stimuli that represent conditions existing prior to implementation of the diffusion process. Nurse planners can categorize the amount of influence environmental stimuli have on the diffusion process by identifying the stimuli as focal, contextual, or residual. A diagnosis reflects the reasons existing practices do not meet the needs of the health care organization. Goals describe adaptive behaviors.

The RAM-RDM uses education to teach potential nurse or patient adopters about an innovation. Nurse planners manage environmental stimuli that influence adopter behaviors. Planners take the adopters' professional and practice characteristics into account and emphasize positive attributes of the innovation as they try to increase the ability of adopters to adapt to the innovation.

Potential adopters adopt or reject the innovation in the decision stage. When they start to use the innovation, planners support them in an effort to solidify adoption decisions. A trial run might cause rejecters to change their minds and might make "true believers" out of lukewarm adopters. The implementation stage ends when the use of the innovation becomes standard practice. The nurse planner's job often ends with evaluation of the diffusion episode and institutionalization of the innovation. In some situations, nurse planners continue to evaluate the extent of adoption over the long term (confirmation stage).

The final section of the chapter presents a case study of a research utilization project that involved the diffusion of an innovation—new practice behaviors—developed from the summary recommendations (protocol) in the Agency for Health Care Policy and Research (AHCPR) clinical practice guideline for the management of cancer pain. The nurse planner formed a small planning committee of nurses from the oncology inpatient unit. When planners assessed prior conditions, they found caregiver practices that did not meet current standards found in the AHCPR guideline on management of cancer pain. They identified the focal stimulus as the development and distribution of the guideline by the agency. The diagnosis summarized the behaviors as an ineffective response to environmental stimuli. Planners set a goal of congruence between the patterns of nurse practice on the oncology unit and the guideline.

The planning committee reviewed professional background information about the caregivers and tailored an educational program for them. Most of the caregivers adopted the innovation during a successful trial run on the oncology unit. The nurse planner formed a new committee to diffuse the innovation in the outpatient unit and in the hospice program administered by the hospital. Continuing evaluation and monitoring of nurse practice patterns demonstrated long-term adoption of the guideline as well as the ways that patients benefitted from its adoption.

References

Agency for Health Care Policy and Research. (1992, January). *AHCPR fact sheet.* Rockville, MD: U.S. Department of Health and Human Services.

Agency for Health Care Policy and Research. (1994, March). *Clinical Practice Guideline Number 9: Management of cancer pain* (AHCPR Publication No. 94-0592). Rockville, MD: U.S. Department of Health and Human Services.

Agency for Health Care Policy and Research. (AHCPR). (1996a, October). [Statement for public release]. Rockville, MD: U.S. Department of Health and Human Services.

Agency for Health Care Policy and Research. (AHCPR). (1996b, November). *AHCPR to help public and private groups develop tools for clinical improvement.* Rockville, MD: U.S. Department of Health and Human Services.

Andrews, H. A., & Roy, C. (1986). *Essentials of the Roy Adaptation Model.* Norwalk, CT: Appleton-Century-Crofts.

Andrews, H. A., & Roy, C. (1991). The nursing process according to the Roy Adaptation Model. In C. Roy & H. A. Andrews (Eds.), *The Roy Adaptation Model: The definitive statement* (pp. 27-54). Norwalk, CT: Appleton & Lange.

Crane, J. (1985a). Research utilization: Nursing models. *Western Journal of Nursing Research, 7,* 494-497.

Crane, J. (1985b). Research utilization: Theoretical perspectives. *Western Journal of Nursing Research, 7,* 261-268.

Havelock, R. G. (1973). *Planning for innovation through dissemination and utilization of knowledge.* Ann Arbor, MI: Center for Research on Utilization of Scientific Knowledge.

Horsley, J. A., Crane, J., Crabtree, M. K., & Wood, D. J. (1983). *Using research to improve nursing practice: A guide.* New York: Grune & Stratton.

Rogers, E. M. (1995). *Diffusion of innovations* (4th ed.). New York: Free Press.

Roy, C. (1984). *Introduction to nursing: An adaptation model.* Englewood Cliffs, NJ: Prentice Hall.

Roy, C., & Anway, J. (1989). Roy's adaptation model: Theories for nursing administration. In B. Henry, C. Arndt, M. DiVincenti, & A. Marriner-Tomey (Eds.), *Dimensions in nursing administration* (pp. 75-78). Boston: Basil Blackwell.

19

Bhola's Configurations
(CLER) Model

BOX 19.1: LOOKING AHEAD

Chapter 19: Bhola's Configurations (CLER) Model
Foundations and History of the Model
The CLER Model: Thinking Through Change
Guidelines for Using CLER

BOX 19.2: KEY WORDS AND PHRASES

— Configuration
— Configuration map
— Expecting/typifying
— Experiencing/correcting
— Grammar of action
— Linkage
— Linkage typing

— Ordering/relating
— Problem setting
— Problem solving
— Social unit
— Systemic model
— Total diffusion

This chapter consists of three parts. After a short discussion of the origin and foundations of Bhola's (1994) Configurations (CLER) Model of planned change, the authors present the model from Bhola's own writings. Suggestions for use of the CLER model follow its presentation.

Foundations and History of the Model

Bhola began work on his CLER model of planned change at the Ohio State University in the early 1960s. Somewhat later, as he worked in a literacy project in his home country of India, he made many observations about social change that informed his later works. Over the years, Bhola has published over 50 articles, book chapters, and Educational Resources Information Center (ERIC) documents that present and explain the model. Scholars in many countries of the world in addition to the United States recognize the CLER model. Bhola's work as a consultant for the United Nations has resulted in the publication of his work in the English, French, Spanish, Arabic, and Persian languages, with a Chinese translation expected. The following presentation of Bhola's (1994) CLER model of planned change is reprinted here in the following section, with minor modifications, from a nursing journal.

The CLER Model:
Thinking Through Change

This section consists of three parts. The first describes conceptual characteristics of the CLER model; the second examines those concepts; the third discusses ways of using CLER to develop strategies.

The acronym *CLER* stands for *configurations* (C) of social relationships within and between systems in the planner and adopter roles, *linkages* (L) to carry communications within and between the planner and adopter systems, *environment(s)* (E) inside and around the systems involved in the change transaction, and *resources* (R) dedicated by the planner system for enabling implementation and to the adopter system for incorporating the change.

The CLER has a 25-year history of development and elaboration but it is likely to be new to nursing professionals (Bhola, 1965, 1977, 1984, 1986, 1988, 1991). While this model is appropriate for nursing, it is not limited by or exclusive to the area of nursing (Major, 1986; Tiffany, 1977). Rather, it is a general model usable in a range of social sectors including education, agricultural extension, family planning, AIDS awareness, business, religion, and a variety of other social marketing situations (Bhola, 1988; Zajc, 1987).

Social reality is marked by complexity and uncertainty (Elster, 1983; Kahneman, Slovic, & Tversky, 1982). As living systems, as open systems, and as systems-in-process, social systems always are making transactions with other systems in the environment. As living systems, they have both *exteriority* (a public life) and *interiority* (a private life). Being dynamic, they are described best as "mental frames put on perpetual flux" and are marked by complexity because reality framed within these systems is multifaceted and multicausal. Because human motivations, human choices, and human responses all are uncertain, social systems exhibit uncertainty.

Change models dealing with living systems cannot promise the model user simplicity, clear causality, certainty, and prediction at the theoretical level, nor a set of formulas or exact steps to be taken in a practical order. Users of such models usually will resonate with the values, assumptions, definitions, and conceptual structure of the model rather than make deductive uses of such models. Open system models will provide their users illumination and insight rather than a set of presuppositions, inviolable instructions, and predetermined choices (Berger & Luckmann, 1967; Richardson, 1984). We also must remember that no model, however comprehensive, is complete and self-contained in and of itself. It can be no more than a template for organizing available knowledge and material resources in relation to a particular social or educational change. No change model can dispense with the need for substantive knowledge about human nature and group process and about people, groups, and institutions actually operating in the real-life setting in which change is taking place.

Conceptual Characteristics of the CLER Model

The CLER model is a general model for problem setting and problem solving within open systems. Some particular characteristics of the CLER model include the following:

1. CLER is a *"modeling model"* used to work with the reality actually faced by the change agent (planner). Rather than let planners "dispense with thinking," it demands that they engage in the exercise of modeling reality in their real-life contexts (Bhola, 1984; Richardson, 1984). Nursing professionals should not expect to come up with one "nursing" model but with models suited to specific situations: nurse-patient relationship, staff development, organizational change, professionalization of nursing.

2. Being a *systemic* model, CLER assumes interrelationships and interdependencies among social entities and social systems in shared and immediate environmental space and accepts all other basic concepts of systems theory. It is dialectical in that it accepts multicausality and mutual shaping of social phenomena existing in interaction. Also, it is constructivist, as it assumes that human beings take an active part in constructing their own reality. Thus it looks at planned change as an experiment in which individuals and institutions engage, as they reconstruct their present reality into a future reality (Bhola, 1991).

3. Although usable in a wide range of value positions from the bureaucratic to the democratic, the CLER value bias is toward collaborative action and participative decision making by planners and adopters. Indeed, the model accommodates the situation where planner and adopter systems overlap and planned change thus becomes self-renewal by individuals and institutions. Nursing as a nurturing profession should find this feature particularly congenial.

4. The CLER model enables the planner both in problem setting (definition and validation of change objectives) and in problem solving (implementation of change). The CLER emphasis on collaboration allows the values of both planners and adopters to come into play in the diagnosis of problems and the development of objectives designed to alleviate problems. Such close collaboration also mandates the incorporation of both scientific and social system knowledge in the strategies and tactics that cause change to occur.

5. Change strategies result from using the four basic categories of the model itself—configurations, linkages, environments, and resources—first to describe the change situation and then to design needed social interventions. The social power for leveraging change is generated through synergistic optimization of C, L, E, and R.

6. Further differentiation of C, L, E, and R (to be elaborated below) provides a taxonomy for the organization of behavioral and social scientific knowledge, and thus offers a "structure of access" to the types and pools of knowledge needed for implementing change. The CLER model also categorizes knowledge as (a) general behavioral and social scientific knowledge, (b) behavioral and social scientific knowledge *specific* to the existential situation in which change is being implemented, and (c) *tacit* knowledge that remains interior to the individual stakeholders engaged in a change situation (Bhola, 1977, 1988).

Elaboration of CLER Concepts

Change can occur in two major ways: (a) *change in transmission,* which takes place through social, institutional, and cultural processes as personal and communal life is lived un-self-consciously, or (b) *change by transformation,* which occurs when an actor self-consciously undertakes the planner role to transform a present social situation into a future situation in terms of sufficiently articulated change objectives. The CLER model is of the latter type.

To use the CLER model effectively, it is necessary to explore the C, L, E, and R components in more detail:

1. A configurational perspective is at the core of the CLER model and asserts that change is not one standard homogeneous phenomenon but that it occurs in many different, often overlapping, configurations. The CLER model includes

TABLE 19.1 Configurational Relationships Between Planners and Adopters

	I	G	IS	CL
I	I-I	I-G	I-IS	I-CL
G	G-I	G-G	G-IS	G-CL
IS	IS-I	IS-G	IS-IS	IS-CL
CL	CL-I	CL-G	CL-IS	CL-CL

SOURCE: From "The CLER Model: Thinking Through Change," by H. S. Bhola, 1994, *Nursing Management, 25*(5), p. 60. Copyright © 1994 by S-N Publications. Reprinted with permission.

four basic social configurations: individuals (I), groups (G), institutions or organizations (IS), and communities, subcultures, and cultures (CL). Each of these can act as a planner or adopter or both. Thus change situations can be described in terms of 16 different configurational relationships between planners and adopters. (See Table 19.1.)

The change agent (enabler of change) must begin by defining the primary relationship between the configurations involved in a change episode. Is it dyadic change (I-I, such as a nurse-patient relationship)? Is it basically interinstitutional change (IS-IS, such as American Medical Association-Food and Drug Administration)? Is it organizational leaders seeking change within the organization (I-IS, such as a nursing administrator in a large hospital)? Is it a charismatic leader seeking to change a whole culture (I-CL, such as a senator going on TV and talking to people about a national health plan)? Or is it an industrialized society seeking to influence a developing nation in the Third World or a particular development sector in that nation (CL-CL, such as the United States seeking to help Thailand in AIDS prevention)?

It is important to define the essential overall configurational relationship of the change in question, remembering that large-scope configurational relationships always are mediated by and through small-scope configurational relationships: For example, a CL-CL relationship necessarily will be mediated by a multiplicity of intermediate and molecular configurational relationships (Bhola, 1986, 1988).

2. The CLER model calls attention to linkages to carry communications both *between* and *within* the planner and adopter systems. It also calls attention to formal and informal linkages—both horizontal and vertical between and among actors (Bhola, 1988).

3. Environment can be seen as the "most outlying" configuration within which all the change transactions are taking place. Environments can be inhibitive, neutral, or supportive, are seldom static, and sometimes may be deliberately

manipulated. Planner and adopter systems engaged in a change transaction will not necessarily be responding to the same single environment (Bhola, 1988).

4. The CLER model elaborates six types of resources: cognitive (aid in understanding substance and process of change), influence (arising from power and goodwill), material (in-kind, cash), personnel, institutional (infrastructures), and time (Bhola, 1988).

Strategizing With CLER

[The concept of power has a central position in the CLER model. Bhola defined *power* as an active principle, an inherent characteristic of every living person. Inequality of power within and among groups and institutions makes possible such societal work as social change. Groups are power fields with multiple power transactions and controls among and between individual members. For Bhola, equating power with coercion and force creates a narrow and negative position (Bhola, 1972, 1973, 1974, 1975, 1991). The definition of change seen below typifies Bhola's stance on power.]

Change can be described as a movement from an existing to a preferred pattern of power relationships. Power is also the instrument for going from an existing to a preferred situation. Change should involve (a) empowering the powerless among those involved in the change relationship and (b) moral use of collective power to bring changes that are good for the collectivity. Significantly, the concept of power in the CLER model has been expanded to include both the exercise of power (A changing B's behavior, with B not necessarily willing) and the experience of power without having to exercise power on another (for example, experiencing the power of utopian imagination, of ideological invention, of sacrifice and service for the powerless and the neglected) (Bhola, 1988).

To use a model means to use the model's vocabulary and definitions and to accept and internalize its underlying conceptual and value structures. The model user must become situated within the value/theory framework of the model. General use of the model may be possible in some settings, while partial use may be adequate in certain situations. If theoretical and research knowledge is used from outside the boundaries of the model, it should be in agreement with the values and theoretical assumptions of the CLER model.

In modeling reality, an ensemble of interrelated components pertains. These interacting components include planners {P}, objectives {O}, and adopters {A}. (See Table 19.2.) In proposing the concept of an ensemble, we are accepting the mutually interactive relationship between and among {P}, {O}, and {A}, and the equality and openness of relationships between {P} and {A}. Change is seen not as something given by {P} to {A}, but as mutually invented. The adopter

TABLE 19.2 The {P} × {O} ×{A} Ensemble

{P}		{O}		{A}
The		The		The
Planner	×	Change	×	Adopter
System		Objective		System

SOURCE: From "The CLER Model: Thinking Through Change," by H. S. Bhola, 1994, *Nursing Management, 25*(5), p. 62. Copyright © by 1994 S-N Publications. Reprinted with permission.

system is seen as one that is enabled to restructure and renew itself. Ideally, the planner system will have changed as well.

At the same time, we are accepting the mutual shaping of {P}, {O}, and {A}, each by the other. Thus we do not accept {O} as immutable, something simply to be transferred into a new setting and inserted within the social fabric of a particular adopter system. Indeed, change objectives must be reinvented within each new context of change—of course, without compromising the integrity of the agreed-upon change objectives.

Conceptualization of the change episode as an ensemble implies also that the boundaries of both {P} and {A} will change more than once because of evolving definitions of change and because of changes in our perceptions and conceptions of the reality in which the change episode is embedded.

After having conceptualized the change situation as an ensemble of {P}, {O}, and {A}, descriptions of entities in the ensemble should be developed. These are called "initial" descriptions because corrections are anticipated, based on feedback and further repetitions of the whole cycle of thinking and doing.

1. Change objectives {O} typically are described in terms such as the following: to restructure, reform, revitalize, renew; to professionalize, to institutionalize, to change the organizational culture; to install a new technology within an organization; to teach a group new norms of collaboration, to help a group develop coherence, or task orientation; to teach individuals new information, attitudes and values, and so on.

Large-scope objectives (restructure, reform, install a new technology, and so on) must be broken into subobjectives, and ultimately into constitutive processes leading to action. The elaboration of objectives of change should lead to three-part "process-locus-indicator" chains that identify the process that will be performed (such as instruction, persuasion, motivation, trust building), the locus of the process (individual, groups, organization, community), and the indicator that will be accepted as evidence that preferred results have appeared.

2. Descriptions of {P} and {A} in the ensemble should be developed in C, L, E, and R terms. The Is, Gs, ISs, and CLs involved either as mediating configurations or as environment should be listed. Then a configurational map

showing overlaps, hierarchies, and other social-structural relationships should be developed. Formal and informal linkages between and within the various configurations should be noted. Together, the configurational maps and linkages will show both the location in the social system network where a planner can enter and the kinds of manipulations of C and L that are possible.

The location of the planner within the configurational map (employee versus consultant, higher versus lower location within the power hierarchy) must be made clear as it will affect both planning and implementation strategies. Resources available to both planner and adopter systems also should be identified clearly.

In conclusion, planning models do not actually discover any new substantive social scientific knowledge. These models are exercises in "the science of the artificial" and merely suggest new and perhaps more adequate ways of organizing existing knowledge so as to bring it to bear on real-life problems of defining and implementing change (Bhola, 1994).

Guidelines for Using CLER

The guidelines given below were adapted from a paper Bhola (1991) presented at a conference. These guidelines describe the phases that Bhola devised for use of the CLER. The chart in Appendix C, section C.2, provides sources of additional information.

When a planner confronts a change situation, he or she thinks first about the identity and social placement of those who will lead the change and those who will adopt the new way of doing things. Bhola advocated making a written description of planners, objectives, and adopters involved in the situation—the $\{P\} \times \{O\} \times \{A\}$ ensemble. As they make descriptions, planners remember that planner and adopter boundaries will change more than once. Some adopters will become planners; some planners might leave. As they work, planners will see the situation differently than they did at first.

Early in the change process, planners describe the objectives of change. They start with an overarching vision that they, together with other stakeholders, "will" invent. Bhola suggested an initial description of plans for change as a crutch to get the dialectical process started. Such a statement might include the identification of the system, a definition of needs, and plans for building conviction. The description will include plans for development of solutions (innovations) and thoughts about implementation of plans. It also will have plans for the evaluation and replanning that will follow as planners apply their plan in the real world.

Collaboration is the most important aspect of the CLER model. In collaboration, planners and adopters function as equals. The CLER model values planners for their scientific knowledge and adopters for their knowledge of the social system; together, these two kinds of knowledge make up what Bhola called a "socio-logic" of processes. Planners start collaboration with representatives of other groups as soon as possible. The fact that they recognize adopters as stakeholders ensures changes in the tentative plans they already have made. Thus planners must prepare themselves mentally and functionally to make several repetitions of the $\{P\} \times \{O\} \times \{A\}$ ensemble as the perceptions of individual planners and adopters develop into collective plans for the change process.

Next, planners, together with adopters, develop an adequate (though not complete) configuration map that shows the social units involved—a graphic representation of the social situation in CLER terms. They picture configurations and linkages that exist among configurations. (See Figure 19.1.) Planners then convert the configuration map into a power map that pictures the types of power (social, economic, political, coercive, persuasive, moral) in the situation. They take care to show linkages among centers of social power. They, in collaboration with all possible stakeholders, discuss the strategies and tactics that would increase the likelihood of change. They think about ways of dealing with linkages (manipulating CLER nets by maintaining, strengthening, cutting, or building linkages) to favor change.

At this point, planners must analyze the implications, for both planners and adopters, of the objectives they devised earlier. For example, the innovation might need a more user-friendly design than originally planned. Planners might need additional knowledge of the local social situation in making specific plans for strategies or in resequencing strategies and tactics. The achievement of objectives might need a slower schedule than they first thought. In their analysis, planners check out their plans with both codified social science knowledge and with the experiential knowledge available from stakeholder groups.

Bhola (1973) advocated the use of a Program Evaluation and Review Technique (PERT) chart for planning change. A PERT chart has a time orientation that allows planners to organize separate actions in an orderly sequence. According to need, planners can develop the chart to include such considerations as individual assignments, performance standards and regulations, expected outcomes of tactics, dates, and costs. Attention to the expected outcomes of actions allows planners to sequence tactics in ways that cause former actions to benefit later actions in a synergistic manner.

To summarize, planners *order* and *relate* elements (the ordering/relating function in the grammar of action) in the change situation through initial configuration mapping and linkage typing. On the basis of collective human wisdom, they *expect typical* behaviors (the expecting/typifying function) from people holding membership in certain groups. As they progress through the activities listed on their PERT charts, they experience the social situation and correct (the experiencing/correcting function) their plans as needed. They can

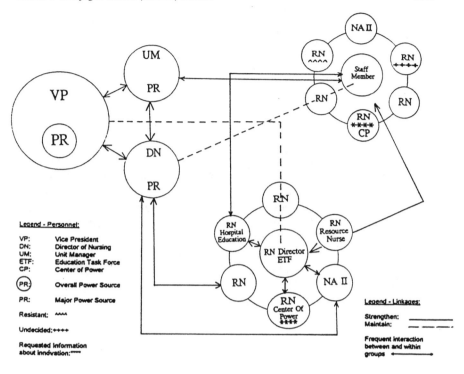

Figure 19.1. Sample Configuration Map for One Hospital Unit

SOURCE: From a configuration map by Katie Wilson, MS, RN, Dayton, OH. Adapted and used with permission of the author.

adjust both the nature of the innovation and the proposed strategies and tactics by which they work toward its adoption (Bhola, 1984). By the very nature of the iterations of the $\{P\} \times \{O\} \times \{A\}$ ensemble, evaluation takes place constantly, from the very beginning of the change effort. Planners evaluate the quality of the objectives for the change episode, the innovations that fulfill the objectives, and the procedures employed for producing change.

Summary

Bhola (1994) designed CLER

as a model for planning and implementing change in interpersonal, institutional, and cultural settings. It is useful for generating other models by modeling reality as actually encountered by planners and adopters. The CLER model is related philosophically to systems thinking (that there is interdependence among social entities), dialectical thinking (that there is mutual shaping among social processes), and constructivist thinking (that human beings take part in creating their own reality). (p. 59).

Bhola (1991) also furnished the following practical guidelines for the use of the CLER model. CLER model users make initial descriptions of planner and adopter systems and think about objectives for the change. They remember that boundaries between planners and adopters will change. Early in the change effort, they invite serious collaboration and think about the necessity of replanning objectives and strategies. They develop a configuration map into a power map as a basis for their strategic and tactical plans. They analyze implications of the objective. A PERT chart helps them provide a workable sequence for the strategies and tactics they plan for the manipulations of what Bhola called CLER nets (linkages). They know that during implementation, they may have to alter the objective of change to fit the reality of the situation. Wise planners provide for evaluation from the beginning of the change event.

References

Berger, P. L., & Luckmann, T. (1967). *The social construction of reality*. New York: Doubleday.

Bhola, H. S. (1965). A theory of innovation diffusion and its application to Indian education and community development. *Dissertation Abstracts International, 27*(01), 135A.

Bhola, H. S. (1972). *Configurations of change: An engineering theory of innovation diffusion, planned change, and development*. Bloomington: Indiana University School of Education.

Bhola, H. S. (1973). *Planning, programming, and administration of functional literacy*. Bloomington: Indiana University. (ERIC Document Reproduction Service No. 901 555)

Bhola, H. S. (1974). *ETV in the Third World: A diffusionist's perspective*. Bloomington: Indiana University. (ERIC Document Reproduction Service No. ED 098 926)

Bhola, H. S. (1975). The design of (educational) policy: Directing and harnessing social power for social outcomes. *Viewpoints, 51*(3), 1-16.

Bhola, H. S. (1977). *Configurations of change: The framework for a research review*. (ERIC Document Reproduction Service No. ED 127 702)

Bhola, H. S. (1984, November). *Tailor-made strategies of dissemination: The story to theory connection*. Paper presented at the Seventh Nationwide Vocational Education Dissemination Conference, Columbus, OH. (ERIC Document Reproduction Service No. ED 253 728)

Bhola, H. S. (1986, October). *Pathways to effective dissemination: Configuration mapping and linkage typing as tools*. Paper presented at the Ninth Nationwide Vocational Education Dissemination Conference, Columbus, OH. (ERIC Document Reproduction Service No. ED 273 781)

Bhola, H. S. (1988). The CLER model of innovation diffusion, planned change, and development: A conceptual update and applications. *Knowledge and Society: An International Journal of Knowledge Transfer, 1*(4), 56-66.

Bhola, H. S. (1991, December). *Designing from the heart of an epistemic triangle: Systemic, dialectical, and constructivist strategies for systems design and systems change.* Paper presented at the Third Annual Conference of Comprehensive Systems Design of Education organized by the International Systems Institute, Asilomar Conference Center, Monterey, CA.

Bhola, H. S. (1994). The CLER model: Thinking through change. *Nursing Management, 25*(5), 59-63.

Elster, J. (1983). *Sour grapes: Studies in the subversion of reality.* Cambridge: Cambridge University Press.

Kahneman, D., Slovic, P., & Tversky, A. (Eds.). (1982). *Judgment under uncertainty: Heuristics and biases.* Cambridge: Cambridge University Press.

Major, M. B. (1986). A configurational analysis of planned change: The professionalization of nursing. *Dissertation Abstracts International, 46*(10), 2992A.

Richardson, J. (1984). *Models of reality.* Mt. Airy, MD: Lamond.

Tiffany, C. H. (1977). Nursing, organizational structure, and the real goals of hospitals: A correlational study. *Dissertation Abstracts International, 38(11),* 5283B.

Zajc, L. (1987). Models of planned educational change: Their ideational and ideological contexts and evolution since the late 1950s. *Dissertation Abstracts International, 48*(05), 1063A.

Analysis and Critique of Bhola's Configurations (CLER) Model

This chapter contains two parts. First, it presents an analysis of Bhola's Configurations (CLER) Model. Second, it provides a critique of the model.

Analysis of the CLER Model

The analysis of the CLER model includes descriptions of the model, the purposes of the model, and relationships among model concepts. The analysis continues with three sections that introduce the three main divisions of the model that stem from systems theory, dialectics, and constructivism.

General Description of the Model

The CLER model is a change-planning model, not a change-watching model. It was devised to help planners design change for social systems. As a model "for all purposive action—to define, to design, to implement and evaluate, in all cultures,

274

in all sectors and at all levels, in conditions of consensus and conflict" (Bhola, 1991, p. 7), this model applies to a wide variety of situations and disciplines.

Purposes of the Model

The explicit objective of the CLER model is to give social activists a tool for planning change. This general objective finds expression in four purposes: definition, design, implementation, and evaluation. The definition purpose directs planners to describe a social situation and to work with its members to determine whether or not the situation demonstrates a need for change. Design concepts guide planners as they work with adopters to develop or choose solutions to social problems. These solutions may be simple and discrete or they may be as complex and extensive as redesigning an institution or overhauling an illness-care delivery system. Third, this model guides implementation; it offers suggestions for the interventions by which social planners help social systems move from old ways to new ways. Last, those who use the model according to its intent will find that they created patterns for evaluation when they carried out definition, design, and implementation activities.

The CLER model contains at least three implicit purposes: to increase the efficiency of planning activities, to prompt planners to think broadly and deeply enough to plan effective change, and to urge planners to invite the collaboration of adopters when planning change.

The CLER model deals with person and environment as these concepts relate to social change. It does not specifically mention health or nursing. Its generality makes it applicable in a wide variety of situations. On a practical level, it either describes real-world events, situations, and processes or provides mechanisms through which planners can make their own descriptions. Model formulation definitely progresses from very broad and abstract ideas to discussions that suggest action-oriented concepts that guide planners in practical ways. The model explains several real-world occurrences related to social interactions, power, and the acceptance of new ideas in a given population. Although it does not offer many predictions, it contains many statements about relationships that provide for predictions. The analysis found in this chapter relates most closely to a paper (1991) in which Bhola described the theoretical roots of his planned change model. It also relates to a paper (1994) he prepared specifically for nurse readers.

Relationships Among Concepts Within the Model

Bhola used selective borrowing. He based the CLER model of planned change on concepts from systems theory, dialectical thinking, and constructivism. These borrowed concepts serve as organizing principles. Concepts in this model are consistent with one another; they do not compete. Definitions for the concepts successfully differentiate among them. In the paper from which this analysis was derived, Bhola (1991) defined most concepts solely by implication, leaving them unclear. Nevertheless, clear definitions for the same concepts exist elsewhere (Bhola, 1972a, 1972b, 1982). Many definitions employ words not usually found in nursing literature, and some narrative examples use ideas not familiar to most nurses. Diagrams, charts, or graphics are in short supply and in several instances seem remote from the experiences of nurse readers.

Relationships in basic structures. The CLER model of planned change contains definite structures formed by explicit relationships. These usually take the form of lists of minor concepts that fall under a major concept. Some relationships connect the systems, dialectics, and constructivism divisions of the model. (See Figure 20.1.) Even the minor concepts assume importance. Some earlier model versions contain concepts not found in the 1991 paper; some of these could be termed peripheral.

The explicit use of standards for diagnosis of social system problems seems absent from presentations of this model, an omission more apparent than real. Bhola's extreme care to include adopters in discussions of means and ends shows his attention to the ownership of the values that engender standards. No one can plan change in the ways mandated by this model without paying attention to the values of both planners and adopters.

The CLER model has many directional relationships, explanatory relationships, and descriptive relationships. Readers could transform some of these into predictions; many could become prescriptions. Almost all relationships show movement from broad to specific and from complex to simple. Most are discrete, but several overlaps provide points of connection between and among concepts stemming from the three foundational theories (systems, dialectics, constructivism). Through systems influence, the CLER model has a great many opportunities for feedback loops. These make the model much more circular than linear in nature.

Structures Organized by Systems Theory

Three structures (the CLER structure, the structure of configurational relationships, and the configuration-mapping/linkage-typing structure) arise from systems theory. The first of these (CLER) contains four major concepts (configurations, linkages, environments, resources), which correspond roughly to the main principles (inputs, processes, outputs, contexts) of systems theory. (Resources and configurations correspond to inputs; linkages relate to processes; objectives [innovations] correspond to outputs; and environments relate to

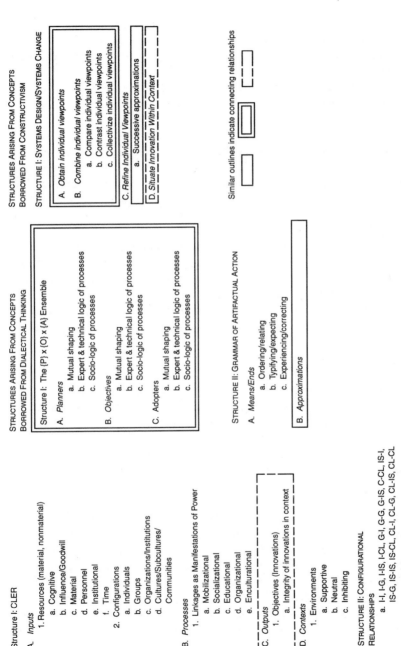

Figure 20.1. Graphic Representation of Relationships Among Concepts in Bhola's CLER Model

Structure I: CLER

A. *Inputs*

 1. Resources (material, nonmaterial)
    a. Cognitive
    b. Influence/Goodwill
    c. Material
    d. Personnel
    e. Institutional
    f. Time
 2. Configurations
    a. Individuals
    b. Groups
    c. Organizations/Institutions
    d. Cultures/Subcultures/
       Communities

B. *Processes*

 1. Linkages as Manifestations of Power
    a. Mobilizational
    b. Socializational
    c. Educational
    d. Organizational
    e. Enculturational

C. *Outputs*
 1. Objectives (Innovations)
    a. Integrity of innovations in context

D. *Contexts*
 1. Environments
    a. Supportive
    b. Neutral
    c. Inhibiting

STRUCTURE II: CONFIGURATIONAL
RELATIONSHIPS
 a. I-I, I-G, I-IS, I-CL, G-I, G-G, G-IS, C-CL, IS-I,
    IS-G, IS-IS, IS-CL, CL-I, CL-G, CL-IS, CL-CL

STRUCTURE III: CONFIGURATION MAPPING/
LINKAGE TYPING

STRUCTURES ARISING FROM CONCEPTS
BORROWED FROM DIALECTICAL THINKING

Structure I: The (P) x (O) x (A) Ensemble

A. *Planners*
    a. Mutual shaping
    b. Expert & technical logic of processes
    c. Socio-logic of processes

B. *Objectives*
    a. Mutual shaping
    b. Expert & technical logic of processes
    c. Socio-logic of processes

C. *Adopters*
    a. Mutual shaping
    b. Expert & technical logic of processes
    c. Socio-logic of processes

STRUCTURE II: GRAMMAR OF ARTIFACTUAL ACTION

A. *Means/Ends*
    a. Ordering/relating
    b. Typifying/expecting
    c. Experiencing/correcting

B. *Approximations*

STRUCTURES ARISING FROM CONCEPTS
BORROWED FROM CONSTRUCTIVISM

STRUCTURE I: SYSTEMS DESIGN/SYSTEMS CHANGE

A. *Obtain individual viewpoints*

B. *Combine individual viewpoints*
    a. Compare individual viewpoints
    b. Contrast individual viewpoints
    c. Collectivize individual viewpoints

C. *Refine Individual Viewpoints*
    a. Successive approximations

D. *Situate Innovation Within Context*

Similar outlines indicate connecting relationships

277

contexts.) Figure 20.1 illustrates this. The second structure contains minor concepts representing 16 possible combinations of configurations. The third structure (configuration mapping and linkage typing) combines elements from the CLER structure and from configurational relationships in a process for making practical descriptions of the local change situation.

Concepts that stem from systems theory generally are broad. The same is true for abstractness; almost all these concepts are quite abstract. Over half of the concepts refer to objects; over a third refer to properties; and only two (configuration mapping and linkage typing) represent an action mandated by the model.

The CLER structure. Two major concepts (resources, configurations) represent *inputs.* Minor concepts identify resources as concerned with cognition, influence, material, personnel, institutions, and time. Bhola divided resources into material and nonmaterial categories. The second major concept, configurations, represents inputs, which range from individuals to groups, institutions (organizations), and cultures.

The model's author chose linkages between and among configurations as a major concept to represent *processes.* Configurations, a static concept, comes alive with the addition of linkages. In keeping with the dynamic nature of systems theory, Bhola proposed several minor concepts that he termed *manifestations of power.* These include *mobilizational, socializational, educational, organizational,* and *enculturational* manifestations. These words name the various ways that planners foster change as they cut, form, maintain, or activate linkages between and/or within configurations.

Bhola designated objectives, which describe the terminal products that innovations produce, as *outputs.* Integrity of the innovation in terms of its context forms a minor concept stemming from the concept of objectives. The idea of integrity-in-context forms a link between concepts that stem from systems theory and those that stem from constructivist thinking.

The major concept of environments corresponds to the systems notion of *contexts.* Minor concepts describe environments as supportive, neutral, or inhibiting.

Configurational relationships. Configurational relationships form the second structure borrowed from systems theory. A configurational relationship is an association or connection between or among two or more configurations. One might take, for example, the relationship between a planner configuration and an adopter configuration. At times, adopters and planners may change roles. The chart provided by the model shows opportunity for 16 configurational relationships. (See Table 19.1.) Although this chart does not propose relationships with three or more configurations, model narrative provides for both dual and more complex relationships under a procedure called configuration mapping and linkage typing.

Configuration mapping and linkage typing. The third structure stemming from systems theory consists of the major concepts of configuration mapping and linkage typing. A configuration map is a diagram that shows social units important to a specific change event. Linkage typing on a configuration map adds lines that show communication linkages. Linkage typing mandates action by planners. Both configuration mapping and linkage typing require reduction of abstract representations of configurations, relationships, and actions into pictures that show important people, communication linkages, and communication actions in change episodes.

Structures Organized
by Dialectical Theory

Dialectics is a system of thinking that involves deliberation, conversation, and discussion. It also stresses the importance of both experience and study. Dialectics recognizes the significance of values held by participants. It prizes knowledge that works in practice. Dialectical thinking covers two basic structures in the CLER model: the $\{P\} \times \{O\} \times \{A\}$ ensemble and the grammar of artifactual action.

Concepts that stem from dialectical theory are slightly more specific and a little less abstract than those related to systems theory. Eight of the twelve concepts refer to objects; none relates to properties; four relate to actions mandated by the model. Concepts borrowed from systems theory tend toward conceptualization; those from dialectics tend toward action.

The $\{P\} \times \{O\} \times \{A\}$ ensemble. The $\{P\} \times \{O\} \times \{A\}$ ensemble forms the first structure that stems from dialectical thinking. It is composed of three major concepts (planners, objective, adopters). This structure also contains two very important minor concepts: the mutual shaping of planners and adopters and the combination of planners' expert knowledge and adopters' practice-oriented knowledge. These notions connect dialectical thinking with constructivism, the third concept Bhola borrowed as a foundation for the model. They require that planners compare, contrast, and fit together ideas that come from adopters, themselves, and other sources.

The grammar of artifactual action. The grammar of artifactual action is a tool that helps planners think logically about the social systems where they plan change. This grammar of artifactual action asks planners to picture people, events, and connections among people. It constitutes the second structure under dialectical theory. The structure contains two major concepts: means-ends and approximations. The means and ends concept contains three minor concepts (ordering/relating, typifying/expecting, experiencing/correcting). In ordering/ relating, planners make mental pictures of the social forces and human organizations involved in the change equation. In expecting/typifying, the planners picture people who are typical to certain kinds of circumstances and think about the actions these groups of people might take. Experiencing/correcting occurs when planners actually carry out some of their plans and correct their expectations so that they fit reality. These three components of the grammar of artifactual action suggest ways for planners to go about organizing situations to increase the likelihood of the occurrence of change. Approximations, the second major concept under the grammar of artifactual action, relates to the feedback loops inherent in systems theory. The approximations idea links dialectical thinking to constructivist thinking by appearing again, as a minor concept, under constructivism.

Structures Organized by Constructivism

Systems design/systems change. Constructivism covers only one structure: systems design/systems change. This structure contains four major concepts. The first of these shows concern for obtaining individual viewpoints, a point of connection between concepts from constructivist thinking and those from dialectical theory. The second major concept prompts planners to combine individual viewpoints. Minor concepts mandate that this occur under three modes of action: comparing ideas, contrasting ideas, and fitting ideas together. This demonstrates the constructivist end of the connection between dialectics and constructivism. The third major concept, repeated refinement of individual viewpoints, shelters the minor concept of a series of successive approximations, a touch point with both dialectics and systems theory. The fourth and last minor concept ensures the fit of the product within the context of the social system under consideration. This also forms a junction with systems theory. Thus concepts borrowed from constructivism exhibit connections with concepts borrowed from dialectics and systems theory.

 Constructivism is a school of thought that proposes the world is both found and made. In practical terms, this means that no planner starts with a totally new slate when planning change. Instead, planners must build from whatever already exists. Working with others in dialogue, they must take what they find in a situation and must make something "new" from it. Concepts that stem from constructivist thinking are slightly more specific and more abstract than those related to systems theory. Only two of the nine concepts refer to objects; none refers to properties; seven relate to actions mandated by the model. This gives the model a definite action orientation.

Assumptions of the Model

Explicit assumptions. The model developer started the 1991 discussion of his model with a dozen explicit assumptions, which he calls statements about "how the world works." They are as follows:

1. Social planning (he used the educational context as an example) has two very important facets: (a) intellectual knowledge as provided by professional planners and (b) social situation knowledge held by the adopting population.
2. Planners must make clear and honest declarations of their intentions.
3. Once they have publicized their values and visions for the future, planners realize that their values and visions must be in line with and respond to the particular setting and the specific historical time in which they work.
4. As they work with adopters, planners engage adopters in discussions about goals and ways of meeting goals.
5. Under this model, new ways of doing things get put into place a little at a time, not all at once. New ways and products come out of the ashes of old ones.
6. The specific placements of planners in social systems limit or increase their capacity to make change.
7. Only the drawing of wide boundaries will enable planners to anticipate all the social, economic, and political influences important to the change episode under consideration. If they fail to draw wide boundaries, problem diagnoses and solutions will miss their marks.
8. Planners must think in terms of systems theory (relationships), dialectical theory (dialogue), and constructivism (moving from what exists to fashion what "should be") as they work together with adopters to plan and carry out a change event.
9. Social systems change constantly.
10. Planners do not have to make choices between the two impossible extremes created by false dichotomies. False dichotomies include the unreal extremes of centralization and decentralization, of national and local purposes, of leadership and followership, and so on.
11. Planners think of themselves as engaging in open-ended encounters with adopters who have psychological, social, and cultural roles.
12. The designs that planners make must include not only the planners and their logic, they also must include the social aspects of adopters' lives and the important aspects of the social structures surrounding the change episode.

Implicit assumptions. This model assumes the ability of planners to conceptualize at a level sufficient to understand and use the concepts of the model. It also assumes that planners possess a reasonable amount of social and political savvy. It has positive regard for social activism and social responsibility. It values and encourages education, skill, and expertise, particularly in the area of social networking and social planning. The model assumes the goodness of the responsible use of social power. It values planning and places high value on collaboration and communication in both planning and intervention.

Critique of the CLER Model

As this section critiques the CLER model, it discusses the completeness and usefulness of the model and reports four nurse authors' requests for a model such as CLER. It also provides a critique of the model from a nonnursing source.

Completeness of the Model

Viewpoints in this book propose that any complete planned change theory has four parts. The four parts include a procedure for the diagnosis of social system problems, a means for either developing or choosing a solution (innovation) for dealing with the problem(s), provision for strategies and tactics, and a scheme for evaluation of the outcomes of the innovation and the quality of the change processes. Each theory part performs a vital function; the absence of one part cripples a theory to a greater or lesser extent. Bhola included all four of these parts in his CLER model of planned change; no serious CLER user can avoid attending to them.

Diagnosis in the CLER model starts when the planner first confronts the change situation. At this stage, the planner uses his or her own standards in developing hunches that a problem exists and in making an initial description of the problem situation to get the dialectical process going. Diagnosis continues as the planner involves adopters in collaborative actions that define needs and build conviction. Innovation choice or development occurs when planners and adopters devise objectives throughout iterations of the planning cycles mandated by the $\{P\} \times \{O\} \times \{A\}$ ensemble. Here, the choice or development of the innovation provides for collaboration between and among planners and adopters.

CLER's call for mapping configurations, typing linkages, making a power map, and developing a Program Evaluation and Review Technique (PERT) chart all verify the presence of a system for choosing and planning strategies and tactics. The experiencing and correcting phases of the grammar of artifactual action provide for implementation of strategies and tactics.

Bhola spun evaluation into the very fibers of the CLER model's warp and woof. Collaboration involves evaluation of worldviews in an integral way. Planners and adopters review objectives and the standards that engendered them throughout the iterations of the $\{P\} \times \{O\} \times \{A\}$ ensemble. Also, the experiencing and correcting phases of the grammar of artifactual action necessitate evaluation.

Usefulness of the Model

Bhola (1991) provided 14 guidelines for the use of the CLER model of planned change. These instructions, taken together with material from Bhola's other writings, assist planners who use the model. Additionally, the model reasonably could serve as a framework for organizational analyses or as a conceptual base for diffusion research or other change-related research. Its use would upgrade any planner's attempts to increase participation of adopters in change events. In logical extensions, this model would combine well with the nursing process, with strategic planning models, and with research utilization models. It also would expedite nurses' efforts to assist patients who have problems complying with treatment regimens and health promotion practices. The model would work well in local situations or in community or national situations. Users of the CLER model who limit its application to simple problem-solving situations will fail to tap the capacity of the model to assist planners in difficult and complex circumstances.

Readers interested in learning to use the CLER model in national, regional, or statewide change projects or in legislative/government situations could start by drawing parallels between the model and the founding of the National Center for Nursing Research (NCNR; now a national institute). Nurse planners could view and analyze the National League for Nursing video production (Moss, 1986) titled *A Case Study in Shaping Health Policy: The National Center for Nursing Research*. As this video depicts the political processes at work in the founding of the center, it shows how key political figures, nurse leaders, and lobbyists shaped the legislation that authorized the center. Viewers could identify configurations (administration, National Institutes of Health, medical community, Congress, nurse leaders, lobbyists, and so on) and linkages within and between configurations. They also could recognize pertinent factors in the environment of change and name the resources necessary for the change to take place. The NCNR situation exemplifies CLER's theoretical foundations—systems theory, dialectics, and constructivism. It also demonstrates the concept of successive approximations inherent in the $\{P\} \times \{O\} \times \{A\}$ ensemble. The award-winning video clearly parallels the concepts of the theory and thus furnishes an efficient learning experience.

Bhola's CLER model, which was presented in Chapter 19, has philosophical roots that relate quite closely to nursing perspectives. Nurses who plan social change would do well to use the power of the CLER model even if its language and conceptualizations at first seem unfamiliar to them.

Nurse Authors Voice a Need

Some nurse authors recently have voiced concerns about the inability of popular change theories to meet nurses' needs. Bircumshaw (1990), Gibbs (1991), and Hawkett and Glen (1991) applied some of the most familiar planned change theories to nursing problems in complex situations. All four authors reported a philosophical and ideological void.

Bircumshaw (1990), in an article on the utilization of research findings in clinical nursing practice, briefly described the Lewin and Rogers theories. As she used these two theories in a local situation, she wrote that they explain change processes in simplistic terms inappropriate to real-world situations. CLER provides for the kinds of situational complexities that Bircumshaw noted. CLER facilitates categorization, codification, and control of change phenomena that otherwise might derail plans for change.

Gibbs (1991) wrote about cultural and political limitations of what he called a rational approach to planned change. He did not dismiss rational approaches, such as those posited by Lewin and Rogers, but observed that their proper application involves a great deal of dialogue. A change theory that follows the suggestions offered by Gibbs would resonate with the dialectical and constructivist foundations of Bhola's CLER model.

Hawkett and Glen (1991), in the same vein, advised nurses to abandon simplistic thinking about planned change. They advocated a truly dialectical approach to the management of change, which they said would allow change planners to combine multiple elements that, on the surface, appear contradictory. Polarized arguments conducted under a dialectical system foster workable and realistic plans for change. Their recommendations suggest a change theory with foundations similar to the dialectical and constructivist roots of the CLER model.

CLER Crosses Disciplinary Boundaries

After an analysis of relevant literature, Havelock (1973) discussed models of dissemination and use of knowledge. In his overview and synthesis, he presented several perspectives assumed by such models. These included the research, development, and diffusion (RD&D) perspective; the social-interaction (S-I) perspective; the problem-solver (P-S) perspective; the concept of linkage; and other perspectives.

In the part of his discussion related to the S-I perspective, Havelock noted that educators then commonly believed that S-I models deal only with individual adopters rather than larger social units such as those found in institutions (like hospitals or health care systems). He considered this belief categorically false and mentioned numerous research instances in which the primary unit of investigation was the social unit rather than the individual. This observation led Havelock (1973) to comment that

> this remarkable consistency of major S-I findings in widely different settings has led Bhola to propose a "configurational theory" of diffusion which permits comparative analysis of patterns of flow and relationships regardless of size and other differing characteristics of the specific adopting units studied. If the configuration is closely similar irrespective of time, circumstances, and unit size, the significance of S-I research findings is enormous, because it means that generalizations from one set of findings in one setting can be applied, at least tentatively, to the analysis of other settings; diffusion research in agriculture and technology can then be used at the very least to make shrewd guesses in medicine, social welfare and education. It is a most significant step toward a general science and an engineering science of D&U processes. (Chap. 11, p. 10)

As Havelock (1973) noted, CLER permits comparisons and analyses of patterns and relationships in change situations. These analyses do not depend on size and types of social units. This characteristic of CLER assures its transferability from one discipline to another. Nurse planners could use the CLER model to advantage.

Summary

Analysis of the CLER model shows that it has three major divisions of concepts. These were borrowed from systems theory, dialectical thinking, and constructivism. The first structure related to systems theory addresses inputs, processes, outputs, and contexts in change situations. The second systems-oriented structure in CLER describes 16 possible relationships among configurations that range from the individual (I) to the culture (CL).

Dialectical thinking furnishes two structures. The first, $\{P\} \times \{O\} \times \{A\}$, mandates planner-adopter collaboration in the development of objectives and the choice of means to reach the ends specified by objectives. The second proposes a series of successive approximations (iterations).

Constructivism provides concepts of systems design and systems change in which planners and adopters obtain individual adopters' viewpoints in a series of successive approximations. The idea of successive approximations links constructivism and dialectics. Concern for the fit of the product of change with the context links constructivism with the outputs mandated by the systems theory foundation.

The CLER model equally values the technical knowledge supplied by planners and the social situation knowledge furnished by adopters. The model also expects planners to operate with clarity and honesty, to make public declarations of intentions, and to provide opportunities for negotiations concerning objectives. The model assumes incremental change specific to the situation at hand.

Further, the model assumes that planners will draw the boundaries of their change efforts widely enough to include whatever configurations are necessary for the success of the effort. It also assumes planners' willingness to think in terms of systems theory, dialectics, and constructivism as they work with the technical and social aspects of the change situation. Implicitly, the model assumes planners' ability to conceptualize in CLER terms. It assumes that the responsible use of social power is good, and it values planning and collaboration.

Examination of the CLER model shows that it contains all four parts considered necessary for a complete planned change theory. The model has wide usefulness in planned change, organizational analyses, and research utilization. It would apply well in management and clinical situations where nurses are dealing with health-related concerns. Several nurse authors have voiced a need for a model such as CLER. Havelock stated that the model possesses broad applicability.

The broadness and generality of the CLER model of planned change are at once its greatest assets and its greatest liabilities. These qualities offer almost limitless possibilities for application; those same qualities may confuse the uninitiated. The model's author employed some words seldom used in nursing textbooks or nursing literature. Nevertheless, the model's values and concepts agree strongly with many nursing values.

References

Bhola, H. S. (1972a). *Configurations of change: An engineering theory of innovation diffusion, planned change, and development.* Bloomington: Indiana University School of Education.

Bhola, H. S. (1972b). Notes toward a theory: Cultural action as elite initiatives in affiliation/exclusion. *Viewpoints, 48*(3), 1-37.

Bhola, H. S. (1982). Planning change in education and development: The CLER model in the context of a mega model. *Viewpoints in Teaching and Learning, 58*(4), 1-35.

Bhola, H. S. (1991, December). *Designing from the heart of an epistemic triangle: Systemic, dialectical, and constructivist strategies for systems design and systems change.* Paper presented at the Third Annual Conference of Comprehensive Systems Design of Education organized by the International Systems Institute, Asilomar Conference Center, Monterey, CA.

Bhola, H. S. (1994). The CLER model: Thinking through change. *Nursing Management, 25*(5), 59-63.

Bircumshaw, D. (1990). The utilization of research findings in clinical nursing practice. *Journal of Advanced Nursing, 15,* 1272-1280.

Gibbs, A. (1991). Cultural and political limitations within a rational approach towards educational change. *Journal of Advanced Nursing, 16,* 182-186.

Havelock, R. G. (1973). *Planning for innovation through dissemination and utilization of knowledge.* Ann Arbor: University of Michigan, Institute for Social Research, Center for Research on Utilization of Scientific Knowledge.

Hawkett, S., & Glen, S. (1991). A corporate college of nursing and midwifery philosophy: A strategy for managing change. *Nurse Education Today, 11,* 327-334.

Moss, L. (Writer/producer). (1986). *A case study in shaping health policy: The National Center for Nursing Research* [Video]. (Available from the National League for Nursing, 350 Hudson Street, New York, NY 10014)

Altering the CLER
Model Square Peg

This chapter consists of three parts: a discussion of ways that key concepts of Bhola's Configurations (CLER) Model of planned change fit with the Roy Adaptation Model (RAM), a translation of concepts from the CLER model from a RAM perspective, and the application of the translated CLER model in nursing situations at two levels—national and local.

Congruence of the CLER Model
With Key Concepts in the RAM

Change theories can enhance nursing theories. A look at the ways that a particular planned change theory coincides with or diverges from a nursing theory has worth because the two types of theories/models have different but valuable purposes. The CLER model, for example, specifically addresses processes of planned change that the RAM does not confront. In doing so, CLER considers concepts of social power, social configurations, communication linkages, innovation development, and resources not found in the RAM. The CLER model asks users to engage in their own model making as they enter a planned change episode; it enables users to design social interactions that encourage social change. The RAM, on the other hand, addresses specific nursing concerns not considered by the CLER. A nurse user would look at the CLER through a nursing perspective that includes nursing's four metaparadigm concepts (person, environment, health, nursing) to picture planned change within the context of the wholeness of an individual in a particular environment. Another basic difference appears in the fact that the CLER model of planned change aligns itself with a simultaneous action worldview while the RAM espouses a reciprocal action worldview.

Although the CLER and the RAM differ, both models focus on wholes and assume that individuals are integrated and organized entities. Moreover, they both view individuals as adaptive as well as holistic. The CLER model, like the RAM, is a systems model; both contain inputs, processes or controls, outputs, and feedback loops.

Person

In the RAM, the person is the recipient of nursing care; the person in the CLER model is the adopter of change. Adopters are recipients of the care or attention provided by nurses, who are the principal planners of change. Individual adopters are configured (C in CLER) into social units such as families, groups, communities, or nursing staff organizations. The notion of configurations is congruent with theoretical work within the RAM that extends the concept of person to pluralities of individuals and interactional units (DiIorio, 1989; Lutjens, 1992, 1994; Roy, 1983, 1984; Roy & Anway, 1989; Schultz, 1988). Roy and Anway (1989) derived a theory to apply the RAM to administration (RAMA) for use in organizations. Communication connects planners to adopters and individuals within social units. Communication linkages (L in CLER) between planners and adopters parallel nurse-client interactions as planner-adopter interactions. Dialogue is critical in both models. Just as planners and adopters are influenced by each other in the CLER model, so too are nurses and clients mutually influenced and shaped by one another.

Environment

The RAM uses the dictionary definition for *environment.* Environment (E in CLER) is similar to environment in the RAM. Inputs include all that is happening in the change environment. The RAM/RAMA categorizes *inputs* as focal, contextual, and residual stimuli in the environment. The *focal stimulus* is the specific situation or event that demands a response. Similarly, the CLER model assumes an event that makes the need for change evident to planners. *Contextual stimuli* are the situations or events that contribute to the occurrence of the focal stimulus. Some of these stimuli are under the control of planners; others are not.

Contextual stimuli can be identified and verified. They contribute to the influencing effect of the focal stimulus on the organization's ability to adapt to change. These stimuli add meaning to organizational behavior. Contextual stimuli can be measured. *Residual stimuli* are hunches, uncertainties, or unknowns. They cannot be or are not measured. Residual stimuli are the beliefs, attitudes, and feelings that potential adopters hold about the prechange situation. The adaptation level is changeable and represents the pooled effect of focal, contextual, and residual stimuli. It reflects the influence of the environment, as a whole, on the capacity of the organization to change.

The physical, role, interpersonal, and interdependence modes categorize ways of coping that characterize organizational behavior. These modes manifest the activity of the stabilizer and innovator adaptive subsystems described in the RAMA. The stabilizer subsystem maintains or provides stability for the organization, whereas the innovator subsystem provides for organizational innovativeness, change, and growth.

Health

Health is the process of moving toward integration and wholeness. According to the RAM, health is a product or state as well as a process. Health is attained when adaptation is effective. From a CLER perspective, adopters and planners proceed through the change process to achieve integrity. Planners and adopters expect that health as an end state will exist when change is fully implemented. Health exists when adopters have adapted to the change and the sense among planners and adopters is that the new situation is good—not perfect—but good.

The goal of nurse caregivers is to promote the adaptation of clients via the nursing process. Similarly, the goal of planners is to promote adaptation of the adopters to the change that has been mutually agreed upon. Planners promote adaptation by optimizing the interaction or communication linkages (L) between planners and adopters and between adopters (C) and the environment (E). The purpose of communication linkages is to attain the goals of the change process. The change process, which requires resources (R in CLER), is the method that planners use to promote adaptation and, thereby, health.

Nursing

Similarities exist between the nursing process described by the RAM and the change process described by CLER. The ensemble of nurses, goals, and clients in the RAM and the ensemble ($\{P\} \times \{O\} \times \{A\}$) of planners $\{P\}$, objectives $\{O\}$, and adopters $\{A\}$ described in CLER parallel one another. Both the nursing process and the change process are problem-solving methods. Both processes are cyclical with overlapping steps. The two steps of the change process according to the CLER model (problem setting and problem solving) are compatible with the six steps of the nursing process according to the RAM (assessment of behavior, assessment of stimuli, nursing diagnosis, goal setting, intervention, and evaluation).

Assessment and diagnosis of a social problem are parts of the problem-setting step in the CLER model. In problem setting, planners assess the behaviors of potential adopters within the social unit (first-level assessment) and make an initial determination as to whether the behaviors are ineffective or adaptive. Behaviors are categorized within the four CLER elements (configurations, linkages, environment, resources) in a way similar to the categorization of organizational behaviors within four adaptive system modes in the RAM applied to administration (RAMA): physical, interpersonal, role, and interdependence. Second-level assessment identifies environmental stimuli influencing the social situation. Assessment provides a description of the social situation that leads to the diagnosis of a social problem.

The goal-setting, implementation, and evaluation steps of the nursing process correspond to the problem-solving portion of the CLER model. Mutual goal setting is a strong value in the CLER model just as it is in the RAM. The CLER, as a constructivist model, uses the change process as a way for people to construct a preferred future; nurses use the RAM to help clients to construct preferred futures. After planners and adopters have mutually devised objectives, they design ways to implement the change. The CLER model encourages planners to empower adopters so that adopters may realize their preferred futures. Likewise, the RAM encourages planners to empower clients for the same purpose. The role of the nurse as client advocate exemplifies the moral use of power described in the CLER model. Evaluation of the success or failure to meet the objectives of the change process is as critical as the evaluation of the success or failure to meet the goals of the nursing process. The information gained from evaluation (*output* in systems terminology) is fed back just as it is in the nursing process. Outcomes of both the change process and the nursing process concern the adaptation of the recipients of "care," whether they are adopters or clients.

In summary, the CLER model is similar in many ways to the RAM. Both hold a worldview of change as inherent, natural, and continuous; both are systems models. Realization of the potential of adopters and clients is emphasized, and progress is valued in both models.

People are viewed in both models as systems capable of adaptation. Both models attend to the environment, although the CLER model devotes effort mainly to the external environment whereas the RAM considers the internal as well as the external environment. Although CLER does not speak of health, it does speak of integrity. Health is defined as integrity in the RAM. Both models have a process to achieve the mutually developed goals of the planner-adopter or nurse-client, and both value mutuality.

Not unlike the RAMA, which extends its view of person to include social units, the CLER model talks about four basic social configurations: individuals (I); groups (G), which could include families; institutions and organizations (IS); and communities, subcultures, and cultures (CL). The CLER model asserts that each of the four configurations can act as planners or adopters, or both. The same can be said within the RAM perspective; nurses can be recipients of care within any of the basic social configurations (units) noted by the CLER and the RAM models. Moreover, the concept of social configurations (C in CLER) is congruent with the concept of the physical adaptive system mode in the RAMA.

A RAM-CLER Change Process

Both the Roy Adaptation Model applied to administration (RAMA) and the CLER view social units as adaptive systems capable of responding positively to change. The RAMA extends the conceptualization of person to pluralities of persons, configured as organizational units (IS configuration in CLER) and communities (CL configuration in CLER). This extension provides a nice fit with the CLER model for planning change by taking advantage of CLER's ability to handle complex social configurations.

The focus of CLER on community and cultures (CL configuration in CLER) as targets for social change fills a void for nurse planners who practice with large and diverse social units and who practice within a multidisciplinary group to deal with multifaceted social problems. This model provides a timely addition to nursing's knowledge base as the practice of nursing moves into the community.

The Problem-Setting Step of the Change Process

Assess behavior. A combined RAM-CLER change process assesses the behaviors of the social unit targeted for change. These behaviors can be categorized within the RAMA adaptive system modes. The physical adaptive system mode includes the configuration of the social unit (C in CLER) and available resources

(R in CLER). The interpersonal adaptive system mode includes the communication linkages (L in CLER) among members of the social unit.

The role adaptive system mode comprises the actions and/or duties of members of the social unit. The interdependence adaptive system mode recognizes the interface and relational behaviors including communication linkages (L in CLER) both within as well as outside the social unit, that is, the environment (E in CLER) in which the social unit is embedded. For example, a nurse who is a member of a planned change team (IS or G configuration in CLER) that desires to make a change in the health of a small tribe (CL configuration in CLER) would assess tribal health behaviors (physical adaptive system mode). Another team member would assess health-related resources such as the waste management system (physical adaptive system mode) that affects health behaviors. The nurse planner also would assess the social behaviors/duties of members of the tribe such as the shaman (role adaptive system mode), how the shaman interacts with tribal members (interpersonal role adaptive system mode), and the congruence between tribal health behaviors, as guided by folk practitioners, and Western health behaviors, as guided by professional practitioners (interdependence adaptive system mode). This step is characterized by the gathering of behavioral data. Planners, in collaboration with members of the social unit, decide whether the identified behaviors, as a whole, constitute an adaptive or ineffective response to the environment. The ongoing and widespread presence of a condition such as dysentery would be indicative, for example, of an ineffective response.

Assess stimuli and diagnose. Second-level assessment challenges the nurse planner to identify environmental stimuli that influence the behavior of the social unit that creates or exemplifies the problem. For example, a high incidence and prevalence of dysentery among tribal members may be the focal stimulus that prompts attention from the health ministry of a developing country. Contextual stimuli may include lack of knowledge of the relationship between hand-washing and disease prevention, or lack of available water for hand-washing. A residual stimulus might be distrust of outsiders, such as the planned change team. The three types of stimuli considered together constitute the adaptation level of the tribe, considered as a whole, and include the four elements of the CLER model. Use of the RAM-CLER change process facilitates the thorough and broad approach necessary for a complex social problem.

The Problem-Solving Step of the Change Process

Set goals. Constructivism accommodates multiple realities fabricated by more than one person in terms of their own individual experiences. It relates to the development of an emerging reality in a situation already partly constructed; the world is both found and made (Bhola, 1991). The CLER, as a constructivist model, uses the change process to help social units construct a better situation, a preferred future.

Dialectics is a method of systematic reasoning that involves dialogue and seeks to resolve internal contradictions by relating human behavior to its historical and social contexts (RAM's environment). Dialectics emphasizes both change (RAMA's innovator subsystem) and stability (RAMA's stabilizer subsystem) but the future takes precedence over the present (Bhola, 1991). When planners and adopters working together in a dialectical exchange try to organize things for the better ($\{P\} \times \{O\} \times \{A\}$ ensemble), they start with goals that vivify the preferred situation. Goals state desired behaviors of members of the social unit.

Intervene. Planners and adopters together devise strategies and tactics (dialectical thinking) to accomplish their mutually developed goals. When working with social units representing cultures unlike that of the planners, planners are especially careful to learn from adopters what interventions will work best and also the best ways to intervene with the particular social unit (dialectical thinking). Strategies and tactics are developed to eliminate, modify, inhibit, or enhance stimuli in the environment, especially the focal stimulus, that contribute to a change occurring in the direction of the mutually preferred future. Planners help adopters help themselves so as to create and sustain the change that will embody the preferred future (constructivism).

Evaluate. Planners and adopters together discuss and evaluate their success with regard to strategies and tactics and progress toward mutually established goals ($\{P\} \times \{O\} \times \{A\}$ ensemble). Some strategies and tactics will need changes and/or refinement. The initial strategies and tactics are considered successive approximations and a natural part of the learning curve. The goals state behavioral changes that constitute an adaptive response. Acceptance and use of the new behaviors indicate adaptation.

The process of change occurs at many different levels in society. The first example seen below recounts a real-life situation at the highest level in the United States and retrofits concepts in the RAM-CLER change process to the situation. The second example applies the RAM-CLER change process to a fictitious situation at a local level.

Application of the RAM-CLER
Process to a National Nursing Situation

The national scene (E in CLER). The Agency for Health Care Policy and Research (AHCPR) was established by the Omnibus Reconciliation Act of 1989 as one of eight agencies of the Public Health Service (PHS) within the Department of Health and Human Services (DHHS). Personnel for the agency included eight doctorally prepared nurses. The agency replaced the National Center for Health Sciences Research and Health Care Technology Assessment (CLER's successive approximation). According to the AHCPR (1990), it has primary responsibility for the Medical Treatment Effectiveness Program (MEDTEP).

MEDTEP is a research program that expands the work of its predecessor, the Patient Outcome Assessment Research Program (POARP). (This represents another successive approximation, in which a new program was fashioned from the old one.) Under the auspices of the national center, studies conducted through the POARP during the past 20 years revealed wide variations in the type and amount of health care provided to apparently similar patients. These practice variations were associated with differences in patient outcomes and/or use of resources. Questions arising from this association between practice variation and patient outcomes prompted the establishment of MEDTEP, which replaced and expanded the POARP. According to AHCPR (1990),

> MEDTEP's major goal is to improve the effectiveness and appropriateness of [health care] practice by developing and disseminating scientific information regarding the effects of presently used health care services and procedures on patients' survival, health status, functional capacity, and quality of life. (p. 1)

Section 901 of Public Law 101-239, the Omnibus Budget Reconciliation Act of 1989, not only established AHCPR but mandated that the Agency Administrator (C in CLER), among other activities, develop clinical practice guidelines (the innovation). AHCPR convened an ad hoc advisory panel of nurses (an IS-G configurational relationship in CLER) six weeks after the creation of the new agency. This panel was to provide the nursing profession's perspective on its role in the overall MEDTEP initiative, with particular emphasis on guideline development.

The Problem-Setting Step of the Change Process

Assess behavior. A congressional review of two decades of studies constituted an assessment of the practice behavior of clinical health care providers, principally physicians. The behaviors indicated ineffective responses to the burgeoning Medicare entitlement program. Moreover, the health care expenditures did not necessarily result in demonstrably positive patient outcomes.

Assess stimuli. The focal stimulus that prompted action by Congress was swelling Medicare expenses. Contextual stimuli that contributed to the expenses included lack of a standard for effective and efficient treatment of common and/or costly health conditions as well as wide variations in practice patterns throughout the nation. Residual stimuli included uncertainty and the practice of "defensive medicine."

Diagnose. For this example, the diagnosis is wide variations in provider practice patterns related to lack of a national standard of care.

The Problem-Solving Step of the Change Process

Set goals. The goal is effective and efficient practice patterns that are consistent throughout the nation as evidenced by greater consistency in provider practice patterns, a decrease in Medicare costs, and demonstrably positive patient outcomes. Because the goal arises from the previous and present situations and sets a preferred national future for health care, it illustrates constructivism. Traditional patient outcomes, primarily viewed from a medical perspective, are morbidity, mortality, hospitalizations, and clinical improvements. Other more directly related patient outcomes produced by nursing interventions include a decrease in occurrence of symptoms, alleviation of symptoms, prolongation of symptom-free periods, improvement in quality of life indicators, increase in patient satisfaction, improvement in health status or well-being, increase in patient satisfaction, and improvement in functional abilities. Nursing research to identify patient preferences, effects of intervening variables such as hardiness and social support, and factors underlying individual responses will yield nursing-sensitive data directly amenable to nursing interventions that are directly attributable to measurable nursing-sensitive patient outcomes.

Intervene. The U.S. Congress acted in the planner role when it created the agency (IS-IS configurational relationship in CLER; also, the creation of a linkage in CLER) and gave it primary responsibility for the MEDTEP program, which included the development of clinical practice guidelines. The strategy called for formation of panels of from 9 to 15 experts (IS-G configurational relationship in CLER) that crossed disciplinary boundaries to develop each guideline. Guidelines were developed for specific conditions and treatments. Criteria included high-risk conditions or treatments, those that affected large numbers of persons or demonstrated wide variations in treatments, and those that included costly services and/or procedures. In 1990, seven panels (G configuration in CLER) were convened; these included nurse and physician adopters as well as consumers. Planners (Congress) and adopters (panel) were interested in the development and dissemination of clinical practice guidelines (the innovation) that would improve the effectiveness and efficiency of clinical practice, thus leading to demonstrably positive patient outcomes at a reasonable cost (mutual shaping as in CLER's {P} × {O} × {A}).

The work of each panel included an extensive review of existing literature (R in CLER) on the condition. The Office of Science and Data Development within MEDTEP, which is responsible for increasing the quality and quantity of data, served as another resource (R in CLER) for panels. The panel synthesized the literature and thus created a research database for each specific guideline. Moreover, summary recommendations—a clinical protocol of sorts—were derived from each database and included in each guideline. In January 1991, three of the panels (pain management, pressure sore, urinary incontinence) submitted initial sets of guidelines to Congress (L in CLER). This communication between the panel and Congress (G-IS configurational relationship in CLER; also, L in CLER) illustrates dialectical thinking as each group mutually shaped and influenced the construction of a preferred national future for health care (constructivism). Panel members consulted (L in CLER) other experts (R in CLER) throughout development of the guidelines. Guidelines were pilot tested in health care organizations (R in CLER) before publication and distribution to the public. The guidelines constitute national standards for specific conditions.

Evaluate. The cost to U.S. taxpayers amounted to approximately $1 million, on average, per guideline. Short-term evaluation of the process of guideline development and distribution includes the quantity of guidelines distributed. Presumably, once the "word" is out, providers will change, albeit slowly, their patterns of practice. Realization of the goal, if at all, will be years in coming.

A major restructuring of the agency's guideline program was announced in April 1996 (AHCPR, 1996a). AHCPR no longer develops clinical practice guidelines as of fiscal year 1997, which runs from October 1996 through September 1997. AHCPR now partners with groups in the private and public sectors by providing evidence reports, decision analyses, literature summaries, and meta-analyses (R in CLER). In a further initiative to reinforce the new role of AHCPR as a science partner, the agency is funding Evidence-Based Practice Centers to produce evidence reports and technology assessments for use by health care organizations (AHCPR, 1996b). This restructuring should decrease the cost of guideline development. It also may facilitate the adoption of guidelines because their development within recognized private and public sector organizations carries more credibility with providers than does the development of guidelines by the government.

Application of the RAM-CLER Model
to a Local Nursing Situation

When providers in health care organizations review a clinical practice guideline and decide to use the research database and summary recommendations to change practice patterns (research utilization) to conform to the national standard, the change process starts anew on another level. The providers in the health care organization who decide to use the guidelines to change practice patterns become the planners, and the clinical providers whose practice they wish to change become the adopters. The change process involves development and dissemination of specific actions developed from a guideline and formatted for use in the specific organization. The specific actions arising from a guideline become the innovation. Thus a research utilization project is developed with the guideline serving as a database and its summary recommendations as a clinical protocol. The goal is for clinical providers to embrace the recommended actions by incorporating them into their practice on a long-term basis. (The Rogers Diffusion Model [RDM] often has been used to guide the dissemination process.) The following example illustrates the continued use of CLER in the change process at a local level.

The local scene (E in CLER). The nurse administrator of a small rural hospice agency noticed, on a regular review of nurses' documentation (a stabilizer subsystem), that pain intensity scores for clients with cancer seemed high (focal stimulus). This situation brought to mind a recently attended workshop that highlighted the recommendations offered in conjunction with the *Clinical Practice Guideline* on cancer pain from the Agency for Health Care Policy and Research (AHCPR).

The Problem-Setting Step
of the Change Process

Assess behavior. The nurse administrator, acting in the role of planner (caregiver), assessed the practice behaviors of the nurses (potential adopters) to manage the clients' pain (I-IS configurational relationship in CLER). The practice behaviors were categorized in the role adaptive system mode. The purpose of the assessment was to determine the degree to which practice behaviors were congruent with recommendations from the guideline (the standard of care). Based on this assessment, the planner concluded that the practice behaviors were ineffective in managing the clients' pain (problem diagnosis in CLER).

Assess stimuli. Dialogue (L in CLER) during a meeting with the planner and potential adopters (I-IS configurational relationship in CLER; an innovator subsystem) revealed the potential adopters' (recipients of care in this example are nurse caregivers) frustration at seeing clients in pain (focal stimulus). They reported that some clients feared addiction; others feared a "drugged" state that would leave them less alert to interact with family and friends (L in CLER). Some potential adopters feared the same things for clients (contextual stimulus). Thus adopter fear supported the clients' fear of addiction. Fear was an environmental factor that could inhibit effective pain management. Others believed that they could be accused of hastening death by liberal use of analgesia (residual stimuli). (Caregivers who withhold analgesia, however well intended, exercise power over clients.) They freely voiced their uncertainty about how to manage cancer pain (contextual stimulus). Additionally, uncertainty in the environment inhibited the effectiveness of pain management.

Diagnose. The planner diagnosed the social problem as ineffective pain management related to lack of knowledge.

The Problem-Solving Step of the Change Process

At this point, the nurse administrator (planner) enlisted the help of a clinical nurse specialist to serve as coplanner. After the meeting, the planner sketched a configuration map to identify caregivers and others in the hospice agency who were sources of informal or formal power. The map included her perspective on their current positions on adopting pain management practices recommended by the *Clinical Practice Guideline.* She identified linkages to be strengthened or retained and noted interaction patterns between, among, and within individuals and groups.

Set goals. Just before meeting with adopters, the planner reviewed the configuration map and thoughtfully planned her actions. When the planner and potential adopters met together, they mutually developed and shaped objectives ($\{P\} \times \{O\} \times \{A\}$), which were to (a) change potential adopters' practice behaviors to be congruent with the guideline and (b) attain, on average, a client score of 4 or less on a 0-10 numeric pain intensity scale.

Intervene. The agency had adequate resources (R in CLER) for offering an educational program to teach potential adopters new practice behaviors (innovation) that would enable them to better manage pain in their clients. The clinical nurse specialist coplanner was knowledgeable about the guideline. The nurse administrator provided released time for her to prepare for and present the program. Moreover, she agreed that the program be offered on work time and caregivers paid "straight time" if they attended on off-duty hours. Typing and other clerical services were provided by a volunteer. The nurse administrator attended the first class to vocalize support for the program. This manifestation of organizational power set a positive tone for the educational program and for adoption of the innovation.

The *Clinical Practice Guideline* on cancer pain, adapted for the hospice agency, and a new plan of care developed for pain management (R in CLER) were used as teaching tools during the program (I-IS). The clinical nurse specialist coplanner used caregivers inclined to adoption as champions for the innovation. She deliberately presented supporting information from credible sources that challenged opinions and beliefs of resistant and undecided caregivers.

Evaluate. Three months after implementation of the educational program, the planner evaluated the adopters' practice behaviors (I-IS) and the clients' pain intensity scores. Nurse adopter behaviors, now more congruent with the guideline, resulted in client pain intensity scores, that were, on average, 4 or less on a 0-10 numeric pain intensity scale. Some inconsistency in behaviors remained. The planner decided to call a meeting to give a progress report that would celebrate success and reinforce areas for continued development and refinement. The planner and adopters agreed that, for the most part, the change objectives $(\{P\} \times \{O\} \times \{A\})$ had been met effectively and that they, as an organizational unit, were professionally healthier. They all agreed to another meeting in six months to provide information on the long-term integrity of the innovation.

This scenario vivifies the interdependence among social entities such as nurse administrators, clinical nurse specialists, caregivers, and clients. Such interdependence is characteristic of systems thinking (Bhola, 1994). It also provides at least two examples of dialectical thinking. The first is the mutual shaping and influencing processes among configurations by the nurse administrator seeking change in the small rural hospice agency (I-IS). The second is the dyadic change between nurse practice behaviors and client expressions of pain intensity (I-I). Constructivist thinking characterizes this scenario in which nurse adopters were instrumental in transforming their practice behaviors to create a preferred client outcome consistent with professional values.

Summary

This chapter pointed out many similarities between Bhola's CLER model for planned change and the Roy Adaptation Model. Both of these systems models focus on wholes, see individuals as parts of social units of varying size, and attend to matters related to the environment. The RAM sees health as a process of moving toward integration; CLER stresses system integrity. Both models value the mutuality that comes from dialogue and shared vision in the construction of a preferred future. The change process espoused by CLER resembles the nursing process; the CLER's problem-setting and problem-solving modes can be viewed as compatible with the six steps of the nursing process.

The chapter ends with an application of the RAM-CLER model in a nurse-related change situation at the national level and another situation, involving a performance discrepancy, at the local level. The first situation retrofits the RAM-CLER change process to a national situation that included nurses as members of a planned change team involving the health care industry. In the second situation, RAM and CLER concepts help a nurse planner devise and implement collaborative planning and a cooperative solution to the problem of ineffective pain management for persons ill with cancer in a hospice setting. The scenario brings to life the interdependence that exists among the various entities in a health care situation. It shows the professional and client-centered benefits of using a nursing perspective in the application of dialectical thinking and constructivism to the solution of a social problem.

References

Agency for Health Care Policy and Research. (AHCPR). (1990, March). *AHCPR program note.* Rockville, MD: U.S. Department of Health and Human Services.

Agency for Health Care Policy and Research. (AHCPR). (1996a, October). [Statement for public release]. Rockville, MD: U.S. Department of Health and Human Services.

Agency for Health Care Policy and Research. (AHCPR). (1996b, November). *AHCPR to help public and private groups develop tools for clinical improvement.* Rockville, MD: U.S. Department of Health and Human Services.

Bhola, H. S. (1991, December). *Designing from the heart of an epistemic triangle: Systemic, dialectical, and constructivist strategies for systems design and systems change.* Paper presented at the Third Annual Conference of Comprehensive Systems Design of Education organized by the International Systems Institute, Asilomar Conference Center, Monterey, CA.

Bhola, H. S. (1994). The CLER model: Thinking through change. *Nursing Management, 25*(5), 59-63.

DiIorio, C. K. (1989). Application of the Roy model to nursing administration. In B. Henry, C. Arndt, M. DiVincenti, & A. Marriner-Tomey (Eds.), *Dimensions of nursing administration: Theory, research, education, practice* (pp. 89-104). Boston: Blackwell Scientific.

Lutjens, L. R. J. (1992). Derivation and testing of tenets of a theory of social organizations as adaptive systems. *Nursing Science Quarterly, 5,* 62-71.

Lutjens, L. R. J. (1994). Hospital payment source and length-of-stay. *Nursing Science Quarterly, 7,* 174-179.

Roy, C. (1983). Roy Adaptation Model. In I. W. Clements & F. B. Roberts (Eds.), *Family health: A theoretical approach to nursing care* (pp. 298-303). New York: John Wiley.

Roy, C. (1984). The Roy Adaptation Model: Applications in community health nursing. In M. K. Assoy & C. C. Ossler (Eds.), *Conceptual models of nursing: Applications in community health nursing: Proceedings of the Eighth Annual Community Health Nursing Conference* (pp. 51-73). Chapel Hill: University of North Carolina.

Roy, C., & Anway, J. (1989). Roy's Adaptation Model: Theories for nursing administration. In B. Henry, C. Arndt, M. DiVincenti, & A. Marriner-Tomey (Eds.), *Dimensions of nursing administration: Theory, research, education, practice* (pp. 75-88). Boston: Blackwell Scientific.

Schultz, P. R. (1988). When client means more than one: Extending the foundational concept of person. *Advances in Nursing Science, 10,* 71-86.

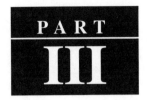

Planned Change
Theory in Practice

Theoretical Underpinnings for Nursing's Planned Change Research

Rather than give an in-depth critique of the specific methodologies used in nursing's planned change research, this chapter introduces ideas about kinds and quality of planned change theory usage in nursing research. The chapter starts with a discussion of general considerations important in the employment of planned change theories and continues with ideas about guidelines for planned change theory use in research situations. Brief reviews of nursing planned change studies follow. The chapter ends by citing planned change models developed by nurses.

Basic Considerations in Planned Change Theory Use

Appropriate planned change theory use starts with an accurate reading and understanding of a theory and its explicit and implicit basic assumptions.

Investigators who read a theory in its original form will find themselves more able to determine the nature of the theory's intent than will those who rely on secondary or tertiary sources for information.

Nurse investigators should select theories that fit their situations; not every planned change theory is appropriate in every situation. For example, nurses should differentiate between theories that watch change (diffusion theories) and theories intended to cause change (engineering theories). (Some diffusion theories provide implications for planning.) Certain theories require collaboration; others have a top-down, authoritarian stance that nurse investigators could find to be at odds with nursing values. Linear-recursive theories might feel comfortable to nurses who use the nursing process extensively. Perhaps a change theory with a gestalt viewpoint will fit best with the realities of the change environment. Researchers also consider units of analysis and levels of organizations when they choose from among planned change theories. Some theories see change as occurring in individuals who would subsequently spread the innovation by means of their influence as members of a group. Other theories see change as occurring in an organization that, in addition to organizational structure and technology, also contains individuals.

Those who use theory for planning change should propose from the start not only to cause change to occur but to evaluate progress toward goals during and after change. Although the development of some evaluation studies occurs after completion of a change, prior planning allows synchronization of evaluations with the initial theory that the planners used.

Guidelines: Planned Change Theory Use in Nursing Research

Nursing literature offers ideas that suggest guidelines for the use of planned change theory in nursing research. Recently, Fawcett (1996) provided four steps for including a conceptual model in a written research report. The steps relate to the identification of the model, the incorporation of concepts and propositions that guided the study, a statement of the influence of the conceptual model on study design, and an assessment of the credibility of the model. Useful before the fact as well as after research completion, Fawcett's discussion of the four steps suggests considerations important to nurses as they develop research projects that incorporate planned change theories.

Earlier, Silva (1986) identified 62 studies based on a total of five nursing models. She found that only 9 (15%) appropriately tested the models/theories. Subsequently, she developed seven criteria for evaluating studies that test nursing theories. Silva's 1986 study had two major strengths. First, it clarified a little-understood term (testing of nursing theory). Second, it distinguished between evaluation criteria for a general determination of the quality of nursing research and criteria for the quality of studies that test nursing theory (Silva & Sorrell, 1992).

Acton, Irvin, and Hopkins (1991) clarified and expanded Silva's seven original criteria in a list that contains 14 criteria for evaluating theory-testing research. When Silva and Sorrell (1992) noted the logical positivist approach of the criteria in both the original and the expanded lists, they presented descriptions of four philosophical approaches that suggest and support evaluation criteria for research designed to verify nursing theory. These include a logical positivist approach, critical reasoning, description of personal experiences, and application of theory to nursing practice. In their article, Silva and Sorrell recognized the expanded list of criteria for quantitative studies by Acton et al. and presented lists of criteria for theory testing under each of the three additional philosophical approaches.

The Fawcett (1996) steps, the Acton et al. (1991) list, and the Silva and Sorrell criteria (1992) all relate to the testing of nursing theories. Nevertheless, they all suggest guidelines for planned change theory usage in nursing research. They do this by delineating specific relationships between the philosophical foundations for the four approaches and the methods they use to link theory to empirical contexts. Nurses interested in planning or evaluating theory-based planned change research may wish to adapt the Acton et al. or Silva and Sorrell criteria that serve their purposes. They will need to make two kinds of adaptations. One concerns changing the name of the kind of theory under consideration from "nursing theory" to "planned change theory." Another adaptation pertains to the purpose of the study. Some studies that use planned change theory test the change theory itself; other studies evaluate the effects of a planned change episode or help in the planning of change. Nurses who develop studies designed to plan change can alter the problem-solving designation to a change-producing designation throughout the seven application-to-practice criteria. For the convenience of readers, three sets of criteria appear in boxes interspersed at appropriate positions throughout the following reviews of nursing planned change research. (The criteria for the critical reasoning approach appear in Box 22.2. None of the nursing research studies reviewed in this chapter used the critical reasoning approach.)

Review of Selected Nursing Planned Change Studies

The following reviews provide general descriptions of the ways that selected nursing studies relate to the guidelines described above. The reviews follow the sequence seen in Table 22.1.

**BOX 22.2: EVALUATION CRITERIA
TO VERIFY TESTING OF NURSING THEORY
THROUGH CRITICAL REASONING**

1. *The underlying philosophic assumptions regarding what constitutes truth in the testing of nursing theory are explicitly stated.*
2. *The testing of nursing theory is congruent with the philosophic assumptions regarding truth.*
3. *The method for testing nursing theory is congruent with the purpose for testing.*
4. *The purpose for testing is clearly stated and significantly advances nursing knowledge or method.*
5. *The testing of nursing theory is based on the simplest method needed to obtain the most valid and powerful results.*
6. *The testing of nursing theory is constructed so that comparable or similar verification can occur.*
7. *The testing of nursing theory lays the groundwork for an applied outcome.*
8. *The overall processes used in the testing of nursing theory exhibit internal consistency, aesthetic unity, and ethical integrity.*

SOURCE: From "Testing of Nursing Theory: Critique and Philosophical Expansion," by M. C. Silva and J. M. Sorrell, 1992, *Advances in Nursing Science, 14*(4), p. 17. Copyright © 1992 by Aspen Publishers. Used with permission of the publisher.

Examples: Research That Evaluates the Effects of a Planned Change Episode

Five diffusion studies (1982-1990). Five studies that evaluated the effects of planned change (Brett, 1987, 1989; Coyle & Sokop, 1990; Delaney, 1989; Kirchhoff, 1982) used selected concepts from the Rogers diffusion model as frameworks. These five studies assessed the impact of dissemination strategies by measuring the extent of the adoption of specified innovations. To a reasonable extent, each researcher followed adaptations of the Acton et al. (1991) criteria for quantitative research (the logical positivist approach). (See Box 22.3.) In all five studies, the authors proposed to evaluate the degree of diffusion of an innovation as a measure of the quality of dissemination strategies. All included, and most named, the Rogers diffusion model; some added concepts from other change models. All gave very brief discussions of the change model they used; some seemed to assume the readers' prior knowledge of the model in question.

TABLE 22.1 Selected Nursing Planned Change Studies

Kinds of Studies	Philosophical/Methodological Approaches to the Use of Planned Change Theory		
	Logical Positivism	Description of Personal Experience	Application to Nursing Practice
Evaluate the effects of a planned change episode	Kirchhoff (1982) Brett (1987, 1989) Delaney (1989) Coyle & Sokop (1990) Geis (1990) Perciful (1990, 1992)* Degerhammar & Wade (1991)* Dufault, Bielecki, Collins, & Willey (1995)* Mahoney (1995)		
Plan a change episode	Degerhammar & Wade (1991)*	Taft & Stearns (1991)	Pearcey & Draper (1996)
Test a planned change theory	Perciful (1990, 1992)* Dufault et al. (1995)*		
Other	McKenna, Parahoo, & Boore (1995)	Bellman (1996)	

*Some studies fall into more than one category.

Probably the strongest criticism of this group of five studies stems from the ways that they used the Rogers diffusion model in conjunction with their research designs and methods. Most of the studies pictured the process of diffusion through one-time data collection snapshots rather than through longitudinal designs. One study attempted a cross-sectional design, which, according to Rogers (1976), ill serves the linear and strongly time-oriented character of his model. Further, some of the researchers used selected organizational aspects of diffusion presented by Rogers without recognizing the fact that organizational concepts do not occupy an integral place in the Rogers diffusion model. Some of the researchers measured differing rates of adoption, a matter central to the Rogers model, without linking adoption rate to any other variable except by conjecture. None made any significant attempt to reconstruct specific message flows in a social system, as advocated by Rogers (1976). In the five studies, the variables

BOX 22.3: EVALUATION CRITERIA TO VERIFY TESTING OF NURSING THEORY THROUGH A LOGICAL POSITIVIST APPROACH

1. *The purpose of the study is to examine the empirical validity of the constructs, concepts, assumptions, or relationships from the identified theoretic frame of reference.*

2. *The theoretic frame of reference must be explicitly described and summarized.*

3. *The constructs and concepts to be examined are theoretically defined.*

4. *An overview of previous studies that are based on the theoretic framework, or that clearly show the derivation of the concepts being tested, must be included in the review of the literature.*

5. *The research questions or hypotheses are logically derived from the definitions, assumptions, or propositions of the theoretic frame of reference.*

6. *The research questions or hypotheses are specific enough to put the theoretic frame of reference at risk for falsification.*

7. *The operational definitions are clearly derived from the theoretic frame of reference.*

8. *The design is congruent with the level of theory described in the theoretic frame of reference.*

9. *The instruments must be theoretically valid and reliable.*

10. *The theoretic frame of reference guided the sample selection.*

11. *The statistics used are the most robust possible.*

12. *The analysis of data must provide evidence for supporting, refuting, or modifying the theoretic framework.*

13. *The research report must include an interpretative analysis of the findings in relation to the theory being tested.*

14. *The significance of the theory for nursing is discussed in the report.*

15. *Ideally, the researcher makes recommendations for further research on the basis of theoretic findings.*

SOURCE: From "Theory-Testing Research: Building the Science," by G. J. Acton, B. L. Irvin, and B. A. Hopkins, 1991, *Advances in Nursing Science, 14*(1), pp. 56-59. Copyright © 1991 by Aspen Publishers. Used with permission of the publisher.

chosen for study and the instruments devised to measure them do flow roughly from the Rogers diffusion model. In summary, all five investigations could have integrated their conceptual frameworks more thoroughly throughout their studies.

Geis (1990). The eclectic, management-oriented framework that Geis used in her diffusion study released her from the restrictions imposed by the Rogers diffusion model. She gave quite a full description of concepts that guided her study. Design and methodology related clearly to concepts in her literature review. (No explicitly named conceptual framework appears in the report.) Perhaps unsure that she had chosen the most important variables, Geis stated her hypotheses as expectations. In this organizational study, Geis measured variables at three levels (organization, local environment, state environment). Her discussion described a planned change in terms of her implied conceptual framework.

Perciful (1990, 1992). Perciful (1990, 1992) studied planning processes for the use of computer-assisted instruction (CAI) in nursing's higher education. She used Lewin's work as the source of her conceptual framework. In her quantitative study, Perciful hoped to discover whether or not a relationship existed between planned change and the successful implementation of CAI. She explicitly named the theory under consideration and described the theory in sufficient depth and breadth to show the relationship between theory and research design. Study hypotheses clearly flow from the theory.

One problem with Perciful's research stems from her selection of concepts from Lewin's microtheories. (Similar problems appear in much nursing literature that uses Lewin's change theories.) First, as explained in an earlier section of this book, Lewin's "deep-freeze" concepts form a very minor part of force field analysis microtheory. The deep-freeze concepts provide change planners and researchers with a method for sequencing change-oriented activities. Perciful used these concepts in additional ways—to organize the purposes, instruments, and analyses of her study. The remainder of force field analysis microtheory calls for the identification, analysis, and measurement of both psychological and nonpsychological data and for the evaluation of balances of forces for and against change in a situation. Only then are activities designed to tip the balance one way or another sequenced appropriately in the deep-freeze complex.

Second, Perciful's instruments measured only the forces that encourage change, not those that discourage it. This deletes any opportunity to employ quasi-stationary equilibria microtheory, mentioned in her conceptual framework but little used in her design. Third, Perciful's study provided some attention to individual-group relationship microtheory but gave this microtheory little emphasis in relating faculty participation in choosing and planning for the innovation to the success of the change effort. Fourth, the conceptual framework mentioned Lewin's channels theory but study procedures did not employ it.

In her study of variables, Perciful used methods appropriate to selected parts of her own conceptual framework. Testing produced some evidence of the appropriateness of change objectives, procedures, and outcomes. The discussion partially supports and explains the effects of the change in terms of the theory. Thus Perciful's research offers some support for Lewin's microtheories and could, in a sense, be called a theory-testing study.

Degerhammar and Wade (1991). Degerhammar and Wade (1991) conducted a dual-purpose study; they planned a change episode and they also evaluated its effects. This study combines concepts from Lewin's action research with normative-reeducation strategies from the writings of Bennis, Benne, and Chin as a foundation for a planned change project and its evaluation. (Readers will remember that Lewin was just getting well started in developing action research when he died; others continued the action research projects after his death.) Degerhammar and Wade announced the theories they intended to use both for planning and for evaluation of the effects of the change. The contents of a chart in their report show clear parallels between the conceptual framework and their project; they properly used Lewin's deep-freeze concepts to sequence their strategies. They aimed to monitor the effects of change, which in a sense assesses the quality of problem diagnosis, innovation, and strategies. Their report names the change theory they employed and discusses it in sufficient depth to show a fairly close relationship between the theory and the project's purposes and design. The evaluators tested the results of the innovation directly and assessed, indirectly, the value of their strategies in terms of the change theory. Their empirical testing supported the appropriateness not only of their change objective but also of the change theory they chose for its implementation. The discussion definitely supported and explained the effects of a planned change in terms of the designated planned change theory.

Dufault, Bielecki, Collins, and Willey (1995). This study also served a dual purpose. It evaluated the effects of a planned change episode and it tests (a very small portion of) a planned change theory. Dufault et al. (1995) combined two concepts from what they called "adoption of innovations" literature with the Conduct and Utilization of Research in Nursing (CURN) model to form a collaborative research utilization model. They used the combination model as an independent variable in a quasi experiment. One problem with this study is the lack of a sufficiently comprehensive delineation of either the CURN or planned change aspects of the theoretic frame of reference. This lack blocked the possibility of fulfilling several of the Acton et al. (1991) criteria for quantitative studies. One reason for the successful performance of the independent variable and the positive outcomes of the experiment lies in the fact that nursing had control over both the independent variable and the context of its implementation. A controversial atmosphere would have called for application of more robust planned change theory concepts that deal with the political contexts of planned change. Even though the quantity of planned change conceptual information included in this study was very small, the direction of the study allows it to serve as a useful example of the combination of a research utilization model and a planned change model as advocated elsewhere in this book.

Mahoney (1995). The purpose of this quantitative pilot study was to determine the extent to which a particular innovation (prescription-writing privileges for nurse practitioners) was adopted. Mahoney employed the theoretical work of Lewin and of Zaltman and Duncan. Study results introduce ideas related to more and different theoretical concepts than the statement of the conceptual framework contains. For example, the report of the study provides a scanty description of Lewin's change-oriented field theory, but the study results address quite a number of ideas associated with Lewinian concepts. Results relate to forces that foster change and that inhibit change, as suggested by Lewin's quasi-stationary equilibria and force field analysis microtheories.

The report has a somewhat fuller description of the Zaltman and Duncan model than of Lewin's theories, but the description fails to address Zaltman and Duncan's "switching rules" that relate to the political dynamics of change situations. A more complete description of the model would have suggested a more powerful exploration of the reasons for nonadoption of prescriptive authority than appears in this report. It might have included a firsthand investigation of some of the crucial political elements present in the context of the study situation, in addition to their naming by nurse subjects. Prescription writing by nurse practitioners does not occur in a vacuum, as the study's report of barrier factors demonstrates. Therefore, examination of the context of practice, in addition to the questioning of nurses themselves, would have made a fuller use of the theories involved. This no doubt would have proved instructive. Readers remember that this was a pilot study; perhaps the study that follows it will make such an examination.

Examples: Research for Planning Change

Although nurse authors often appeal to planned change theories in their planning, they rarely use research methods in that planning. Three exceptions follow.

One study that used planned change theory for planning purposes (Degerhammar & Wade, 1991) had a dual purpose. (Because both purposes were addressed in the discussion above, the study was not reviewed here.) The Degerhammar and Wade study, like all the other studies reported above, used quantitative research methods. One of the following studies (Taft & Stearns, 1991) used a qualitative research approach that aligns most closely with the

BOX 22.4. EVALUATION CRITERIA TO VERIFY TESTING OF NURSING THEORY THROUGH DESCRIPTION OF PERSONAL EXPERIENCES

1. *A purpose of the study is to verify the relationship of the described personal experiences to the specific philosophical beliefs and assumptions that underlie the developing nursing theory.*
2. *Identification of the research question(s) is based on an attempt to provide elaboration of concepts related to the developing nursing theory.*
3. *The primary data sources include sufficient in-depth descriptions of personal experiences to capture the essence of the phenomenon under investigation.*
4. *Simplicity, ethical integrity, and aesthetic presentation are integral characteristics of the described personal experiences.*
5. *Analysis of data incorporates a sense of wholeness of the described personal experiences.*
6. *Formative hypotheses and/or theory are derived inductively from qualitative analysis of the described personal experiences.*
7. *Multiple personal experiences of an individual and/or similar personal experiences of several individuals about a particular phenomenon are used to validate the derived hypotheses.*
8. *Analytic procedures of data analysis and fit of the generated concepts to the personal experiences provide indirect evidence of the validity (or lack thereof) of the developed nursing theory.*
9. *Findings are discussed in terms of how they relate to the developed nursing theory.*
10. *If an existing nursing theory is used to frame a theory that is to be developed and tested inductively, both the developed and existing theories must be internally consistent and congruent with one another.*

SOURCE: From "Testing of Nursing Theory: Critique and Philosophical Expansion," by M. C. Silva and J. M. Sorrell, 1992, *Advances in Nursing Science, 14*(4), pp. 18-19. Copyright © 1992 by Aspen Publishers. Used with permission of the publisher.

personal experiences set of evaluation criteria (see Box 22.4) described by Silva and Sorrell. The Pearcey and Draper (1996) study used an application to nursing practice approach in an effort to plan a change episode.

Taft and Stearns (1991). Taft and Stearns (1991) used research methods in a large-scale type of planning that nurses must consider when turbulent environments prevail in health care systems. They addressed a single change-planning function with research methodologies that assessed readiness for nurse-instigated planned change strategies in a group of hospitals.

Taft and Stearns employed Nadler and Tushman's (1980) congruence model of organizational behavior to analyze facilitating and barrier factors related to change making by nurses. Their open-ended questions gave opportunities for hospital leaders to provide information based on their individual experiences as executives in hospitals. The leaders' responses captured the essence of the phenomena under investigation. Their descriptions of personal experiences, as presented in the report, displayed simplicity, integrity, and an aesthetic quality. The researchers used the high number of responses they received to develop a simple model of organizational change that conveys a sense of wholeness. This model and the parent organizational behavior model both exhibit internal consistency and congruence with one another. The discussion points out the need for nursing studies to focus on organizations as a whole and to assume a systems viewpoint so that nurses can create change successfully in multifaceted health care situations.

Pearcey and Draper (1996). The Pearcey and Draper (1996) study probably fits best under the application-to-nursing-practice approach. (See Box 22.5.) The abstract for this study claimed that it employed selected ideas from action research to plan and facilitate research-based nursing practice and used concepts from the Rogers diffusion model to depict and analyze the change process. The report printed a copy of the graphic representation of the Rogers diffusion model but the text of the report does not present or explain either the action research approach or the Rogers diffusion model. Further, the claim for congruence of action research and the Rogers model ignores the fact that these two approaches have widely differing philosophical foundations. Some varieties of action research do favor the development of an innovation from within, but the Rogers model makes no such provision; it expects planners to demonstrate concern and compassion for adopters, but it also expects planners to provide the innovation destined for adoption. The report also includes an examination of prior conditions in the knowledge stage; in the Rogers model, prior conditions precede the knowledge stage. Time limitations caused this study to end with the decision stage, which prematurely terminated the use of the Rogers diffusion model for data collection and analysis. It also canceled opportunities for the researchers to discover the results of their efforts. The research plan for this study specified interesting, important, and ethical problems, and repetition of the study under a more carefully devised plan and more favorable research conditions would provide an interesting example of the application of a planned change theory to nursing practice.

BOX 22.5. EVALUATION CRITERIA TO VERIFY TESTING OF NURSING THEORY THROUGH APPLICATION TO NURSING PRACTICE

1. *A purpose of the application is to demonstrate the problem-solving effectiveness of a designated nursing theory for nursing practice.*
2. *The nursing theory is explicitly stated as the framework for the application process.*
3. *The plan for implementation identifies specific problems targeted for solution through application of the nursing theory.*
4. *The problems to be addressed represent interesting, important, and ethical problems for nursing practice.*
5. *Outcomes are measured in terms of problem-solving effectiveness of the applied nursing theory.*
6. *Problem-solving effectiveness is determined in comparison with applications in which the nursing theory is not used.*
7. *Findings are discussed in terms of how the nursing theory was instrumental in defining and implementing problem-solving strategies.*

SOURCE: From "Testing of Nursing Theory: Critique and Philosophical Expansion," by M. C. Silva and J. M. Sorrell, 1992, *Advances in Nursing Science, 14*(4), p. 20. Copyright © 1992 by Aspen Publishers. Used with permission of the publisher.

Examples: Research That Tests a Planned Change Theory

Two studies (Dufault et al., 1995; Perciful, 1990, 1992) made limited or indirect tests of planned change theories by means of quantitative research; reviews appear in an earlier section.

Example: An "Other" Kind of Planned Change Theory Use

McKenna, Parahoo, and Boore (1995). The McKenna et al. (1995) study offers an interesting example of an "other" use of a planned change theory in research. In this quantitative study, the researchers used a planned change theory to position an independent variable (a specific nursing model) for their quasi experiment. They did not use the change theory as a foundation for their research design or to guide their data collection procedures. The planned change theory simply offered an efficient method for putting the independent variable in place in a way that did not contaminate the data they collected.

This type of study implicitly addresses the ability of the change theory to effect change, thus yielding a secondary, practical test of the theory. Even though the researchers did not directly relate any of the data they collected to the efficacy of the planned change theory, the success of the independent variable may demonstrate the viability of the change theory. In such situations, researchers should remember the importance of using the planned change theory carefully. In some instances, they could collect data to test both the effects of the independent variable and the integrity of the planned change theory.

Bellman (1996). Bellman (1996) used the personal experience approach to research. Like McKenna et al., Bellman employed a planned change perspective (action research) to put a specific nursing model in place. Unlike McKenna et al., Bellman collected qualitative data that related to both the planned change model and the nursing model.

Bellman mentioned the Silva and Sorrell (1992) criteria for the personal experience approach in her report. No doubt, this attention fostered her sensitivity to the appropriate set of evaluation criteria. Bellman definitely designed her study to test the validity of a particular nursing theory. She attempted to verify the relationship of described personal experiences to beliefs and assumptions of the nursing model in question. Study objectives related closely to the nursing theory concepts. Nevertheless, the nursing theory and the action research approach she selected have enough similarities that the empowerment she hoped to observe through recitation of personal experiences might stem from either theoretical approach.

The descriptions of personal experience in this study do capture the essence of the phenomena under study, sometimes negatively, sometimes positively. Descriptions exhibit simplicity, ethical integrity, and an aesthetic quality. Data analysis called another change theory—Lewin's force field analysis—and a change process evaluation tool into play. In this study, results of analytic procedures may fit the findings more to action research than to the nursing theory under study.

Nurses and Planned Change Model Making

The Tiffany, Cheatham, Doornbos, Loudermelt, and Momadi (1994) survey of nursing periodical literature (and hundreds of related items) revealed seven nurse-generated planned change models. Most of the models are linear-recursive problem-solving models similar in form to the nursing process. Several provided useful information regarding planned change in health care situations. None of the nurse model developers claimed that they had tested the models they developed.

Bille (1981) called his model a "strategy for change." He chose an eclectic foundation that includes ideas from the work of Lionberger, Kübler-Ross, Bloom, Knowles, Maslow, Lewin, Knox, and others. His short statement of the model provided lean descriptions of model content intended to enable users to cause social change. In this linear-recursive model, the author advocated partici-pation—when and if it is possible. He paid some attention to social power when he discussed resistance and facilitating forces. Model language confuses the concepts of problem diagnosis, change, and innovation. The model gives some attention to each of the four components of a complete planned change model (diagnosis, choice or development of an innovation, strategies and tactics, and evaluation of results of the innovation and of the processes of change). Thus the model is complete but displays restricted depth. The statement of the model could be amplified and its language clarified to increase its usefulness.

Brooten, Hayman, and Naylor (1978) claimed to have developed a pragmatic problem-solving model. They adapted information from a number of sources (Lewin, Maslow, Herzberg, Beckhard) in developing their model. Brooten et al. intended their model to provide a basis for planning change. This linear model with a top-down flavor places a major emphasis on classical definitions of social power. Its terminology is quite clear. Like some of the theorists whose work they used, Brooten et al. slighted some aspects of planned change—notably diagnosis and the choice or development of the innovation. Thus the model starts working at a late stage in the change cycle. Its goals concern a limited selection of strategies and it confines evaluation to judging the quality of those strategies.

In a "model for collaboration," Archer, Kelly, and Bisch (1984) provided lean, yet clear, descriptions of the ways that planners can achieve a particular social outcome through collaborative planning. These authors based their gestaltist model on Bisch's research. They referred to systems theory and focused on the intersystem, a conceptualization borrowed from Chin. This model assumes that persons in the target system diagnose the social problem and choose the change objective. Collaborative dialectics and constructivism provide the strategies. The model attends to the matter of the resources necessary for making a change. Limited in scope and depth, the model pays little attention to social power. It presents a creative gestalt that incorporates many of the same concepts that appear in Bhola's (CLER) Configurations Model.

Stevens (1975, 1977, 1983) made no claim for the development of a model. Nevertheless, assembling several of her change-related writings provides the necessary components. Stevens garnered the change concepts for this top-down model from the writings of Lewin, Herzberg, and R. Lippitt. The model pays moderate attention to issues of social power. It assumes that the planners' diagnosis, if carefully done, represents reality and that planners can choose an appropriate innovation without adopter input. Although model language sometimes confuses definitions of innovation, change, and resources, it contains a clear discussion of strategies and tactics. It provides useful information regarding evaluation of a change episode. The model emphasizes a problem-solving approach at the strategy/tactic stage. When taken together, the pieces of this linear model of restricted depth offer useful insights on change from a nurse administrator's standpoint.

Claus and Bailey (1977, 1979) did claim model status for their "tool." They claimed that it adheres to scientific methods, shows a systematic and integrated structure, supports critical analysis, and defends action choices. Developed over a six-year period, this model finds its base in systems theory, operations research, and design engineering. It also incorporates some of Lewin's force field analysis concepts. This model combines linear and gestalt properties. It contains a feedback loop that provides for comparison of results with goals and allows modification of the change plan.

Claus and Bailey used clearly worded statements to describe their leader-oriented model. Further, they said that linearity is a convenient and useful conceptual fiction. The fullness of model description varies from concept to concept. They paid little attention to social power, but adding their 1977 statements on the topic of power greatly strengthens the model. More attention to the diagnosis of social problems would make the model more useful. The authors' discussion of choice or development of the innovation, their strong emphasis on strategies and tactics, and their thoughtful consideration of evaluation help to make this model a useful addition to nursing's change literature.

Spradley (1980, 1985) claimed model status for the change formulation that she based on the work of Lewin, Zaltman and Duncan, R. Lippitt, and Hersey and Blanchard. She intended that this linear, mostly top-down model would help planners to cause change to occur. She advocated force field analysis and included all four components needed for a planned change model. Although her discussions provide unclear distinctions between "change" and the innovation (solution), this problem-solving model offers some useful concepts for nurse planners.

In the process of using Nadler and Tushman's organizational dynamics model in a research study, Taft and Stearns (1991) developed a graphic representation and a short verbal explanation for the processes of social change. Perhaps due to the brevity of their presentation, Taft and Stearns did not emphasize social power or specify whether change came from the top or from the grass roots of an organization. They used very clear terminology to describe only a little information regarding the diagnosis of social problems. They centered their work on the choice or development of the innovation and on strategies for its implementation. Evaluation received scant attention in this problem-solving cycle with a systems flavor.

Summary

This chapter on nursing's planned change research did not attempt to furnish in-depth critiques of methodologies in nursing's existing planned change research. Instead, the aim of the chapter was to provide ideas about appropriate ways to use planned change theories in nursing research and change planning. It stressed the importance of firsthand knowledge of planned change theories and of accurate theory use.

Silva (1986) offered seven criteria for the evaluation of research that tests nursing theories. Acton et al. (1991) amplified and refined the original Silva criteria and related them closely to research in the logical positivist tradition. Then Silva and Sorrell (1992) offered three additional approaches for the evaluation of theory-testing research. This chapter provided ideas about the adaptation of the four sets of criteria to serve in the evaluation of planned change theory usage in nursing research situations. These situations could include theory-based evaluation of the effects of planned change, theory-based change planning, and the testing of a planned change theory.

The chapter provided a review of 14 nursing studies that relate to the kinds of evaluation approaches and planned change theory usage discussed. It also gave some information regarding selected planned change models that nurses have presented; most have a problem-solving approach with a linear-recursive worldview. Some display gestaltist outlooks or systems connotations. One nurse-generated model describes change.

References

Acton, G. J., Irvin, B. L., & Hopkins, B. A. (1991). Theory-testing research: Building the science. *Advances in Nursing Science, 14*(1), 52-61.

Archer, S. E., Kelly, C. D., & Bisch, S. A. (1984). *Implementing change in communities: A collaborative process.* St. Louis: Mosby.

Bellman, L. M. (1996). Changing nursing practice through reflection on the Roper, Logan, and Tierney model: The enhancement approach to action research. *Journal of Advanced Nursing, 24,* 129-138.

Bille, D. A. (1981). Managing the process of change. *Hospital Topics, 59*(6), 21-28.

Brett, J. L. L. (1987). Use of nursing practice research findings. *Nursing Research, 36,* 344-349.

Brett, J. L. L. (1989). Organizational integrative mechanisms and adoption of innovations by nurses. *Nursing Research, 38,* 105-110.

Brooten, D. A., Hayman, L. L., & Naylor, M. D. (1978). *Leadership for change: A guide for the frustrated nurse.* Philadelphia: J. B. Lippincott.

Claus, K. E., & Bailey, J. T. (1977). *Power and influence in health care: A new approach to leadership.* St. Louis: C. V. Mosby.

Claus, K. E., & Bailey, J. T. (1979). Facilitating change: A problem-solving/decision-making tool. *Nursing Leadership, 2*(2), 32-39.

Coyle, L. A., & Sokop, A. G. (1990). Innovation adoption behavior among nurses. *Nursing Research, 39,* 176-180.

Degerhammar, M., & Wade, B. (1991). The introduction of a new system of care delivery into a surgical ward in Sweden. *International Journal of Nursing Studies, 28,* 325-336.

Delaney, C. W. (1989). Nurse educators' acceptance of the computer in baccalaureate nursing programs. *Computers in Nursing, 3,* 129-136.

Dufault, M. A., Bielecki, C., Collins, E., & Willey, C. (1995). Changing nurses' pain assessment practice: A collaborative research utilization approach. *Journal of Advanced Nursing, 21,* 634-645.

Fawcett, J. (1996). Putting the conceptual model into the research report. *Nurse Author and Editor, 6*(2), 1-4.

Geis, M. J. (1990). Diffusion of associate degree nursing programs among U.S. community colleges. *Journal of Nursing Education, 29,* 176-182.

Kirchhoff, K. T. (1982). A diffusion survey of coronary precautions. *Nursing Research, 31,* 196-201.

Mahoney, D. F. (1995). Employer resistance to state authorized prescriptive authority for NPs: Results from a pilot study. *Nurse Practitioner, 20*(1), 58-61.

McKenna, H. P., Parahoo, K. A., & Boore, J. R. P. (1995). The evaluation of a nursing model for long-stay psychiatric patient care. Part 1: Literature review and methodology. *International Journal of Nursing Studies, 32,* 79-94.

Nadler, D. A., & Tushman, M. A. (1980, Autumn). A model for diagnosing organizational behavior. *Organizational Dynamics,* pp. 35-51.

Pearcey, P., & Draper, P. (1996). Using the diffusion of innovation model to influence practice: A case study. *Journal of Advanced Nursing, 23,* 714-721.

Perciful, E. G. (1990). The relationship between planned change and successful implementation of computer-assisted instruction (CAI) within higher education in nursing as perceived by faculty. *Dissertation Abstracts International, 52*(05), 2504B. (University Microfilms No. AAC91-29261)

Perciful, E. G. (1992). The relationship between planned change and successful implementation of computer assisted instruction. *Computers in Nursing, 10,* 85-90.

Rogers, E. M. (1976). Where are we in understanding the diffusion of innovations? In W. Schramm & D. Lerner (Eds.), *Communication and change: The last ten years—and the next* (pp. 205-222). Honolulu: University Press of Hawaii.

Silva, M. C. (1986). Research testing nursing theory: State of the art. *Advances in Nursing Science, 9*(1), 9-11.

Silva, M. C., & Sorrell, J. M. (1992). Testing of nursing theory: Critique and philosophical expansion. *Advances in Nursing Science, 14*(4), 12-23.

Spradley, B. W. (1980). Managing change creatively. *Journal of Nursing Administration, 10*(5), 32-37.

Spradley, B. W. (1985). *Community health nursing: Concepts and practice* (2nd ed.). Boston: Little, Brown.

Stevens, B. J. (1975). Effecting change. *Journal of Nursing Administration, 5*(2), 23-26.

Stevens, B. J. (1977). Management of continuity and change in nursing. *Journal of Nursing Administration, 7*(4), 26-30.

Stevens, B. J. (1983). *First-line patient care management* (2nd ed.). Rockville, MD: Aspen.

Taft, S. H., & Stearns, J. E. (1991). Organizational change toward a nursing agenda: A framework from the Strengthening Hospital Nursing Program. *Journal of Nursing Administration, 21*(2), 12-21.

Tiffany, C. R., Cheatham, A. B., Doornbos, D., Loudermelt, L., & Momadi, G. G. (1994). Planned change theory: Survey of nursing periodical literature. *Nursing Management, 25*(7), 54-59.

Planned Change Theories and Research-Based Nursing Practice

Technology, in the sense used in this chapter, concerns the use of knowledge in the service of the human race. This entire chapter emphasizes the importance of encouraging nursing's technology—the use of research-based knowledge in the practice of nursing. The discussion starts by addressing the general concerns of technology and nursing. It continues with information about knowledge use in planned change literature and in nursing. The main part of the chapter describes seven approaches to research-based nursing practice. The last part makes observations about the need for planned change theories in programs designed to implement research-based nursing practice.

Technology and Nursing

Technology includes much more than machines and tangible products. *Technology,* in a broad sense, refers to the use of research-based scientific knowledge in the service of humankind. Technology development and dissemination are political processes that require social change. According to Dickson (1975, pp. 63-95), technology and social patterns reinforce each other. Social control often takes the form of control over the development and dissemination of technology. The invention of clocks, for example, enabled leaders in monasteries to exert control over hours of labor and of prayer; later, clocks helped Josiah Wedgewood, a founder of modern capitalism, to discipline his workforce. Early in the industrial revolution, the owners of certain kinds of manufacturing equipment gathered machines together in factories more as a means of controlling workers than as a business necessity.

Perrow's (1967) technology construct contains an implicit dimension—knowledge (Lynch, 1974). As applied to nursing, this knowledge dimension concerns knowledge of human beings, knowledge of how to deal with humans, and knowledge of how to obtain needed information (through research and other methods) when exceptional cases arise. The use of research-based scientific knowledge to accomplish nursing goals contributes greatly to the development and employment of nursing's technology. Society has not always valued nursing technology. Control over technology has profound implications for nursing, particularly in these days of economic uncertainty in health care.

Knowledge Use in Planned Change Literature

General change literature. In 1973, Havelock described knowledge use as a crude art that had emerged in the 1960s and then occupied only a handful of scholars in a few learning centers. Many forces in society were combining to create a knowledge explosion, and the populace carried the expectation that new knowledge would be harnessed in the service of humankind. These conditions called for the creation of systems to link those who generate knowledge with those who use it. Glaser (1973, 1986) and Glaser, Abelson, and Garrison (1983) wrote extensively about knowledge utilization.

Knowledge use in four change theories/models. Lewin "feared that the seeds of totalism might grow to destroy democracy in the United States. This outcome could be forestalled if the forces of research, education, and action could be united in the elimination of social injustice and minority self-hatred and in the wise resolution of intergroup conflicts" (Benne, 1985, p. 273). Bennis, Benne, and Chin (1985) maintained that the extent to which planners and adopters can use knowledge effectively depends largely upon the kind of relationship that planners and adopters develop. For this reason, they emphasized the social dynamics of knowledge use in the planning of change. The Rogers (1995) diffusion model contains an entire stage devoted to knowledge. Conceptual resources and their use feature prominently in Bhola's CLER model (1982).

Knowledge Use and Nursing

Historically, control over the technology of healing took a dark turn from Germany to England in the fifteenth and sixteenth centuries, where the work of midwives tended toward empirical medicine and male physician practice relied heavily upon tradition. Catholic and Protestant churches, with physicians who saw their hegemony over the practice of medicine threatened by midwives, joined hands with civil authorities to institute witch hunts. Local authorities were instructed in the "legal" ways to conduct witch hunts by the *Malleus Malefi-carum* (Hammer of Witches), a document written in 1484 by two clergymen (Dickson, 1975; Ehrenreich & English, 1973). A conservative estimate puts the number of witches executed at 100,000, with 85% of the victims female. The witch-craze scourge was so severe that two German villages had only one surviving female apiece (Barstow, 1994).

Control over technology still has profound implications for nursing and the consuming public. Health care institutions that allow the technology of nursing to advance have better patient outcome statistics than do those that devalue nursing technology (Knaus, Draper, Wagner, & Zimmerman, 1986). Nursing technology itself can reorganize health care for the betterment of patient care. Lynaugh (1990), for instance, attributed organization of care according to acuity (rather than by medical specialty) to the acquisition and reshuffling of expert knowledge by nurses.

Utz and Gleit (1995) raised a vital issue when they warned that the very existence of the profession of nursing soon will come into question if nurses do not provide scientific evidence regarding the efficacy of nursing care. Unless nurses move toward research-based practice, continued nursing autonomy remains in doubt. Utz and Gleit advocated nursing technology—a systematic, research-based approach to nursing interventions. This approach can take the form of a national effort or a series of local efforts.

Approaches to Research-Based Nursing Practice

Nursing technology has had an impact at the national level. Nurses have a strong hand in the development of the guidelines disseminated by the Agency for Health

Care Policy and Research (AHCPR), an agency established in 1989 by Congress to improve the quality of health care in the United States. Agency personnel identify specific patient-care problems that reveal wide national variations in the type and amount of health care provided to apparently similar patients. Then a panel of experts reviews the literature on a problem, such as pressure sores or urinary incontinence, to develop a research database that serves as a foundation for clinical practice guidelines and recommendations for care.

After pilot testing, the AHCPR clinical practice guidelines appear in booklet form, and the effort moves from a national to a local level. Health care organizations now take responsibility to augment nursing technology. They do this as they design a nursing practice innovation; conduct clinical trials to evaluate the innovation; decide on adoption, modification, or rejection of the innovation; disseminate the innovation; and ensure its long-term survival.

Just as the implementation of the AHCPR recommendations occurs at the local level, so nurses devise or manage critical paths in some local institutions. Janken (1995) wrote that the development of critical pathways without reference to research constitutes common practice. She urged the formation of research-based critical pathways and attention to patient-oriented outcomes. Not only do these concerns have human value, they exert an impact on the financial standing of health care organizations. Other approaches to research-based nursing practice include research utilization models.

Research utilization (RU) models, in essence, are models for the refinement and implementation of nursing technology (the use of—nursing's—research knowledge in the service of humans). These models fall into two general classes—models that encourage both the development and the dissemination of nursing's technology and those that focus mainly on dissemination. Short descriptions of several nursing RU models (WICHE, NCAST, CURN, Iowa, Stetler, UNC, Oxford) and the ways that they deal with planned change theories appear in the following sections.

Western Interstate Commission for Higher Education (WICHE) Model

Precursor articles. As the director of WICHE's Regional Program for Nursing Research Development, Lindemann wrote a series of articles (Lindemann, 1973, 1975a, 1975b, 1984; Lindemann & Krueger, 1977) that served as precursors to the WICHE RU model. In these articles, Lindemann stressed the need for a multifaceted nursing research program. This program would support collaborative research endeavors among nurses through a large-scale structural approach with three purposes. First, the program would foster the generation of research hypotheses by practicing nurses. Second, it would identify nursing research priorities. This identification would support the development of valid and reliable nursing research instruments. Third, the program would provide for use of research findings. If this model works as intended, it has the capacity to assist in the development and implementation of nursing's technology.

Demonstration project. Planners at WICHE designed a demonstration project that they hoped would create general models for overcoming barriers to research use (Krueger, 1977). They felt that they had the resources needed for research utilization, and they assumed the existence of practicing nurses with the personal characteristics and political connections needed for instituting change. Planners worked to form a link between practicing nurses and the resources the planners themselves could provide.

Change theory content. The WICHE plan consisted of five phases. In the first phase (recruitment), planners sent preparatory informational materials to prospective participants. They included nurses in rural as well as urban areas and ensured the inclusion of persons of color. In the second phase, participants came to a workshop city for three days of intensive instruction in the critical evaluation of research, the selection of valid research findings, and change theory. Change theory content consisted mainly of concepts from Lewin's force field analysis and quasi-stationary equilibria microtheories along with an introduction to Lewinian concepts that place change activities in the unfreeze, move, and freeze phases. With workshop staff guidance, participant pairs refined their descriptions of the patient-care problems to which they would later apply research findings. They also developed implementation plans.

Phase three lasted five months. Participants, in telephone and letter contact with WICHE planners, implemented the clinical change projects in their own employment situations. For phase four, participants again gathered in workshop format for two days to report outcomes of their interventions. This phase included analysis of the model and recommendations for changes. The continuation phase of the project (phase five) lasted from three to six months. Participants made follow-up reports as they kept in telephone and letter contact with project staff.

Workshop procedures. The WICHE planners repeated the workshop sequence three times, testing their five-phase model with pairs of nurses who participated in one of three sites (San Francisco, Seattle, Denver). For two main reasons, planners could not compare the results of the three sequences. First, they had held the demonstration workshops sequentially in the three sites so that the second workshop could profit from feedback gathered during and after the first; the third took advantage of feedback from both the second and the first. Thus, heeding feedback changed the nature of each workshop sequence.

Conceptual frameworks. Second, WICHE planners tested a different conceptual framework for each of the three workshop sequences. In the first sequence (San Francisco), planners featured a problem-solving framework, "based on the assumption that if a problem were identified, all possible resources could be used toward its solution" (Krueger, Nelson, & Wolanin, 1978). This assumption proved erroneous; nurse participants had great difficulty locating appropriate research findings to apply to their problem situations.

The second sequence (Seattle) used a diffusion model approach. This assumed that participants, in their own employment surroundings, had the status and power necessary to effect change toward research-based nursing practice (Krueger et al., 1978). Participants were to match research-based solutions with nursing care problems. Participants still had difficulty locating appropriate research findings (Krueger, 1978).

The third workshop sequence had a research, development, and dissemination (RD&D) basis. WICHE planners had listened to participant feedback and made observations about the difficulty earlier participants encountered in finding and understanding applicable research. The WICHE staff responded by offering semipackaged innovations in the form of bibliographies that listed groups of research studies (Krueger, 1978).

Publication results. In addition to the results published by WICHE planners, Krueger et al. (1978) listed several publications and presentations that came from the three regional workshops, in addition to the results published by WICHE planners. Participants' publications included a generalized RU model that Dracup and Breu (1977) developed and applied to a specific clinical situation. Other publications and/or presentations involved structured preoperative teaching, diabetes care, and bowel control in the elderly.

WICHE planners saw themselves as planners who would influence nurse participants to adopt the use of research findings in their practices back home. Their reports demonstrate what Rogers (1995, pp. 285, 286) called a two-step flow model of communication. They used the workshop setting to convey modernizing messages (the use of research findings in nursing practice) to opinion leaders from outlying communities in the expectation that these opinion leaders, in turn, would influence the actual practice of nursing.

Nursing Child Assessment
Satellite Training (NCAST) Model

King, Barnard, and Hoehn (1981) reported a project funded by the Division of Nursing, Bureau of Health Resources, and, later, by the Harris Foundation of Chicago. The first phase of the project demonstrated the feasibility of using a nonnursing technology (satellite communication) to help nurses implement nursing's technology. The project was intended to furnish nurses in various geographic areas with information regarding the importance of assessments of caregiver-infant interactions and of infants' environments. In a second phase, the project taught nurses specific procedures for assessing the quality of an infant's animate and inanimate environment, a phase oriented toward the implementation of actual assessment procedures. Nurses received manuals with articles and study guides for use in this phase.

Project components. The NCAST project had four major components (recruitment of nurse learners, translation of research findings into an understandable form, dissemination of research information, formative and summative evaluation). It tested four communication modes. According to Krueger (1979), the NCAST group tried to answer the question, "How much direct interaction does the learner need to gain knowledge, develop attitudes, and change behavior?" (p. 73). Nurse participants in the *duplex mode* had both two-way visual and two-way audio transmission as they interacted with nurse researchers and instructors in Seattle. One-way visual transmission and two-way audio transmission characterized the *simplex mode.* The *videotape mode* allowed learners to view the instructors but gave learners no opportunity for direct communication with them. Learners in the *conventional mode* had only reference lists and other written documents (King et al., 1981).

Crane (1985) cited a third NCAST phase, in which project leaders taught public health nurses how to use a protocol for following preterm infants. This project, called Nursing Systems Toward Effective Parenting-Premature (NSTEP-P), provided both workshop instruction and supervised clinical practice. All three NCAST project phases emphasized the translation of research findings into terms appropriate for the practicing nurse; all attempted to persuade nurse participants to value research use in practice. Crane (1985) noted that none tried to influence practice settings or use nurse participants as agents to change the practice of other nurses.

Diffusion model and plans. King et al. (1981) described two ways that the NCAST project used concepts from the Rogers diffusion model. First, project leaders classified potential nurse participants along the innovativeness dimension described by Rogers and Shoemaker (1971). Then they segmented their total audience into homophilous subaudiences so that they could devise appropriate messages for each. Crane (1985, pp. 495, 496) wrote that project leaders used diffusion model concepts that deal with communication flow through various types of channels and with stages of the diffusion process. Thus workshop planners used a diffusion model for structuring workshop procedures, but not as content to help workshop participants cope with the political realities they would meet in their own practice situations. Procedures in the third NCAST project reflected changes introduced in the 1983 version of the Rogers diffusion model.

Even before the outset of the NCAST projects, Rogers and Shoemaker (1971) described what they called the one-step (hypodermic needle) model of communication flow. In this model, communicators assume that (mass) media exert rapid and direct effects on large numbers of people with no interference from sociological factors. The two-step communication model allows for peer communication but remains too simplistic to explain reality. Readers will note that both the WICHE and NCAST RU projects used (but did not reference) either the one-step (hypodermic needle) or two-step communication flows described by Rogers and Shoemaker (1971). The NCAST model assumed that contact by nurse leaders (nurse researchers) with powerful media (satellite television and so on) would convey messages to individual adopters (practicing nurses) who then would make behavior changes (pp. 284, 285). As early as 1971, Rogers and Shoemaker cited the hypodermic model as too simple and too mechanistic to offer adequate explanations for the effects of mass media (pp. 203, 204). They also described the inadequacies of the two-step flow model of communication (pp. 206-208) to explain communication processes.

Conduct and Utilization of Research in Nursing (CURN) Model

CURN received support from a 5-year Division of Nursing grant awarded the Michigan State Nurses Association by the Department of Health, Education, and Welfare. Nurses participated in replication studies at 12 Michigan hospital intervention (experimental) sites. Scientific work occurred at the University of Michigan's School of Nursing and Institute for Social Research and at the Michigan State University School of Nursing. After completion of the project, Pelz and Horsley (1981) measured the extent to which research utilization activities introduced during the CURN project had survived.

Introductory information. In the introductory chapter of the guide to CURN use, the authors (Horsley, Crane, Crabtree, & Wood, 1983) stated that the purpose of the project was to assist nurses in their efforts to institute research-based nursing in their places of clinical practice. The authors saw research and research utilization as complementary processes, each necessary to the other. Research identifies problems and refines solutions; research utilization puts those solutions to use in a series of practical activities. An innovation protocol translates research into clinical language and considers the usage context of research-based solutions; research utilization requires planned change processes.

Planned change theory in CURN. The CURN model tells users how to employ planned change concepts in research use programs in employment situations. The model provides instruction about dealing with political entities and the importance of having strong nurse leaders who possess political savvy. It tells how to evaluate the research-based protocol with respect to its potential for adoption, how to plan steps to diffuse the innovation beyond the trial unit, and how to develop mechanisms that maintain the innovation over time.

The CURN model's integral inclusion of planned change theory shows the influence of one of Havelock's colleagues at the Center for Research on Utilization of Scientific Knowledge at the University of Michigan. Pelz collaborated with the CURN project team. (Havelock, 1973, referenced publications by Pelz in his volume on the dissemination and use of knowledge.) The CURN project also drew upon change information from sources in addition to Havelock's linking model. Pelz and Horsley wrote (1981) that for development of the CURN model, knowledge about the process of research utilization

> was drawn from a wide literature on the innovating process, particularly Havelock's (1969) formulation of a "linkage model" of knowledge use. A major concern was to minimize the risk of misutilization. . . . Accordingly, a comprehensive process of research utilization (RU) was designed, under the guideline that *knowledge generated in a controlled, scientific context may not be valid when used in an uncontrolled, clinical context.* (pp. 126, 127)

Evidence that the CURN team consulted sources (Aiken & Hage, 1968; Rogers, 1983; Rogers & Agarwala-Rogers, 1976; Rothman, 1974; Sieber, 1968; Zaltman & Duncan, 1977) in addition to Havelock's linking model appears not only in the 1983 guide but in a related publication by Horsley and Crane (1986).

Action plans. The research utilization process used in the CURN project identified seven steps that relate to the use of research outcomes, the employment of research methods, and the incorporation of planned change processes. Because their developers envisioned feedback from clinicians to researchers, these steps have the capacity to foster not only the dissemination of nursing's technology but also its development. The first step, systematic identification of patient-care problems, involves the use of research methods and planned change processes. This step emphasizes data-based decision making. The second step combines planned change concepts with previously obtained patient-care data to assess and select research-based protocols (solutions, innovations). Nurse model users must assess and understand the nature and quality of an original research report and a resulting clinical protocol to avoid clinical misuse of the research.

The third step calls for a careful and detailed assessment of a research-based protocol and its original research base for the purpose of understanding the limits of the research base. This step determines whether a protocol can both meet unique organizational requirements and maintain the integrity of its research base. In the fourth step, nurse model users employ research methodologies and planned change processes to implement a nursing practice innovation in a small segment of an organization, such as a clinical unit. They evaluate the effectiveness of the innovation in solving a patient-care problem.

The fifth step, a decision to adopt, alter, or reject an innovation, requires an understanding both of its research base and of planned change concepts. Upon adoption of an innovation, the sixth step provides for its dissemination beyond the trial unit. Finally, model users develop mechanisms to maintain innovation usage over time, for example, by incorporation of the innovation into the quality improvement program to ensure ongoing evaluation and monitoring.

Project culmination. CURN, the most extensive of the research utilization projects reported in this chapter, started in the late 1970s and continued into the 1980s. Workshops and seminars in participating agencies preceded replications and development of innovation protocols. The CURN project culminated in the development of 10 research-based innovation protocols that appeared in a series of 10 small books along with a guide to their use (Horsley et al., 1983). Utz and Gleit (1995) wrote that the "CURN project provided the first example of research-based nursing interventions" (p. 9) and that nurse researchers currently are building on the CURN work. As an example, Beaudry, VandenBosch, and Anderson (1996) followed CURN procedures to summarize an existing research base and to develop guidelines for fever screening in afebrile adult patients. Their research-based guidelines could favorably affect patient outcomes in redesigned clinical work situations.

The Iowa Model

Although White, Leske, and Pearcy (1995) listed the Iowa model as a separate RU model, they wrote that the Iowa and CURN RU models exhibit remarkable similarities, and listed seven ways that they are alike. Important differences surface when one looks at the ways that the models deal with planned change and the environmental context of research use. For example, with reference to the Iowa model, Titler et al. (1994) noted that the adoption of research-based practice requires administrative support, but they did not employ any planned change theory that would tell model users how to obtain that support. On the other hand, the CURN model references and uses the work of several change theorists and CURN literature shows a step-by-step linking process of organizational change in keeping with a diffusion-of-innovation view.

The Titler et al. descriptions paint a broad picture of a practice environment that enhances the effectiveness of stimuli that encourage inquiry and critical thinking. The gestalt that emerges shows a milieu so strongly supportive of inquiry and critical thinking that any nurse within it who fails to adopt a scholarly mode of practice might feel ostracized. The practice environment that Titler et al. described certainly would value the development and use of nursing's technology.

The Iowa descriptions of an inquiry-friendly environment and inquiry-related stimuli constitute the model's unique features and greatest strengths. These lists would provide many useful ideas to nurses who want to instigate research-based practice. Nevertheless, the Iowa model pictures the "ideal" environment without telling readers how to obtain it. Not all nurses who value research-based nursing practice can work where others value such practice. What nurses in many situations need is a strong planned change theory that gives them conceptual tools to analyze their political situations and to go about planning in realistic ways for change to a research-friendly environment. Conceptual handles can help them grasp concepts related to centers of social power, communication linkages, resources necessary for making change, and placement of important change components within environments.

The Stetler Research Utilization (RU) Model

The Stetler (1994) model relates more to use of research findings by individual nurses than to use by groups of nurses or an institutional RU program. The model was developed initially by a dyad rather than by a group. Readers can trace the evolution of the recent Stetler (1994) model through the earlier model formulation by Stetler and Marram (1976) and a subsequent series of articles on the topic of research utilization. Stetler and Marram saw the need for more than an appraisal of a research study's quality of design in making a determination of its fitness for application in practice. They developed and published a model that asks nurse research users to look at feasibility and the congruence of research findings with a theoretical base for nursing practice. Stetler later published articles and chapters that discussed the responsibility and involvement of nurses in research activities (1983) and ways that nursing research fits into a service setting (1984). In additional articles, Stetler also defined the concept of research utilization (1985) and gave nursing instructors a strategy (1989) for teaching research use. She and DiMaggio (1991) published a report that described research use among clinical specialists. More recently, Stetler, Bautista, Vernale-Hannon, and Foster (1995) evaluated the impact of research utilization forums for clinical nurse specialists.

Conceptual framework. As it now stands, the Stetler RU model finds its base in the field of knowledge utilization. Stetler applied knowledge utilization to individual practitioners but acknowledged that, at times, planned institutional change may become necessary. Stetler (1994) stressed three forms of research utilization: instrumental (direct and concrete application), conceptual (understanding, increased enlightenment), or symbolic (political application). According to Anderson (1994), this emphasis on three forms of research utilization represents a nontraditional model of use now valued by both social scientists and nurses. Anderson reasoned that conceptual use of research can influence the level of professionalization of nursing practice as surely as instrumental usage can. The Stetler model uses system concepts (environmental inputs, internal throughputs, utilization outputs) to furnish broad descriptions of research use.

Six model phases. Nurse model users employ a series of six phases when they use the Stetler (1994) model. In the first phase, users make a purposeful research review. They might need to solve a clinical problem, update a knowledge base, validate or revise an existing procedure, or prepare an educational program. In the second phase, users engage in an "accept/reject" research critique. If they accept a study, they make a statement of the degree of applicability of study findings. This statement reflects what study statistics probably mean to future clients and to daily nursing activities.

Comparative evaluation requires users to compare the setting of the study with the setting in which it might find use. Three "Rs" pertain: risk, resource requirements, and the readiness of others in the practice situation to accept application of the research findings. In this phase, the nurse user also must consider the effectiveness of current practice and make a determination regarding whether the proposed change would improve, maintain, or worsen the practice situation. Users also must seek substantiating evidence for the research in terms of additional research and reliable nonresearch literature. A meta-analysis is preferred to a conglomeration of miscellaneous literature sources.

Decisions, in the fourth phase, can take the form of use, consideration for use, delay, or rejection. The fifth phase requires the nurse user to transform research findings into actions, a process made easier by studies with concrete concepts. The user must think of practice implications; these might extend far beyond study findings. In evaluation, the last phase, the user compares outcomes with the purposes established in the first phase and differentiates formal from informal applications. The Stetler model concentrates more effectively on the dissemination of nursing's technology than on its development.

The Stetler model and planned change. Stetler recognized the fact that some research application projects require the employment of planned change concepts, but she consciously chose not to incorporate these in her model.

The University of North Carolina (UNC) Model

When they presented the University of North Carolina (UNC) model for improving the dissemination of research, Funk, Tornquist, and Champagne (1989) made an effort to complement other research use models, not to supplant them. They wished to lessen the gap between nursing research and the practice of nursing. They cited problems that included the disparity between the styles of research-oriented and practice-oriented nursing journals, the presentation of research findings in a manner too technical for practitioners, and the inadequate dissemination of research on any one topic of interest to clinicians. With a grant from the National Center for Nursing Research, they developed a three-pronged approach to the problems listed above.

Design of the model. The UNC model concerns qualities of the research, attributes of its communication, and aids to research use. It furnishes guidelines for three avenues for research communication that include research conferences, research monographs, and research information centers. Funk et al. (1989) followed each practice-oriented research conference with an accompanying monograph. The main flow of information in the three avenues progresses from researcher to clinician, causing the model to stress the dissemination of nursing's technology more strongly than its development. To avoid fragmentation, both the conference and the monograph focused on one important and clinically applicable theme. Each theme concerned an area over which nurses have control in practice. Each concerned a research-practice gap and each had available research. The research included for the conference and the monograph must possess scientific merit, significance, and readiness for practice.

Conferences provide opportunities for researchers to interact with clinicians. Conference presenters are expected to cite only relevant literature, eliminate overly technical jargon, provide simple descriptions of research processes, and supply copies of instruments for participants. They use statistics only as adjuncts to their explanations and give in-depth discussions of implications for clinical practice. The conferences also feature strategies for implementation of research and provide opportunities for demonstration sessions and dialogue.

Researchers submit clearly stated research reports for inclusion in a monograph that follows the conference theme and structure. Each conference participant receives a copy of the monograph. A major book company publishes each monograph.

In the UNC model, an information center acts as a clearinghouse by providing a newsletter, consultations, and referrals that support the conferences and monographs. Both researchers and clinicians contribute to newsletters that carry information on strategies for research utilization in addition to the research concerns addressed in the conferences and monographs.

Planned change theory and the UNC model. The UNC model features three main components of the process of disseminating research—qualities of the research, characteristics of the communication process, and methods used to facilitate use. The initial statement of the model takes a very nurse-oriented and nurse-controlled view of all three of these components. This viewpoint does little to address the environment of research-based practice in the politically oriented manner that a strong planned change theory suggests.

The Oxford Model for Integrating Nursing Research and Practice

History of the model. The Oxford model (Kitson, Ahmed, Harvey, Seers, & Thompson, 1996) for integrating nursing research and practice strongly advocates a thorough integration of the deductive and inductive phases of the research spiral. Such an integration creates the potential for both the development and the dissemination of nursing's technology.

In 1991, the National Health Service in the United Kingdom acted to close the gap between research and practice. Nurses involved in the effort noted several emerging themes in nursing literature. These themes recognized the organizational overtones in research use; stressed the importance of strong research; emphasized the planning of educational, audit, and change management interventions; highlighted the evaluation of the impact of research-based interventions; and commented on the scarcity of models that successfully combine research and practice. The model developers hoped to devise an organizational model that answered these five concerns.

Kitson et al. (1996) felt that a combination of the deductive and inductive portions of the inquiry spiral would serve as a stronger base for their model than would either portion taken alone. For example, the deductive phase of the inquiry spiral separates the development of knowledge from its implementation and evaluation. Under ideal circumstances, deduction, the "traditional" mode of inquiry, provides a well-tested intervention. A drawback exists in the fact that the deductive model, by itself, suggests little observation of or information about how to introduce change.

The inductive approach generates theory through careful descriptions of everyday practice combined with a thorough analysis and interpretation of the events. The processes inherent in practice often remain implicit, but encouraging practitioners to make explicit descriptions of processes helps them to systematize and formalize what they see in practice situations. This enables them to pin down underlying concepts as they work to develop theories. The difficulty with induction includes the problems associated with persuading practitioners to describe everyday events in ways that demonstrate principles. Lack of rigor often characterizes this approach.

Blueprint for the model. Although research use projects based on both the deductive and the inductive models have occurred, Kitson et al. (1996) sought to combine the positive features of both approaches and to avoid their limitations by developing an integrated model. In the Oxford model, National Institute for Nursing members assist clinical staff as they describe and analyze their practice in the hypothesis-generating phase. Next, staff systematically test hypotheses (interventions) and formally implement them. By the time they have evaluated the interventions, they have completed one cycle on the inquiry spiral. Model developers described three projects (community hospital, Northampton ward, and a project they called ODySSSy) as examples of the integration approach. The model also calls for the establishment of a number of national and international practice development research centers.

The Oxford model and planned change theory. Kitson et al. (1996) fell short of recommending the inclusion of planned change theory concepts in their model. They did write that an important element in getting research into practice involves dealing with contextual issues because many extraneous factors can hinder the implementation of research-based interventions. The important matters they noted include the development of staff nurses' descriptive, analytical, and research capabilities.

(For a summary of the attributes of various approaches to research-based nursing practice, see Table 23.1.)

Planned Change Theory and
Research-Based Nursing Practice

Almost two decades ago, Ketefian (1980) wrote that

> it may be necessary . . . to have a new cadre of nurses whose sole function would be to identify worthy research, evaluate it, examine feasibility for a given setting, test its validity, and in collaboration with nurses of concern, plan and implement the suggested change effort systematically, utilizing appropriate change strategies. (p. 431)

That suggestion still pertains and sees partial fulfillment in the call for unification of the deductive and inductive portions of the research spiral. It also resonates with the development, dissemination, and use of the recommendations that accompany the Agency for Health Care Policy and Research guidelines.

The fact remains that many organizations will not cherish, or perhaps even tolerate, nursing's research use activities in the absence of politically oriented

TABLE 23.1 Approaches to Research-Based Nursing Practice

	Approach						
Dimensions	*WICHE*	*NCAST*	*CURN*	*IOWA*	*STETLER*	*UNC*	*OXFORD*
Level of abstraction:							
Abstract							X
Concrete	X	X	X	X	X	X	X
Purpose:							
Integrate deduction and induction	X		X	X		X	X
Make research knowledge accessible	X	X	X	X		X	X
Implement research-based practice innovations	X	X	X	X	X	X	X
Method:							
Regional conferences, workshops, consultations, information centers	X	X				X	X
Media activities (e.g., print, satellite TV)		X				X	
Unit/institutional planned change			X	X			
Individual or small group efforts	X	X			X		
Demonstration projects	X	X	X	X		X	X
Social system addressed:							
Individual nurse, small group	X	X			X		
Unit, institution			X	X			
State/region/nation						X	X
Planned change concepts:							
Thoroughly integrated			X				
Moderately integrated	X						X
Absent				X	X	X ·	
Used to structure workshop, not used as content for participants		X					

interventions such as those planned under the guidance of a robust planned change theory. Recent publications confirm this assertion. For example, in mid-1990, Reedy, Shivnan, Hanson, Haisfield, and Gregory (1994) started the first application of the Stetler-Marram research utilization process by clinical nurses to a clinical problem. They developed an innovation (nursing protocol),

recognized the presence of configurations (i.e., the Nursing Research Committee), formed linkages (i.e., sent recommendations to the Nursing Research
Committee), engaged in a series of successive approximations (refined their
approach as they sought approvals from multiple groups), and confronted the
need for resources (time, knowledge, support). This group planned and implemented communication and educational strategies and conducted evaluations of
both the processes of change and the results of the innovation. Reedy et al. (1994)
remarked that the factors they met caused implementation of their program to
be a "much longer and more difficult process than was anticipated" (p. 719). A
sound planned change theory or model could not have eliminated all the
difficulties they encountered, but consulting it early would have forewarned
them regarding some of the political exigencies they would meet. It would have
enabled them to make timely and proactive plans for the political strategies
necessary for meeting the goals of their project.

In a companion project, Hanson and Ashley (1994) described the role of
advanced practice nurses who use the Stetler (1994) research utilization model.
The results of their work in formal research use programs demonstrated the need
for resource persons such as expert clinical nurses to help staff nurses achieve
comfort and facility with research critiques. A planned change theory that
emphasizes attention to resources would have helped them foresee the need for
knowledge resources.

In a more recent publication, Tornquist, Funk, and Champagne (1995)
reported on results achieved by implementation of the UNC research utilization
model. Although five well-attended conferences and five highly acclaimed
research volumes resulted from their project, outcomes showed little impact on
the research-practice gap. A few notable exceptions, such as the first Thunder
Project of the American Association of Critical Care Nurses, emerged. (Readers
may wish to note that a second Thunder Project is now under way.)

In discussing the disheartening results, Tornquist et al. wrote that "it makes
no sense to talk about the use of research in practice if the practice setting neither
values nor rewards research or research use" (p. 108). They continued by writing
about the need for administrative support, a democratic climate, and positive
expectations of nurses. Nursing educational programs must change by teaching
students to value research as a viable foundation for practice and by abandoning
outmoded formats for theses and dissertations. Nursing must connect researchers
and clinicians as equals. The Tornquist et al. (1995) summary recommendations
resonate with and add to the top barriers to research use that a sample of nurse
clinicians had identified earlier (Funk, Champagne, Wiese, & Tornquist, 1991).
The recommendations align with the intent of planned change theories designed
to guide the diagnosis and management of just such social problems as those
they described. The thesis of this chapter states that nurses who wish to embark

on a program for the use of nursing research need viable planned change theories to employ in conjunction with nursing's research use models.

Summary

After a brief discussion of knowledge use, technology, and social control issues, this chapter described several nursing models for encouraging research-based nursing practice. The chapter ended with discussions of relationships between some of nursing's approaches to knowledge use and selected planned change theories.

The WICHE demonstration project in three western cities provided intensive instruction in the evaluation of research for practice and included some information about Lewin's change strategies. Because a problem arose with the inaccessibility of pertinent research, the workshop content and format changed to include the provision of research study bibliographies. Some publications resulted from the WICHE workshops.

The NCAST RU project tested four communication modes with differing degrees of interaction. A later NCAST project, called NSTEP-P, taught public health nurses how to use a protocol for following preterm infants. This project employed some Rogers diffusion model concepts in the selection of participants and in communicating with them.

The CURN RU project was sponsored by the Michigan State Nurses Association and funded for five years by the Department of Health, Education, and Welfare. Planned change concepts form such integral parts of this model that it could be considered a planned change model of sorts. The CURN projects involved extensive research and resulted in the development of 10 research-based nursing protocols and a guide to their use. The model assumes that research and research use form complementary parts of a whole.

The Iowa model, much like CURN, differs in one very important aspect—its way of dealing with planned change theory. The CURN model makes integral use of planned change theory; the Iowa model mentions it. A major strength of the Iowa model lies in its descriptions of environmental factors that encourage inquiry and critical thinking. It lacks a planned change theory base that tells model users how to go about the political work of creating such an environment.

Stetler intended that her RU model serve individual nurses rather than institutions. Stetler depicted instrumental, conceptual, and symbolic forms of research utilization and described six phases in the research use process. This model, with its base in the field of knowledge use, lays no claim to a planned change theory, but it could be combined with change theory for use in organizational situations. Of the models described in this chapter, CURN and the Stetler model have, at this point, found the most frequent usage.

Funk, Tornquist, and Champagne developed and tested a model for research knowledge dissemination that involved carefully orchestrated conferences. Each conference generated a monograph published by a major book publisher and was followed by information center activities that included a newsletter, consultations, and referrals.

The Oxford model from the United Kingdom seeks to close the research-practice gap. The Oxford model developers used illustrations and applications of the deductive-inductive phases of the research spiral to illustrate their model, which advocates a thorough integration of the two research phases. After the trial of the model in three projects, model developers noted the need for attention to the political context of practice.

Almost 20 years ago, Ketefian wrote that nurses should view knowledge utilization as planned change. This chapter's review of RU models highlights the relative inattention of some RU models to planned change theory. The "state of the art" of planned change theory when these models were developed explains this lack only in part; Havelock's work, so prominent in the CURN model, appeared before any of nursing's RU models took full shape.

Society does not always realize the value of nursing's technology. Therefore, the inclusion of appropriate planned change theory concepts in nursing's efforts to foster research-based nursing practice would encourage the development of nursing technology, would move nursing toward research-based practice, and consequently would benefit the consuming public.

References

Aiken, M., & Hage, J. (1968). *The relationship between organizational factors and the acceptance of new rehabilitation programs in mental retardation* (Report of Project RD-1556-6). Washington, DC: Rehabilitation Services Administration (formerly the Vocational Rehabilitation Administration).

Anderson, J. E. (1994). The "you" in research utilization. In *Research utilization: A compilation of articles from the Michigan Nurse.* Okemos: Michigan Nurses Association.

Barstow, A. L. (1994). *Witchcraze: A new history of European witch hunts.* San Francisco: Pandora, c/o HarperCollins.

Beaudry, M., VandenBosch, T., & Anderson, J. (1996). Research utilization: Once-a-day temperatures for afebrile patients. *Clinical Nurse Specialist, 10*(1), 21-24.

Benne, K. D. (1985). The process of re-education: An assessment of Kurt Lewin's views. In W. G. Bennis, K. D. Benne, & R. Chin (Eds.), *The planning of change* (4th ed., pp. 272-283). New York: Holt, Rinehart & Winston.

Bennis, W. G., Benne, K. D., & Chin, R. (1985). *The planning of change* (4th ed.). New York: Holt, Rinehart & Winston.

Bhola, H. S. (1982). Planning change in education and development: The CLER model in the context of a mega model. *Viewpoints in Teaching and Learning, 58*(4), 1-35.

Crane, J. (1985). Research utilization: Nursing models. *Western Journal of Nursing Research, 7,* 494-497.

Dickson, D. (1975). *The politics of alternative technology.* New York: Universe.

Dracup, K. A., & Breu, C. S. (1977). Strengthening practice through research utilization. In M. Batey (Ed.), *Communicating nursing research: Vol. 10. Organizing environments for health: Nursing's unique perspective* (pp. 339-353). Boulder, CO: Western Interstate Commission on Higher Education.

Ehrenreich, B., & English, D. (1973). *Witches, midwives, and nurses: A history of women healers.* Old Westbury, NY: Feminist Press.

Funk, S. G., Champagne, M. T., Wiese, R. A., & Tornquist, E. M. (1991). Barriers to using research findings in practice: The clinician's perspective. *Applied Nursing Research, 4,* 909-995.

Funk, S. G., Tornquist, E. M., & Champagne, M. T. (1989). A model for improving the dissemination of nursing research. *Western Journal of Nursing Research, 11,* 361-367.

Glaser, E. M. (1973). Knowledge transfer and institutional change. *Professional Psychology, 4,* 434-444.

Glaser, E. M. (1986). Planned organizational change. *Knowledge: Creation, Diffusion, Utilization, 2,* 260-269.

Glaser, E. M., Abelson, H. H., & Garrison, K. N. (1983). *Putting knowledge to use: Facilitating the diffusion of knowledge and the implementation of planned change.* San Francisco: Jossey-Bass.

Hanson, J. L., & Ashley, B. (1994). Advanced practice nurses' application of the Stetler Model for Research Utilization: Improving bereavement care. *Oncology Nursing Forum, 21,* 720-724.

Havelock, R. G. (1969). *Planning for innovation through dissemination and utilization of knowledge.* Ann Arbor, MI: Center for Dissemination and Utilization of Scientific Knowledge, Institute for Social Research.

Havelock, R. (1973). *Planning for innovation through dissemination and utilization of knowledge.* Ann Arbor, MI: Center for Research on Utilization of Scientific Knowledge.

Horsley, J. A., & Crane, J. (1986). Factors associated with innovations in nursing practice. *Family and Community Health, 9*(1), 1-11.

Horsley, J. A., Crane, J., Crabtree, M. K., & Wood, D. J. (1983). *Using research to improve nursing practice: A guide.* New York: Grune & Stratton.

Janken, J. K. (1995, November-December). What critical pathways are not. *Tar Heel Nurse,* pp. 36, 37.

Ketefian, S. (1980). Using research in practice: Selected issues in the translation of research to nursing practice. *Western Journal of Nursing Research, 2,* 429-431.

King, D., Barnard, K. E., & Hoehn, R. (1981). Disseminating the results of nursing research. *Nursing Outlook, 29,* 164-169.

Kitson, A., Ahmed, L. B., Harvey, G., Seers, K., & Thompson, D. R. (1996). From research to practice: One organizational model for promoting research-based practice. *Journal of Advanced Nursing, 23,* 430-440.

Knaus, W. A., Draper, E. A., Wagner, D. P., & Zimmerman, J. E. (1986). An evaluation of outcome from intensive care in major medical centers. *Annals of Internal Medicine, 104,* 410-418.

Krueger, J. C. (1977). Using clinical research findings in practice: A structured approach. In M. Batey (Ed.), *Communicating nursing research: Vol. 9. Nursing research in the bicentennial year* (pp. 381-394). Boulder, CO: Western Interstate Commission on Higher Education.

Krueger, J. C. (1978). Utilization of nursing research: The planning process. *Journal of Nursing Administration, 8*(1), 6-9.

Krueger, J. C. (1979). Research utilization: What is it? *Western Journal of Nursing Research, 1,* 72-75.

Krueger, J. C., Nelson, A. H., & Wolanin, M. O. (1978). *Nursing research: Development, collaboration, and utilization.* Germantown, MD: Aspen.

Lindemann, C. A. (1973). Nursing research: A viable component of nursing practice. *Journal of Nursing Administration, 3*(2), 18-21.

Lindemann, C. A. (1975a). Nursing practice research: What's it all about? *Journal of Nursing Administration, 5*(3), 5-7.

Lindemann, C. A. (1975b). Priorities in clinical nursing research. *Nursing Outlook, 23,* 693-698.

Lindemann, C. A. (1984). Dissemination of nursing research. *Image: The Journal of Nursing Scholarship, 16,* 57-58.

Lindemann, C. A., & Krueger, J. C. (1977). Increasing the quality, quantity, and use of nursing research. *Nursing Outlook, 25,* 450-454.

Lynaugh, J. (1990). Four hundred postcards. *Nursing Research, 39,* 254-255.

Lynch, B. P. (1974). An empirical assessment of Perrow's technology construct. *Administrative Science Quarterly, 19,* 338-356.

Pelz, D., & Horsley, J. A. (1981). Measuring utilization of nursing research. In J. A. Ciarlo (Ed.), *Utilizing evaluation: Concepts and measurement techniques* (pp. 125-149). Beverly Hills, CA: Sage.

Perrow, C. (1967). A framework for the comparative analysis of organizations. *American Sociological Review, 32,* 194-208.

Reedy, A. M., Shivnan, J. C., Hanson, J. L., Haisfield, M. E., & Gregory, R. E. (1994). The clinical application of research utilization: Amphotericin B. *Oncology Nursing Forum, 21,* 715-719.

Rogers, E. M. (1983). *Diffusion of innovations* (3rd ed.). New York: Free Press.

Rogers, E. M. (1995). *Diffusion of innovations* (4th ed.). New York: Free Press.

Rogers, E. M., & Agarwala-Rogers, R. (1976). *Communication in organizations.* New York: Free Press.

Rogers, E. M., & Shoemaker, F. F. (1971). *Communication of innovations: A cross-cultural approach.* New York: Free Press.

Rothman, J. (1974). *Planning and organizing for social change.* New York: Columbia University Press.

Sieber, S. D. (1968). Organizational influences on innovative roles. In T. L. Eidell & J. M. Kitchell (Eds.), *Knowledge production and utilization in educational administration* (pp. 120-142). Eugene: University of Oregon, Center for Advanced Study of Educational Administration.

Stetler, C. B. (1983). Nurses and research: Responsibility and involvement. *Journal of the National Intravenous Therapy Association, 6,* 207-212.

Stetler, C. B. (1984). *Nursing research in a service setting.* Reston, VA: Reston.

Stetler, C. B. (1985). Research utilization: Defining the concept. *Image: The Journal of Nursing Scholarship, 17,* 40-44.

Stetler, C. B. (1989). A strategy for teaching research use. *Nurse Educator, 13*(3), 17-20.

Stetler, C. B. (1994). Refinement of the Stetler/Marram model for application of research findings to practice. *Nursing Outlook, 42,* 15-25.

Stetler, C. B., Bautista, C., Vernale-Hannon, C., & Foster, J. (1995). Enhancing research utilization by clinical nurse specialists. *Nursing Clinics of North America, 30,* 457-473.

Stetler, C. B., & DiMaggio, G. (1991). Research utilization among clinical nurse specialists. *Clinical Nurse Specialist, 5,* 151-155.

Stetler, C. B., & Marram, G. (1976). Evaluating research findings for applicability in practice. *Nursing Outlook, 24,* 559-563.

Titler, M. G., Kleiber, C., Steelman, V., Goode, C., Rakel, B., Barry-Walker, J., Small, S., & Buckwalter, K. (1994). Infusing research into practice to promote quality care. *Nursing Research, 43,* 307-313.

Tornquist, E. M., Funk, S. G., & Champagne, M. T. (1995). Research utilization: Reconnecting research and practice. *AACN Clinical Issues, 6,* 105-109.
Utz, S. W., & Gleit, C. J. (1995). Current developments in research-based interventions: Enhancing and advancing the CNS role. *Clinical Nurse Specialist, 9*(1), 8-11, 22.
White, J. M., Leske, J. S., & Pearcy, J. M. (1995). Models and processes of research utilization. *Nursing Clinics of North America, 30,* 409-420.
Zaltman, G., & Duncan, R. (1977). *Strategies for planned change.* New York: John Wiley.

Appendix A: Glossary

This glossary gives definitions germane to usage in the text of this book. The chapter number that follows a definition indicates the first chapter in which a significant usage of the word appeared.

Abstraction. A representation or expression of the qualities of an object or process that is not associated with any specific instance of the object or process. (Chapter 2)

Action research. Community-oriented research that confronts current social problems. Lewin and his staff defined four types of action research: diagnostic action research designed to produce a needed plan of action, participant action research that involved members from a community in need, empirical descriptions of daily experiences, and experimental action research with controlled experiments in almost identical social situations. (Chapter 5)

Adaptation. "A process of responding positively to environmental changes in such a way as to decrease responses necessary to cope with the stimuli and increase sensitivity to respond to other stimuli" (Roy, 1984c, p. 37). (Chapter 9)

Adaptation level. "A changing point (of response), influenced by the demands of the situation and the person's internal resources including capabilities, hopes, dreams, aspirations, motivations, and all that makes the person constantly move toward mastery" (Andrews & Roy, 1991a, p. 6). (Chapter 9)

Adaptive. "The capacity to adjust effectively to changes in the environment and, in turn, affect the environment" (Andrews & Roy, 1991a, p. 10). (Chapter 9)

Adaptive modes. Coping methods that demonstrate the activity of the regulator and cognator mechanisms (Andrews & Roy, 1991a). Roy's four adaptive modes include the physiological, self-concept, role function, and interdependence modes. (Chapter 9)

Adaptive system modes. Modes of action that "encompass the relevant phenomenon in the nurse administrator's universe" (Roy & Anway, 1989, p. 81). Adaptive system modes include the interdependence, physical, and role adaptive system modes. (Chapter 9)

Adopter. The person who accepts and uses an innovation. The person's adoption decision might be relatively permanent or might be short-lived. (Chapter 6)

Adoption. The choice to accept and use an innovation. (Chapter 16)

Adoption curve. The S-shaped cumulative curve or bell-shaped frequency curve that results from a time-oriented plotting of adopters in a social system. Tarde (see Rogers, 1983) and Ryan and Gross (1943) demonstrated the adoption curve; Rogers made it famous. (Chapter 16)

Affiliated change agent. Change agents (planners) who belong, through employment or some kind of consulting arrangement, to the systems they try to change. (Chapter 7)

Applied research. Research planned to confront a specific practical problem. (Chapter 5)

Blame the victim. A mind-set in which a person censures or condemns another for the negative results of wrongs the other has suffered and could not prevent. (Chapter 4)

Centralization. The concentration of power, authority, and accountability in positions at the top of an organization's social structure. (Chapter 16)

Change agent. An "individual who influences clients' innovation-decisions in a direction deemed desirable by a change agency" (Rogers, 1995, p. 27). (Chapter 18)

Channel. A path along which new ideas, practices, or products flow into a social system. Food channels include grocery stores and gardens. Information channels include the media, libraries, and so on. (Chapter 7)

Channels microtheory. A Lewin microtheory that depicts the ways that messages pass gates and gatekeepers and travel through specific passageways in entering and traveling through a social system. (Chapter 7)

Classical theories of change. Change theories that explain social changes that span thousands of years. (Chapter 2)

Clinical protocol. "A written document that transforms the individual studies in a research base into a synthesized whole, translates research jargon into clinical jargon, and addresses issues surrounding the use of the new knowledge in practice" (Horsley, Crane, Crabtree, & Wood, 1983, p. 2). (Chapter 18)

Cognator subsystem. Mechanism that "responds through four cognitive-emotive channels: [p]erception and information processing, learning, judgment, and emotion" (Andrews & Roy, 1991a, p. 14). (Chapter 9)

Collaboration. A joint venture, typically of an intellectual nature, into planning and decision making. Collaborators enter into the collaborative process willingly, see themselves as team members, offer their expertise, share responsibility and power, and recognize the contributions of others. Collaboration is a process that occurs between individuals. It is not accommodation or compromise. (Chapter 3)

Competence credibility. The degree to which adopters believe that the person who provides information about an innovation possesses accurate knowledge and expertise related to the innovation. (Chapter 16)

Conceptual ordering. The mental process whereby planners categorize entities such as the people, places, things, timing, motives, and conditions of a change situation for purposes of organizing plans and actions. (Chapter 1)

Configuration. In CLER model terms, a social unit (individual, group, institution, or culture [I, G, IS, or CL]) in which individual persons play a variety of social roles. (Chapter 19)

Configuration map. A diagram showing social units and linkages among them that are important to a planned change episode. (Chapter 19)

Confirmation stage. A stage in the Rogers diffusion model in which the adopter looks for reasons to continue the use of an innovation that he or she already has adopted. (Chapter 16)

Conflict. A state characterized by clashes in values. Lewin's microtheories say that conflict occurs when two or more force fields overlap and have forces of about equal strength. (Chapter 10)

Constructivism. A philosophy that helps planners include, in their plans for change, serviceable elements that already exist in the environment. (Chapter 2)

Context (of a change or nursing practice situation). The physical, psychological, emotional, social, geographic, economic (and so on) environment of a change or nursing practice situation. (Chapter 1)

Contextual stimuli. "All the environmental factors that present to the person from within or without, but which are not the center of the person's attention and/or energy" (Andrews & Roy, 1991a, p. 9). (Chapter 9)

Correspondence of forces. A Lewin term for the origin of the forces that correspond to a person's own needs, the induced forces that correspond to another's wishes, and the impersonal forces that correspond to objective sources. (Chapter 10)

Criterion-referenced standards. Standards that compare performance with fixed reference points. These standards do not recognize aptitude or growth. (Chapter 5)

Data-based strategies. Planned change strategies that rely on the collection, analysis, interpretation, and application of information for the making of planned change. (Chapter 7)

Data-based strategies with initiatory aims. Data-based strategies directed at the development of a problem-identification and problem-solving climate for the making of planned change. (Chapter 7)

Data-based strategies with pragmatic aims. Data-based change strategies developed with the objective of finding and applying solutions appropriate to social problems. (Chapter 7)

Destructive power. A type of social power described by Boulding that involves threat, defiance, counterthreat, flight, disarming behavior (and possibly fight). Sometimes destructive power has productive results, as when cutting down a tree produces lumber for houses. (Chapter 3)

Developmental approach. A broad classification of nursing knowledge that draws upon such disciplines as psychology, biology and physics, and sociology to provide claims about the nature of human beings. These claims address growth, development, and maturation; change; direction of change; identifiable states; forms of progression; forces; and potentiality. (Chapter 9)

Developmental category of nursing knowledge. See "developmental approach." (Chapter 9)

Dialectical theory. A theory that describes a system of conscientious dialogue for putting opposing thoughts together and, through reasoning, resolves the ensuing conflict. (Chapter 7)

Dialectics. Orderly reasoning that combines diverse ideas and works toward resolution of the resultant conflict. (Chapter 2)

Dialogic relationship. A relationship characterized by respectful and serious dialogue among the parties involved in a change episode. (Chapter 5)

Diffuser. An adopter (or other individual) who receives an incentive, such as a monetary payment, to persuade another to adopt an innovation (Rogers, 1995, pp. 219, 220). (Chapter 18)

Diffusion. A process that includes "both the planned and the spontaneous spread of new ideas" (Rogers, 1995, p. 7). In diffusion, a social unit includes an innovation in its life in a relatively stable way. (Chapter 2)

Diffusion theories. Change theories that trace the adoption of a particular innovation, over time, through a social system. (Chapter 2)

Directive role. The guise or character in which a person commands or mandates specific actions on the part of others. (Chapter 4)

Discipline. Body or branch on knowledge, characterized by collective knowledge development among persons within a common interest area. (Chapter 9)

Doctor-nurse game. The rigid power hierarchy of the illness-care culture that expects nurses to make recommendations about patient care in ways that cause their suggestions to appear as physicians' ideas and in which physicians are expected to ask for nurses' opinions without appearing to solicit them. (Chapter 3)

Domain of the professional nurse. The theoretical and practice sphere of a learned and expert nurse. This domain has stable elements but it responds to situations in other spheres. For example, nursing would respond to politics as well as to social science knowledge of planned change theories that tell how to deal with political situations. With respect to flexibility and time, current professional concerns do not limit the boundaries of a professional domain. (Chapter 1)

Driving force. A force that leads to locomotion toward a goal that has a positive valence for the person or away from a goal that has a negative valence for the person. (Chapter 10)

Economic power. A type of social power that generates income and is characterized by production and exchange. Economic power always includes some elements of threat power and integrative power. (Chapter 3)

Engineering theory. A theory designed to give guidance and instruction to change planners. (Chapter 2)

Environment. In RAM terms, "all conditions, circumstances, and influences that surround and affect the development and behavior of the person" (Andrews & Roy, 1991a, p. 18). (Chapter 9)

In CLER terminology, the total of the physical, social, and intellectual forces where social units are located. Environments can be supportive, neutral, or inhibitive with respect to a specific planned change. (Chapter 19)

Epistemology. Philosophical inquiry about the nature and origins of knowledge. (Chapter 13)

Espoused theory. The theory chosen, but not yet used, to provide guidance in a particular change episode. (Chapter 2)

Expecting/typifying. A CLER term for the process by which planners use previous knowledge to develop expectations regarding the nature and likelihood of behaviors typical to a particular individual or group. (Chapter 19)

Experiencing/correcting. A CLER term for the process of testing expectations regarding typical behaviors against reality and then making the needed adjustments. (Chapter 19)

Field. A Lewin term for the total life space (environment) of an individual or group, as perceived by that individual or group. (Chapter 10)

Field theory. A Lewin theory for building scientific constructs and theory. (Chapter 10)

First-level assessment. "Gathering data about behavior in each adaptive mode by skillful observation, accurate measurement of responses, and communicative interviewing" (Roy, 1984d, p. 43). (Chapter 9)

Focal stimulus. "The internal or external stimulus most immediately confronting the person; the object or event that attracts one's attention" (Andrews & Roy, 1991a, p. 6). (Chapter 9)

Force. A tendency toward locomotion (i.e., resources, ability, peer pressure) at a given point in the life space (field). This tendency has strength and direction. See "correspondence of forces," "driving force," "force field," "restraining force," "resultant force." (Chapter 10)

Force field. The properties of the field as a whole; the total of the influences toward change or away from change in the physical and social environment of a person or group. (Chapter 3)

Force field analysis. A careful, preferably measured, estimation of the strength of influences for and against change in a particular situation. (Chapter 10)

Force field analysis microtheory. A Lewin microtheory for the measurement, in a social system, of forces for and against a particular course of action. (Chapter 7)

Formalization. The degree to which members of an organization rely on rules and procedures in doing their work. (Chapter 16)

Formative evaluation. Evaluation that occurs during the development and conduct of a planned change event. (Chapter 8)

Freeze. A Lewin term for the process by which "new" ideas or practices become relatively fixed in individual or group functioning. (Chapter 10)

Gantt chart. A chart that displays the tasks and names of responsible persons in row stubs and the time frames in columns. Lines drawn through the cells formed by intersections of the rows and columns show the progress of the work. This chart preceded the PERT chart. (Chapter 7)

Gate. A device for controlling the entry or flow of ideas, practices, or goods (i.e., promotion committees, administrative positions, ANA council memberships) in a social system. (Chapter 10)

Gatekeeper. A person who formally or informally controls the flow of ideas, practices, or goods into and throughout social system channels. Examples include nurse executives, medical librarians, and procedure committees. (Chapter 10)

Generalization. A process in which observers examine the characteristics of a class of items of interest and then make extrapolations to other items of the same class. (Chapter 2)

Gestalt. A configuration, an organized whole, in which the functional whole cannot be derived from the sum of its parts. (Chapter 10)

Gestalt psychology. A system of psychology that considers an individual's perception and behavior in light of configurational wholes. (Chapter 10)

Goal. In Lewin terms, a goal is a force field where all forces go in the same direction. (Chapter 10)

Goal-based evaluation. Determination of the degrees to which the conduct and outcomes of planned change events meet the objectives of planner and adopter groups. (Chapter 8)

Goal-free evaluation. Determination of the degrees to which the conduct and outcomes of planned change events coincide with the values of the people who furnish evaluation information. These people may be involved in either informal or formal ways with the change episode. (Chapter 8)

Goal of nursing. "Promotion of adaptation in each of the four modes, thereby contributing to the person's health, quality of life, and dying with dignity" (Andrews & Roy, 1991a, p. 20). (Chapter 9)

Goals of the human system. These include survival, growth, reproduction, and mastery. (Chapter 9)

Grammar of action. A CLER term for social action organized by ideas about the relationship between means and ends (strategies and outcomes). (Chapter 19)

Growth-oriented standards. Standards that plot an individual's or group's past and present achievement as growth points over time. They ignore both aptitude and absolute reference points. (Chapter 5)

Health. "A state and a process of being and becoming an integrated and whole person . . . a reflection of adaptation" (Andrews & Roy, 1991a, p. 19). (Chapter 9)

Heterophily. The property by which persons differ with respect to their belief systems, customs, and social backgrounds. (Chapter 16)

Holism. A view that considers the total, not the parts. Mind, body, and spirit are one and different than the sum of the parts. (Chapter 9)

Homophily. The property by which individuals are the same with respect to their belief systems, customs, and social backgrounds. (Chapter 16)

Hypothesis. A statement of a diagnosis of a social system problem most reasonably expected from the information currently available. (Chapter 5)

Impersonal force. See "correspondence of forces." (Chapter 10)

Incentive. "Direct or indirect payments of either cash or in kind that are given to an individual or a system to encourage some overt behavioral change" (Rogers, 1995, p. 219). (Chapter 18)

Individual-blame bias. A viewpoint that places blame for a problem on individuals more readily than it places blame on the social system around them. (Chapter 8)

Individual-group relationships microtheory (I-G). A Lewin microtheory that explains the steps by which individual and group experiences work together in setting new standards for group and individual functioning. (Chapter 10)

Induced force. See "correspondence of forces." (Chapter 10)

Ineffective response. Behavior that "does not promote integrity or contribute to the goals of adaptation" (Andrews & Roy, 1991a, p. 12). (Chapter 9)

Innovation. A practice, device, or idea that is new to the social system where it is introduced; a solution to a social system problem. (Chapter 4)

Innovation-decision process. A series of stages that includes five phases (knowledge, persuasion, decision, implementation, confirmation) in the diffusion of an innovation. This process forms the basic structure of the Rogers diffusion model. (Chapter 4)

Innovation in nursing. "Implies changes in practice that are new to those using them and that are intended to benefit clients" (Horsley et al., 1983, p. 120). (Chapter 18)

Innovativeness. The degree to which individuals or organizations adopt innovations more or less readily than do their peers. (Chapter 16)

Innovator. In planned change terms, a change agent, a planner. He or she may or may not be the inventor of the innovation under consideration. (Chapter 6)

Innovator subsystem. Structures and processes that enable organizational growth. These may be new technologies, task forces, educational programs, or problem-solving methods. (Chapter 9)

Integrative power. Love and respect combined with small but complex elements of threat and exchange power. (Chapter 3)

Interaction approach. A broad classification of nursing knowledge that draws upon such disciplines as psychology, biology and physics, and sociology to provide claims about the nature of human beings. These claims address social acts and relationships, perception, communication, role, and self-concept. (Chapter 9)

Interaction category of nursing knowledge. See "interaction approach." (Chapter 9)

Interdependence adaptive mode. "The close relationships of people that involve the willingness and ability to love, respect, and value others, and to accept and respond to love, respect, and value given by others" (Tedrow, 1991, p. 386). (Chapter 9)

Interdependence adaptive system mode. Involves "both private and public contacts that result in interpersonal relationships established both intra- and interorganizationally" (Roy & Anway, 1989, p. 81). (Chapter 9)

Interpersonal adaptive system mode. "Reflects how people and . . . [individuals and groups in organizations] perceive themselves because of environmental feedback" (Roy & Anway, 1989, p. 81). (Chapter 9)

Laboratory learning. Staff-supervised and supported learning in a residential setting designed to increase participants' authenticity and ability to attend to others' concerns. (Chapter 13)

Level of generality. Degree of abstractness. (Chapter 2)

Levers of nurse power. A means for the application of energy or ability that nurses can use to create social change. (Chapter 3)

Linear. Pertaining to or consisting of lines. (Chapter 9)

Linkage. A CLER term for the communication network connections that enable social units to send or receive information from each other. Formal or informal linkages exist between and within social units. (Chapter 19)

Linkage typing. A CLER term for a process that uses a diagram to show communication linkages important to a change event. Linkage typing shows which linkages should be built, maintained, or cut. (Chapter 19)

Linking-pin concept. An idea structure developed by Likert to describe connections among work groups for purposes of increasing communication in organizations. (Chapter 7)

Locomotion. A Lewin term for the movement from one position to another that occurs when the sum of forces exceeds zero. (Chapter 10)

Logical positivism. See "positivism." (Chapter 13)

Macrotheory. A theory that deals with phenomena on a grand scale that includes vast amounts of time, space, or numbers of people. Related words include "grand," "molar," and "holistic." (Chapter 2)

Matrix of discovery. A chart composed of columns and rows with headings and stubs pertinent to a situation under study. The utility of the chart comes from the combination of the ideas represented by the column heads and row stubs associated with each cell; each cell displays a unique combination. (Chapter 5)

Measurement method. A technique or procedure for assessment of the amount of a factor present in a data collection situation. (Chapter 5)

Metaparadigm concepts. Person, environment, health, and nursing (actions). (Chapter 9)

Metatheory. A theory that concerns theory and theory development. (Chapter 2)

Microtheory. A theory that deals with only narrowly selected phenomena. Related words include "atomistic" and "molecular." (Chapter 2)

Model. Kaplan (1964) likened models to structural analogies. Models are representations of reality that find expression in words, pictures, mathematics, or physical forms. (Chapter 2)

Morphology. A study of the structure and form of a class of things. Nutt (1985) presented a conceptual scheme for use in studying planning processes; he called his scheme a morphology. (Chapter 13)

Move. A Lewin term for the action phase during which an individual or social system changes position from one point to a different state or condition. (Chapter 10)

Need. A state of dissatisfaction or frustration that occurs when one's desires or wants outweigh what one actually has (Rogers, 1995). (Chapter 18)

Need creation. The process by which planners employ strategies of persuasion or publicity to develop, in a target population, a desire or demand for the product that the planners wish the population to use. (Chapter 5)

Need recognition. A process by which persons in or connected with a social system recognize a social problem. (Chapter 5)

Network. A set of individuals and groups linked together in a pattern of communication and exchange. (Chapter 16)

Nomenclature. The system of terms used in a particular science or profession. (Chapter 5)

Normative-reeducative strategy. A planned change strategy that rests on the assumption that humans are rational, intelligent, social beings who change in response to altered norms and new knowledge. (Chapter 4)

Normative standards. Standards that relate performance to that of a particular reference group. These standards ignore aptitude and "absolute" reference points. (Chapter 5)

Nursing (actions). "Assess behavior and factors that influence adaptation level and intervene by managing the focal, contextual, and residual stimuli" (Roy, 1984a, p. 13). (Chapter 9)

Nursing diagnosis. "Judgment process resulting in a statement conveying the person's adaptation status" (Andrews & Roy, 1991b, p. 37). (Chapter 9)

Nursing intervention. Management of stimuli that "involves altering, increasing, decreasing, removing, or maintaining" focal, contextual, and residual stimuli (Andrews & Roy, 1991b, p. 37). (Chapter 9)

Objective approach. See "quantitative approach." (Chapter 5)

Opinion leader. An "individual who influences other individuals' attitudes or overt behavior informally in a desired way with relative frequency" (Rogers, 1995, p. 27). (Chapter 18)

Ordering/relating. A CLER term for the intellectual process of "getting a handle on" (the mental structuring of) a social situation. The person doing this ordering/relating (modeling) establishes time and social space boundaries and relationships for social subsystems and assigns causes and effects. (Chapter 19)

Organizational behavior. The ways people act when they group themselves together to accomplish purposes they cannot fulfill alone. (Chapter 5)

Organizational structure. The ways people align themselves in groups designed to accomplish purposes they cannot fulfill alone. (Chapter 1)

Own-needs force. See "correspondence of forces." (Chapter 10)

Person. "Holistic adaptive system" (Andrews & Roy, 1991a, p. 6). (Chapter 9)

Persuasion. The act or process of inducing, influencing, or swaying a person or persons toward a particular view or course of action. (Chapter 4)

Persuasion stage. A stage in the Rogers diffusion model in which an individual forms attitudes about an innovation, not necessarily in the direction desired by planners. In the Rogers model, persuasion does not mean an attempt by planners to influence potential adopters. (Chapter 16)

PERT. See "Program Evaluation and Review Technique." (Chapter 16)

Physical adaptive system mode. "Basic operating resources and conditions without which an organization cannot maintain even rudimentary functioning" (Roy & Anway, 1989, pp. 80, 81). (Chapter 9)

Planned change theory. A set of logically related concepts that explain, in a systematic way, how planned social change occurs, that predict how various forces in the environment will react in specified situations, and that help planners control variables that increase or decrease the likelihood of the occurrence of change. (Chapter 1)

Position. A Lewin term for one point within the social space of a group. (Chapter 10)

Positivism. An orientation that stresses fact as the object of knowledge while denying that knowledge has any other object. Positivism prefers data to theory, theory to speculation, physical data to psychological data, formal logic to informal logic, and deduction to induction. (Chapter 13)

Power as ability. The natural or acquired capacity to reason and implement plans. (Chapter 3)

Power as compliance. The natural or acquired capacity to cause others to follow one's own plans. (Chapter 3)

Power-coercive strategies. Integrated sets of plans intended to compel persons to make social changes they do not wish to make. (Chapter 3)

Power field. In Lewin language, values are constructs with the same psychological dimension as power fields. Thus power fields (values) bring on (induce) force fields but do not act as force fields. (Chapter 3)

Power trap. A deceptive technique that catches unaware persons and diminishes their social power. Examples include getting caught by the image rather than the substance of power (i.e., a macho image) and group infighting. (Chapter 3)

Practice innovation. Specific nursing actions administered to patients that are derived from a clinical protocol (Horsley et al., 1983, p. 2). (Chapter 18)

Problem setting. The process of defining and validating change objectives. (Chapter 19)

Problem solving. Implementation of change plans. (Chapter 19)

Program Evaluation and Review Technique (PERT). A procedure designed to help managers use charts that list and prioritize tasks as they plan and monitor activities connected with and crucial to a specific change episode. (Chapter 7)

Pro-innovation bias. A viewpoint that automatically considers an innovation better than the concept, tool, or skill it replaces. (Chapter 8)

Protocol. A plan for the transformation of research results into a practice innovation for use by professional practitioners. (Chapter 6)

Qualitative approach. A system of belief that sees situations and entities in the world as subjective and therefore views data collection as requiring some kind of participation in the situation under observation. (Chapter 5)

Quantitative approach. A system of beliefs that sees situations and entities in the world as objective and therefore views data collection as an activity in which the observer must remain detached from the situation under observation. This approach sees situations and entities as measurable and emphasizes numerical measurement and statistics. (Chapter 5)

Rational-empirical strategies. Strategies that rely on reasoning and on the ability of people to choose the good for themselves. (Chapter 7)

Reaction worldview. A worldview (weltanschauung) that sees humans as bio-psycho-social-spiritual beings who react to external environmental stimuli in a linear, causal manner. "Change occurs only for survival and as a consequence of predictable and controllable antecedent conditions. Only objective phenomena that can be isolated, defined, observed, and measured are studied" (Fawcett, 1995, p. 15). (Chapter 9)

Reciprocal interaction worldview. This worldview sees humans as holistic beings and views parts only in the context of the whole. Humans are active, with reciprocal interactions between themselves and their environments. Reality is multidimensional, context dependent, and relative. Change comes as a result of multiple antecedent factors. Change is probabilistic and may be continuous or only for survival. This worldview espouses study of both objective and subjective phenomena through both quantitative and qualitative methods. It emphasizes empirical observations, methodological controls, and inferential analyses (Fawcett, 1995, p. 16). (Chapter 9)

Reformulation. Translation of a theory by "redefining concepts and restating propositions that do not reflect the preferred world view or category of nursing knowledge, so that all ideas presented in the conceptual model are consistent" (Fawcett, 1995, p. 58). (Chapter 9)

Regulator subsystem. "Responds automatically through neural, chemical, and endocrine coping processes" (Andrews & Roy, 1991a, p. 14). (Chapter 9)

Research base. A common conceptual area obtained through the identification and synthesis of multiple research studies (Horsley et al., 1983, p. 2). (Chapter 18)

Research utilization model. A systematic overall plan for the employment of the results of scientific inquiry in a practical situation. (Chapter 1)

Residual stimuli. Factors "having an indeterminate effect on the person's behavior; their effect has not or cannot be validated" (Andrews & Roy, 1991b, p. 35). (Chapter 9)

Resistance. Any actions that people use to keep a situation or practice the way it was before a planner introduced an innovation. (Chapter 7)

Resources. The assets (time, money, intelligence, land, goodwill, knowledge, legal mandates, political connections, water, soil, space, and so on) needed for the dissemination and adoption of an innovation. (Chapter 6)

Restraining force. A physical or social obstacle or barrier that prevents locomotion by influencing the effects of driving forces. (Chapter 10)

Role adaptive system mode. "Relates to job performance" (Roy & Anway, 1989, p. 81). (Chapter 9)

Role function adaptive mode. Focuses specifically on the roles the person occupies in society. (Chapter 9)

Sacrifice trap. A situation in which an enabler, caught in enabling cycles, has difficulty recognizing that he or she makes sacrifices in vain. (Chapter 3)

Safety credibility. The degree to which adopters believe that they can trust the person who provides information about an innovation. (Chapter 16)

Second-level assessment. "Identification of the focal, contextual, and residual factors that influence the person" (Roy, 1984d, p. 43). (Chapter 9)

Segmentation. The analysis and division of a population according to characteristics that relate to the likelihood of their responses to planned change. (Chapter 7)

Self-concept adaptive mode. "Composite of beliefs and feelings that one holds about oneself at a given time, formed from perceptions particularly of others' reactions, and directing one's behavior" (Driever cited in Andrews, 1991, p. 270). (Chapter 9)

Simultaneous action worldview. A worldview that sees human beings as identified by pattern and as beings in rhythmical interchange with their environments. "Human beings change continuously and evolve as self-organized fields. Change is unidirectional and unpredictable as human beings move through stages of organization and disorganization to more complex organization. Phenomena of interest are personal knowledge and pattern recognition" (Fawcett, 1995, p. 17). (Chapter 9)

Social mandate. The bidding of society that directs an individual or group to carry out certain functions deemed valuable in that society. (Chapter 1)

Social network. See "network." (Chapter 16)

Social power. See "power." (Chapter 3)

Social structure. The form taken by arrangements people make among themselves to accomplish a specific purpose, such as work. (Chapter 7)

Social unit. A configuration (I, G, IS, CL) is an individual, group (which may be as small as a dyad), institution, or culture that, in CLER terms, forms part or all of a configuration. (Chapter 19)

Space allocation. The allotment of physical working space in an institution or organization. (Chapter 3)

Stabilizer subsystem. Refers to "the structures and processes aimed at system maintenance" (Roy & Anway, 1989, p. 79). (Chapter 9)

Standard. A criterion or model set up as an ideal. (Chapter 5)

Strategy. A plan of action that is congruent with a particular planned change theory or model (example: reeducation). A strategy is less general than a theory or model but not as specific as a tactic. (Chapter 7)

Subjective approach. See "qualitative approach." (Chapter 5)

Successive approximation. One of a series of increasingly successful attempts to reach a goal. (Chapter 5)

Summative evaluation. An evaluation that determines the worth of a completed change episode according to some system of values. (Chapter 8)

Systemic model. A planned change model founded, at least in part, on systems theory. (Chapter 19)

Systems approach. A broad classification of nursing knowledge that draws upon such disciplines as psychology, biology, physics, and sociology to provide claims about the nature of human beings. These claims address integration of parts; systems; environment; open and closed systems; boundaries; tension, stress, strain, and conflict; equilibrium and steady state; and feedback. (Chapter 9)

Systems category of nursing knowledge. See "systems approach." (Chapter 9)

Tactic. A specific maneuver used to further the aims of a particular strategy (example: appointing a member of the opposition to a vital committee). (Chapter 7)

Task analysis. The breakdown of an activity into component parts for the purpose of providing instruction about the best way to conduct the activity. (Chapter 6)

Technology. Application, to human enterprises, of scientific knowledge of raw materials and of processes for dealing with raw materials. (Chapter 5)

Technology cluster. A bundle of innovations that fit together. Adoption of one of the innovations invites (sometimes mandates) adoption of some or all of the others. (Chapter 6)

Technostructural strategy. A strategy that alters technology for the purpose of changing social structure or that alters social structure or the physical environment for the purpose of changing technology. (Chapter 7)

Teleological. Relating to design or purpose as seen in natural phenomena. (Chapter 13)

Theory-in-use. The theory being put into operation by change planners. (Chapter 2)

Threat power. A type of power with largely destructive overtones and small amounts of economic power and integrative power. This is the least potent of Boulding's (1989) three types of social power. (Chapter 3)

Total diffusion. A situation that exists when a social unit seeks and values an innovation and can provide the skills and resources needed to maintain its adoption by a new member. In total diffusion, not every member of the social unit must adopt the innovation. (Chapter 19)

Transformation, change by. The general category of change that occurs by conscious design. (Chapter 1)

Transmission, change by. Evolutionary change that occurs as culture passes without design from one generation to another. (Chapter 1)

Triangulation. The employment of two or more instruments, and, if possible, measurement modes, to the measurement of a thing under consideration. (Chapter 5)

Unaffiliated mode. A kind of operation in which planners have no formal ties with the social system that is the object of change. (Chapter 4)

Unfreeze. The process of softening toward change in a social system. (Chapter 10)

Unit of analysis. The part, element, or segment of a social situation, group, or organization chosen for study. (Chapter 5)

Utilitarian standard. A standard that relates performance to the pragmatic concerns of safety, effectiveness, and efficiency rather than to the performance of others or a fixed standard. (Chapter 5)

Valence. The degree of attractiveness (positive valence) or repulsion (negative valence) of an activity, social position, or other possible goal in a person's life space. (Chapter 10)

Worldview. "Philosophic claims about the nature of human beings and the human-environment relationship" (Fawcett, 1993b, p. 56). (Chapter 9)

Appendix B:
The Tiffany-Lutjens
Planned Change Theory
Evaluation Procedure

Tiffany, Cheatham, Doornbos, Loudermelt, and Momadi (1994) conducted an 11-year survey of nursing periodical literature that deals with planned change. As they looked at ways that nurse authors use planned change theories, they noted an almost total lack of theory evaluation. The evaluation that did occur used no systematic classification or ranking methods. In response, Tiffany and Lutjens (Tiffany et al., 1995) developed a procedure, which appears below, for informally rating a planned change theory according to its goodness of fit with nursing perspectives. Readers can use this procedure either as a guide to learning about a particular planned change theory or as a decision-making tool in the choice of a theory for planning a change episode.

Scoring Procedure

After they have acquired sufficient knowledge about a planned change theory, theory users can choose one of two scoring methods. Users with little time employ the subscale headings as anchor points and the specific questions as

AUTHORS' NOTE: This theory evaluation procedure carries a copyright by Sage Publications, 2455 Teller Road, Thousand Oaks, CA 91320. Please ask permission before using it. Also, please give credit to the developers. They request and appreciate reports of the use of the procedure.

prompters. Those who have more time can answer all the questions to obtain an estimation of how well a planned change theory fits the intended situation.

Short Method

Users see the individual questions as prompters to help themselves think about the characteristics of planned change theories. (They don't assign any score for the 54 individual questions.) Each section heading gets a score of 0-4. When users add the scores together, the total score ranges from 0 to 24. A high score indicates that a theory is well suited to nursing purposes; a low score means that a theory is poorly suited to nursing purposes.

Long Method

Users assign a score of 0-4 for each individual question. (They don't assign any score for the headings). When they add all scores, the total score ranges from 0 to 216. A high score indicates that a theory is well suited to nursing purposes; a low score means that a theory is poorly suited to nursing purposes.

I. Significance

1. The planned change theory addresses targets for change.
2. The theory has an assessment process that could help a change agent identify a problem in a social system.
3. The theory has a clear process for evaluating the total change event.
4. The theory accounts for emerging problems and/or goals throughout the change process.
5. The theory prompts nurse change agents to ask if the proposed change is important for nursing.
6. The theory encourages the ethical use of power.
7. The theory encourages close cooperation between change agents and target population.
8. The theory encourages change agents to help people in the target population make informed decisions.
9. The theory stresses social justice.
10. The theory looks at the world as a whole.
11. The theory views the world as changing rather than nonchanging.
12. The theory prompts change agents to consider whether the strategies they plan will agree with expectations of the social unit targeted for change.

II. Clarity and Consistency

13. The theory has a clear process for planning change.
14. The theory has a clear process for implementing change (causing change to occur).
15. The theory clearly defines planned change.
16. The definition of planned change fits with the remainder of the content of the theory.
17. Key ideas are clearly defined.
18. Relational statements are clearly stated.
19. Key ideas and relational statements avoid unnecessary repetition.
20. Key ideas are consistently used as defined throughout the theory.
21. The theory clearly states what it accepts as truth (assumptions).
22. Key ideas are related to one another.
23. Any diagrams offered increase the reader's understanding of planned change and its processes.
24. The planned change theory contributes to an understanding of planned change beyond what could be obtained from everyday experience or formal study of other planned change theories.

III. Generality

25. The planned change theory could help change agents plan change.
26. The theory focuses only on the processes of planned change, not on unplanned change.
27. The purpose of the theory allows a change agent to carry out plans for change in any one of a number of clinical settings rather than in one specific setting or area.
28. The theory could apply to individuals.
29. The theory could apply to groups.
30. The theory could apply to communities.
31. The theory could apply to society.
32. The theory could apply to different cultures within and outside the United States.
33. Nurses could use this theory as a foundation for research.
34. The theory could be tested through research.
35. Testable hypotheses could be developed from the theory.
36. Key ideas and processes of the theory can be observed in the real world.

IV. Practicality

37. The theory prompts change agents to consider time frames.

38. The theory prompts change agents to consider the people (including experts) available to make the change.
39. The theory prompts change agents to consider space, equipment, and supplies.
40. The theory prompts change agents to consider financial resources.
41. The theory prompts change agents to consider organizational support.
42. The theory prompts change agents to consider whether they can obtain needed political resources for implementing change.
43. The theory prompts change agents to consider whether they can obtain needed legal resources for implementing change.

V. Applicability

44. Nurse change agents could use this theory to create change in clinical settings.
45. Nurse change agents could use this theory to create change in nursing education.
46. Nurse change agents could use this theory to create change in nursing administration.

VI. Foresight

47. The theory helps change agents to foresee possible procedural pitfalls in planning change.
48. The theory helps change agents to foresee possible cultural pitfalls in planning change.
49. The theory suggests ways to deal with possible procedural pitfalls in planning change.
50. The theory suggests ways to deal with possible cultural pitfalls in planning change.
51. The theory helps change agents to foresee immediate resistance to change.
52. The theory helps change agents to foresee long-term resistance to change.
53. The theory helps change agents to foresee immediate results of adoption of proposed solutions.
54. The theory helps change agents to foresee long-term results of adoption of proposed solutions.

A Quantitative Evaluation

Tiffany and Lutjens developed their planned change theory evaluation procedure to assess the goodness of fit between a planned change theory and nursing perspectives.

This scale contains 54 items divided into six subscales (significance, clarity and consistency, generality, practicality, applicability, and foresight). Scores earned by a planned change theory can range from 0, for a totally "unfit" theory, to 216, for a "perfect" theory—both unlikely extremes. In an initial reliability and validity study, 390 subjects evaluated Lewin's theories in response to a five-page synopsis. The mean of the scores they assigned equaled 144, which puts nurse evaluation of Lewin's theories by 395 nurses in active practice at about 63% of the possible score. Preliminary testing indicates that nurses score Lewin's theories at neither the lowest nor the highest point in relation to other planned change theories.

References

Tiffany, C. R., Cheatham, A. B., Doornbos, D., Loudermelt, L., & Momadi, G. G. (1994). Planned change theory: Survey of nursing periodical literature. *Nursing Management, 25*(7), 54-59.

Tiffany, C. R., Lutjens, L. R. J., Dwyer, L., Watson, C., Weitor, B., & Willison, S. (1995). Development and initial assessment of the Tiffany/Lutjens Planned Change Evaluation Instrument. *Nursing Administration Quarterly, 19*(2), 75-76.

Appendix C:
Sources of Key
Planned Change Concepts

C.1. Sources of Key Concepts
in Lewin's Microtheories

This book highlights the change writings produced by Lewin; Bennis, Benne, and Chin; Rogers; and Bhola. Benne, Bennis, and Chin and Rogers collected their work in books with comprehensive tables of contents and indexes. This is not the case with either Lewin or Bhola; hence the need for this appendix to assist readers in finding original sources of their writings.

Lewin lacked concern for authorship credit. Some or what he wrote appears under the names of his students or coworkers; the true extent of his writings remains unknown. Bhola has written extensively on planned change topics but at this date his writings remain scattered. The Appendix C charts were organized to reflect the literature placement and publication dates of Lewin's and Bhola's writings regarding specific planned change concerns. The charts will help readers access reliable sources of Lewin and Bhola literature of interest to nurse planners.

C.1. Lewin

CHART C.1. Sources of Key Concepts in Lewin's Planned Changed Writings

Writings by Lewin

	Background Concepts	Channels Theory	Comments by Others	Quasi-Stationary Equilibria	Field Theory	Force Field Analysis	Individuals-Groups	Jewish Situation	(Re)Education	Research Methods	Time Orientations
Lewin, K. (1935A). *A dynamic theory of personality: Selected papers* (D. K. Adams & K. E. Zener, Trans.). New York: McGraw-Hill.	X			X					X	X	
Lewin, K. (1935B). Psycho-sociological problems of a minority group. *Character and Personality, 3,* 175-187.								X			
Lewin, K. (1936A). *Principles of topological psychology.* New York: McGraw-Hill.	X			X	X					X	
Lewin, K. (1936B). Some social-psychological differences between the United States and Germany. *Character and Personality, 4,* 265-293.	X			X	X		X		X		
Lewin, K. (1939A). Experiments in social space. *Harvard Educational Review, 9,* 21-32.							X			X	
Lewin, K. (1939B). Field theory and experiment in social psychology: Concepts and methods. *American Journal of Sociology, 44,* 868-897.					X					X	
Lewin, K. (1939C, September). When facing danger. *Jewish Frontier.*							X	X			
Lewin, K. (1940A). The background of conflict in marriage. In M. Jung (Ed.), *Modern marriage* (chap. 4). New York: F. S. Crofts.	X						X				

C.1. Lewin

CHART C.1. *(continued)*

	Background Concepts	Channels Theory	Comments by Others	Quasi-Stationary Equilibria	Field Theory	Force Field Analysis	Individuals-Groups	Jewish Situation	(Re)Education	Research Methods	Time Orientations
Lewin, K. (1940B). Bringing up the Jewish child. *Menorah Journal, 28,* 29-45.	X						X	X			
Lewin, K. (1940C). Formalization and progress in psychology. *University of Iowa Studies in Child Welfare, 16(3),* 9-42.	X				X						
Lewin, K. (1941A). Appendix: Analysis of the concepts whole, differentiation, and unity. *University of Iowa Studies in Child Welfare, 18,* 226-261.	X										
Lewin, K. (1941B). Regression, retrogression, and development. In R. Barker, T. Dembo, & K. Lewin, *Frustration and aggression* (chap. 1 and Appendix), *University of Iowa Studies in Child Welfare, 18(1),* 1-43.	X										
Lewin, K. (1941C). Self-hatred among Jews. *Contemporary Jewish Record, 4,* 219-232.							X	X			
Lewin, K. (1942A). Field theory of learning. *Yearbook of the National Society for the Study of Education, Part II, 41,* 215-242.	X				X				X		X
Lewin, K. (1942B). Time perspective and morale. In Goodwin Watson (Ed.), *Civilian morale* (Second yearbook of the Society for the Psychological Study of Issues, chap. 4). Boston: Houghton Mifflin.	X						X				X

C. 1. Lewin

CHART C.1. *(continued)*

Reference	Background Concepts	Channels Theory	Comments by Others	Quasi-Stationary Equilibria	Field Theory	Force Field Analysis	Individuals-Groups	Jewish Situation	(Re)Education	Research Methods	Time Orientations
Lewin, K. (1943A). Cultural reconstruction. *Journal of Abnormal and Social Psychology, 38,* 166-173.	X										
Lewin, K. (1943B). Defining the "field at a given time." *Psychological Review, 50,* 292-310.	X				X					X	X
Lewin, K. (1943C). Forces behind food habits and methods of change. *Bulletin of the National Research Council, 108,* 35-65.		X		X	X						
Lewin, K. (1943D). Psychology and the process of group living. *Journal of Social Psychology, 17,* 113-131.	X										
Lewin, K. (1943E, Winter). The special case of Germany. *Public Opinion Quarterly,* pp. 555-566.	X			X		X	X			X	
Lewin, K. (1944A). Constructs in psychology and psychological ecology. *University of Iowa Studies in Child Welfare, 20,* 1-29.	X				X				X	X	
Lewin, K. (1944B). The solution of chronic conflict in industry. *Proceedings of Second Brief Psychotherapy Council* (pp. 36-46). Chicago: Institute for Psychoanalysis.	X						X				
Lewin, K. (1946A). Action research and minority problems. *Journal of Social Issues, 2,* 34-36.										X	

C. 1. Lewin

CHART C.1. *(continued)*

Reference	Background Concepts	Channels Theory	Comments by Others	Quasi-Stationary Equilibria	Field Theory	Force Field Analysis	Individuals-Groups	Jewish Situation	(Re)Education	Research Methods	Time Orientations
Lewin, K. (1946B). Behavior and development as a function of the total situation. In L. Carmichael (Ed.), *Manual of child psychology* (pp. 918-970). New York: John Wiley.	X			X	X	X	X			X	X
Lewin, K. (1947A). Frontiers in group dynamics I. *Human Relations, 1,* 5-42.	X			X	X	X				X	X
Lewin, K. (1947B). Frontiers in group dynamics II. *Human Relations, 1,* 143-153.	X			X	X	X				X	X
Lewin, K. (1949). Cassirer's philosophy of science and social science. In P. A. Schlipp (Ed.), *The philosophy of Ernst Cassirer* (pp. 271-288). New York: Tudor.	X			X	X	X				X	X
Lewin, K. (1958). Group decision and social change. In E. E. Maccoby, T. M. Newcomb, & E. L. Hartley (Eds.), *Readings in social psychology* (3rd ed., pp. 197-211). New York: Holt.		X		X		X	X			X	X
Lewin, K. (1961). Quasi-stationary social equilibria and the problem of permanent change. In W. G. Bennis, K. D. Benne, & R. Chin (Eds.), *The planning of change* (pp. 235-238). New York: Holt, Rinehart & Winston.		X		X		X	X			X	X
Lewin, K. (1964). Group dynamics and social change. In A. Etzioni & E. Etzioni (Eds.), *Social change: Sources, patterns, and consequences* (pp. 354-361). New York: Basic Books.		X		X		X	X			X	X

C. 1. Lewin

CHART C.1. *(continued)*

Reference	Background Concepts	Channels Theory	Comments by Others	Quasi-Stationary Equilibria	Field Theory	Force Field Analysis	Individuals-Groups	Jewish Situation	(Re)Education	Research Methods	Time Orientations
Lewin, K., & Grabbe, P. (1945). Conduct, knowledge, and acceptance of new values. *Journal of Social Issues, 1,* 53-63.							X		X		
Writings by Others											
Benne, K. D. (1985). The process of reeducation: An assessment of Kurt Lewin's views. In W. G. Bennis, K. D. Benne, & R. Chin (Eds.), *The planning of change* (4th ed., pp. 272-283). New York: Holt, Rinehart & Winston.			X				X		X		
Cartwright, D. (Ed.). (1951). *Field theory in social science: Selected theoretical papers by Kurt Lewin.* New York: Harper.			X								
De Rivera, J. (1976). *Field theory as human science: Contributions of Lewin's Berlin group.* New York: Gardner.	X		X		X					X	
Lewin, G. W. (1948). *Resolving social conflicts: Selected papers on group dynamics by Kurt Lewin.* New York: Harper.			X								
Marrow, A. J. (1969). *The practical theorist.* New York: Basic Books.			X								
Stivers, E., & Wheelan, S. (1986). *The Lewin legacy.* New York: Springer.	X	X	X	X	X	X		X		X	

371

The Lewin literature listed below falls into six categories: selected early writings, writings collected and published by others in 1948, writings collected and published by others in 1951, reprints of selected Lewin monographs, commentaries by others on Lewin's theories and legacy, and miscellaneous selections. (Uppercase letters after dates in the references refer to original publications listed in the table above.)

Selected Early Writings

Lewin, K. (1935A). *A dynamic theory of personality: Selected papers* (D. K. Adams & K. E. Zener, Trans.). New York: McGraw-Hill.

Lewin, K. (1936A). *Principles of topological psychology.* New York: McGraw-Hill.

Writings Collected and Published by Others in 1948

Lewin, K. (1935B). Psycho-sociological problems of a minority group. *Character and Personality, 3,* 175-187.

Lewin, K. (1936B). Some social-psychological differences between the United States and Germany. *Character and Personality, 4,* 265-293.

Lewin, K. (1939A). Experiments in social space. *Harvard Educational Review, 9,* 21-32.

Lewin, K. (1939C, September). When facing danger. *Jewish Frontier.*

Lewin, K. (1940A). The background of conflict in marriage. In M. Jung (Ed.), *Modern marriage* (chap. 4). New York: F. S. Crofts.

Lewin, K. (1940B). Bringing up the Jewish child. *Menorah Journal, 28,* 29-45.

Lewin, K. (1941C). Self-hatred among Jews. *Contemporary Jewish Record, 4,* 219-232.

Lewin, K. (1942B). Time perspective and morale. In Goodwin Watson (Ed.), *Civilian morale* (Second yearbook of the Society for the Psychological Study of Issues, chap. 4). Boston: Houghton Mifflin.

Lewin, K. (1943A). Cultural reconstruction. *Journal of Abnormal and Social Psychology, 38,* 166-173.

Lewin, K. (1943E, Winter). The special case of Germany. *Public Opinion Quarterly,* pp. 555-566.

Lewin, K. (1944B). The solution of chronic conflict in industry. *Proceedings of Second Brief Psychotherapy Council* (pp. 36-46).

Lewin, K. (1946A). Action research and minority problems. *Journal of Social Issues, 2,* 34-36.

Lewin, K., & Grabbe, P. (1945). Conduct, knowledge, and acceptance of new values. *Journal of Social Issues, 1,* 53-63.

Writings Collected and Published by Others in 1951

Lewin, K. (1939B). Field theory and experiment in social psychology: Concepts and methods. *American Journal of Sociology, 44,* 868-897.

Lewin, K. (1940C). Formalization and progress in psychology. *University of Iowa Studies in Child Welfare, 16*(3), 9-42.

Lewin, K. (1941A). Appendix: Analysis of the concepts whole, differentiation, and unity. *University of Iowa Studies in Child Welfare, 18,* 226-261.

Lewin, K. (1941B). Regression, retrogression, and development. In R. Barker, T. Dembo, & K. Lewin, *Frustration and aggression* (chap. 1 and Appendix), *University of Iowa Studies in Child Welfare, 18*(1), 1-43.

Lewin, K. (1942A). Field theory of learning. *Yearbook of the National Society for the Study of Education, Part II, 41,* 215-242.

Lewin, K. (1943B). Defining the "field at a given time." *Psychological Review, 50,* 292-310.

Lewin, K. (1943C). Forces behind food habits and methods of change. *Bulletin of the National Research Council, 108,* 35-65.

Lewin, K. (1943D). Psychology and the process of group living. *Journal of Social Psychology, 17,* 113-131.

Lewin, K. (1944A). Constructs in psychology and psychological ecology. *University of Iowa Studies in Child Welfare, 20,* 1-29.

Lewin, K. (1946B). Behavior and development as a function of the total situation. In L. Carmichael (Ed.), *Manual of child psychology* (pp. 918-970). New York: John Wiley.

Lewin, K. (1947A). Frontiers in group dynamics I. *Human Relations, 1,* 5-42

Lewin, K. (1947B). Frontiers in group dynamics II. *Human Relations, 1,* 143-153.

Reprints of Selected Lewin Monographs

Lewin, K. (1958). Group decision and social change. In E. E. Maccoby, T. M. Newcomb, & E. L. Hartley (Eds.), *Readings in social psychology* (3rd ed., pp. 197-211). New York: Holt.

Lewin, K. (1961). Quasi-stationary social equilibria and the problem of permanent change. In W. G. Bennis, K. D. Benne, & R. Chin (Eds.), *The planning of change* (pp. 235-238). New York: Holt, Rinehart & Winston.

Lewin, K. (1964). Group dynamics and social change. In A. Etzioni & E. Etzioni (Eds.), *Social change: Sources, patterns, and consequences* (pp. 354-361). New York: Basic Books.

Commentaries on Lewin's Theories and Legacy

Benne, K. D. (1985). The process of reeducation: An assessment of Kurt Lewin's views. In W. G. Bennis, K. D. Benne, & R. Chin (Eds.), *The planning of change* (4th ed., pp. 272-283). New York: Holt, Rinehart & Winston.

Marrow, A. J. (1969). *The practical theorist.* New York: Basic Books.

Stivers, E., & Wheelan, S. (1986). *The Lewin legacy.* New York: Springer.

Miscellaneous Selections

De Rivera, J. (1976). *Field theory as human science: Contributions of Lewin's Berlin group.* New York: Gardner.

Lewin, K. (1949). Cassirer's philosophy of science and social science. In P. A. Schlipp (Ed.), *The philosophy of Ernst Cassirer* (pp. 271-288). New York: Tudor.

C.2. Bhola

CHART C.2. Sources of Key Concepts in Bhola's Configurations (CLER) Model

Reference	Plan for Participation	Make Power Map	Formulate Diagnosis	Think of Implications	Redefine Objectives	Plan Grammar of Action	Choose Actions	Negotiate Actions	Create Action Sequence	Implement Plans	Evaluate Change Event
Bhola, H. S. (1972). Notes toward a theory: Cultural action as elite initiatives in affiliation/exclusion. *Viewpoints, 48*(3), 1-37.	X	X	X	X			X	X			
Bhola, H. S. (1973). *The organizational and the interpersonal in an international development education project.* Bloomington: Indiana University. (ERIC Document Reproduction Service No. ED 084 674)							X	X			
Bhola, H. S. (1973). *Planning, programming, and administration of functional literacy.* Bloomington: Indiana University. (ERIC Document Reproduction Service No. ED 091 555)	X	X	X		X		X	X	X		
Bhola, H. S. (1974). *ETV in the Third World: A diffusionist's perspective.* Bloomington: Indiana University. (ERIC Document Reproduction Service No. ED 098 926)	X	X	X	X	X		X	X		X	X
Bhola, H. S. (1975). The design of (educational) policy: Directing and harnessing social power for social outcomes. *Viewpoints, 51*(3), 1-16.		X									
Bhola, H. S. (1975). *The grammar of artifactual action.* Bloomington: Indiana University. (ERIC Document Reproduction Service No. ED 109 830)	X					X	X				

C.2. Bhola

CHART C.2. *(continued)*

	Plan for Participation	Make Power Map	Formulate Diagnosis	Think of Implications	Redefine Objectives	Plan Grammar of Action	Choose Actions	Negotiate Actions	Create Action Sequence	Implement Plans	Evaluate Change Event
Bhola, H. S. (1975). *Power: The anchor of stability, the lever of change: Notes toward a general theory of being and society.* Bloomington: Indiana University. (ERIC Document Reproduction Service No. ED 117 828)		X									
Bhola, H. S. (1975). *Some introductory lessons on "Organizational Literacy" for functional literacy workers.* Bloomington: Indiana University. (ERIC Document Reproduction Service No. ED 107 938)							X				
Bhola, H. S. (1976). *Institutional approaches to innovation and change: A review of the Esman model of institution building.* Washington, DC: Agency for International Development, Department of State. (ERIC Document Reproduction Service No. ED 117 820)							X				
Bhola, H. S. (1976). *Institutional approaches to innovation and change (II): The configurational perspective on institution building.* Bloomington: Indiana University. (ERIC Document Reproduction Service No. ED 122 454)							X				
Bhola, H. S. (1979). *Curriculum development for functional literacy and nonformal education programs* (pp. 77-107). Bonn, FRG: German Foundation for International Development. (ERIC Document Reproduction Service No. ED 239 819)	X		X		X		X	X			

C.2. Bhola

CHART C.2. *(continued)*

Reference	Plan for Participation	Make Power Map	Formulate Diagnosis	Think of Implications	Redefine Objectives	Plan Grammar of Action	Choose Actions	Negotiate Actions	Create Action Sequence	Implement Plans	Evaluate Change Event
Bhola, H. S. (1979). *Evaluating functional literacy.* Teheran, Iran: International Institute for Adult Literacy Methods. (ERIC Document Reproduction Service No. ED 169 498)	X	X									X
Bhola, H. S. (1981). Conceptualizing the use of learning resources in community education: A general model of strategy design. *Viewpoints in Teaching and Learning, 57*(4), 50-64.	X						X				
Bhola, H. S. (1981). Planning rural vocational and adult education: A multi-framework mega model. *Viewpoints in Teaching and Learning, 57*(3), 91-101.					X		X				
Bhola, H. S. (1984). *Tailor-made strategies of dissemination: The story and theory connection.* Bloomington: Indiana University. (ERIC Document Reproduction Service No. ED 250 458)					X		X				
Bhola, H. S. (1986). *Pathways to effective dissemination: Configuration mapping and linkage typing as tools.* Columbus: Ohio State University. (ERIC Reproduction Service No. ED 273 781)		X									
Bhola, H. S. (1989). Training evaluators in the Third World: Implementation of the action training model (ATM) in Kenya. *Evaluation and Program Planning, 12,* 249-258.	X			X			X	X			X

C.2. Bhola

CHART C.2. *(continued)*

	Plan for Participation	Make Power Map	Formulate Diagnosis	Think of Implications	Redefine Objectives	Plan Grammar of Action	Choose Actions	Negotiate Actions	Create Action Sequence	Implement Plans	Evaluate Change Event
Bhola, H. S. (1990). *Evaluating "literacy for development": Projects, programs, and campaigns.* Hamburg, Germany: UNESCO Institute of Education. (Order from Publications Office, UNESCO, Paris.)	X	X									X
Bhola, H. S. (1991, December). *Designing from the heart of an epistemic triangle: Systemic, dialectical, and constructivist strategies for systems design and systems change.* Paper presented at the Third Annual Conference of Comprehensive Systems Design of Education organized by the International Systems Institute, Asilomar Conference Center, Monterey, CA.			X	X	X	X	X	X	X		
Bhola, H. S. (1992). A model of evaluation planning, implementation, and management: Toward a "culture of information" within organizations. *International Review of Education, 38*(2), 103-115. (ERIC Document Reproduction Service No. ED 328 590)								X		X	X

Appendix D:
Planned Change Literature
in Nursing Periodical Articles

The following lists were derived from the survey conducted by Tiffany, Cheatham, Doornbos, Loudermelt, and Momadi (1994) with the help of Andrews University graduate students. As no new trends were noted in the literature during the 11 years of the survey, continuing the survey into the years beyond 1992 would not have been a good use of our resources. Another research team might consider resurveying the nursing literature 10 to 15 years after publication of this book.

D.1. Lewin Literature in Nursing Periodical Articles

1992

Bushy, A. (1992). Managing change: Strategies for continuing education. *Journal of Continuing Education in Nursing, 23,* 197-200.

Conger, M. M. (1992). Application of change theory to a clinical problem. *Nursing Management, 23*(10), 89, 90.

Haynes, S. (1992). Let the change come from within: The process of change in nursing. *Professional Nurse, 10,* 635-638.

Hinkle, J. L. (1992). Development of an acute stroke unit. *Journal of Neuroscience Nursing, 24*(2), 113-116.

Perciful, E. G. (1992). The relationship between planned change and successful implementation of computer assisted instruction. *Computers in Nursing, 10,* 85-90.

1991

Aliberti, L. C. (1991). Managing change: A practical perspective for the gastroenterology laboratory. *Gastroenterology Nursing, 13,* 162-165.

Blakeslee, J. A., Goldman, B. D., Papougenis, D., & Torell, C. A. (1991). Making the transition to restraint-free care. *Journal of Gerontological Nursing, 17*(2), 4-8.

Caramanica, L., & Rosenbecker, S. (1991). A pilot unit approach to shared governance. *Nursing Management, 22*(1), 46-48.

Comack (Fenton), M., Smith, S. D., Bowman, A., Gillow, K., Hunt, M., Snell, L., Thomsen, F., & Turner, D. (1991). Planning change in scheduling practices: A theoretical perspective. *Canadian Journal of Nursing Administration, 4*(1), 17-21.

Degerhammar, M., & Wade, B. (1991). The introduction of a new system of care delivery into a surgical ward in Sweden. *International Journal of Nursing Studies, 28,* 325-336.

Harris, M. G., & Bean, C. A. (1991). Changing the role of the nurse in the hematology-oncology outpatient setting. *Oncology Nursing Forum, 18*(1), 43-46.

Kaplan, S. M. (1991). The nurse as change agent. *Dermatology Nursing, 3,* 419-422.

Muller, O., Bierman, J., & van Loggerenberg, M. (1991). Change! *Nursing RSA Verpleging, 6*(11-12), 9-11.

Schutzenhofer, K. K. (1991). Scholarly pursuit in the clinical setting: An obligation of professional nursing. *Journal of Professional Nursing, 7,* 10-15.

Sella, S., & MacLeod, J. A. (1991). One year later: Evaluating a changing delivery system. *Nursing Forum, 26*(2), 5-11.

Smeltzer, C. H. (1991). The art of negotiation: An everyday experience. *Journal of Nursing Administration, 21*(7-8), 26-30.

Smith, J. (1991). Changing traditional nursing home roles to nursing case management. *Journal of Gerontological Nursing, 17*(5), 32-39.

1990

Bircumshaw, D. (1990). The utilization of research findings in clinical nursing practice. *Journal of Advanced Nursing, 15,* 1272-1280.

Clark, P., & Hall, H. S. (1990). Innovations probability chart: A valuable tool for change. *Nursing Management, 21*(8), 128V-128X.

Kaplan, S. M. (1990). The nurse as change agent. *Pediatric Nursing, 16,* 603-618.

Morse, G. G. (1990). Resurgence of nurse assistants in acute care. *Nursing Management, 21*(3), 34-36.

Neatherlin, J. S. (1990). Presidential address: Change. *Journal of Neuroscience Nursing, 22,* 207-208.

Sheehan, J. (1990). Investigating change in a nursing context. *Journal of Advanced Nursing, 15,* 819-824

1989

Davidhizar, R., & Kuipers, J. (1989). How to plan and implement change. *Advancing Clinical Care, 4*(3), 38, 39.

Fine, E. L. (1989). Community hospital merger: The challenge to nursing management. *Nursing Management, 20*(12), 30-34, 36.

Jennings, B. M., & Rogers, S. (1989). Using research to change nursing practice. *Critical Care Nurse, 9*(5), 76, 78, 80-82, 84.

Ouelett, L. L., & Rush, K. L. (1989). Forces influencing curriculum evaluation. *Nurse Education Today, 9,* 219-226.

Sauter, M., & Nodine, F. (1989). Using the change process to implement nursing diagnosis. *Journal of Nursing Staff Development, 5,* 211-217.

Schwartz, L. A., & Lowe, D. (1989). Applying a theoretic framework for reducing medication errors in intensive care units. *Focus on Critical Care, 16,* 438-443.

Shidler, H., Pencak, M., & McFolling, S. D. (1989). Professional nursing staff: A model of self-governance for nursing. *Nursing Administration Quarterly, 13*(4), 1-9.

Stark, J. L. (1989). Research reflections: A multiple-strategy based research program for staff nurse involvement. *Journal of Nursing Administration, 19*(9), 7-8.

Walsh, K. C. (1989). Using planned change to implement a pressure sore program. *Journal of Neuroscience Nursing, 21,* 245-249.

1988

Burkman, K. (1988). Effecting change: You can do it. *Neonatal Network, 6*(6), 41-43.

Knollmueller, R. N. (1988). Reshaping supervisory practice in home care. *Nursing Clinics of North America, 23,* 353-362.

Van Servellen, G. M., Lewis, C. E., & Leake, B. (1988). Nurses' response to the AIDS crisis: Implications for continuing education programs. *Journal of Continuing Education in Nursing, 19,* 4-8.

1987

Ellis, D. J. (1987). Change process: A case example. *Nursing Management, 18*(4), 14-19.

Lahti, J. T. (1987). Challenging change. *Health Care Supervisor, 5*(3), 55-60.

Lawler, T. F. (1987). Effecting change in a community hospital: Implications for staff development. *Journal of Continuing Education in Nursing, 18,* 59-63.

Yura, H., & Young, S. (1987). The nurse supervisor charged with change. *Health Care Supervisor, 5*(3), 12-27.

1986

Everden, J. J. (1986). Preparing for change: An investigation into the attitudes of assessors to ward-based assessments as a preliminary to continuing clinical assessments. *Journal of Advanced Nursing, 11,* 713-718.

Huckabay, L. M. D. (1986). Computerization of nursing department and force field theory. *Nursing Administration Quarterly, 10*(2), 75-86.

Hurst, J. D., & Stullenbarger, B. (1986). Implementation of a self-care approach in a pediatric interdisciplinary phenylketonuria (PKU) clinic. *Journal of Pediatric Nursing, 1,* 160-163.

Lunney, M. (1986). Implementing an educational program on nursing diagnosis. *Journal, New York State Nurses' Association, 17*(4), 28-34.

McGovern, W. N., & Rodgers, J. A. (1986). Change theory. *American Journal of Nursing, 86,* 566-567.

Monaco, R., & Nayagam, T. (1986). Implementation of family-centered care at Harbor-UCLA Medical Center. *EMPHASIS: Nursing, 2*(1), 18-25.

Monger, M. (1986). An ED nursing documentation tool and the process of planned change. *Journal of Emergency Nursing, 12,* 370-377.

Proctor, D. M., & Rhodes-Auton, V. S. (1986). Documenting care in the medical intensive care unit: Change theory in action. *Critical Care Nurse, 6*(5), 82-86.

Schutzenhofer, K. K., & Spikes, J. M. (1986). Setting the stage for change: Using elective courses to create social and political awareness. *Nurse Educator, 11*(4), 20-23.

Skeoch, M. (1986, December). Implementing change in the O.R. setting. *Canadian Operating Room Nursing Journal,* pp. 16-21.

1985

Crane, J. (1985). Research utilization: Theoretical perspectives. *Western Journal of Nursing Research, 7,* 261-268.

Wianko, D. C. (1985, August). Primary nursing: A program for change. *Canadian Nurse,* pp. 33-35.

Wright, S. G. (1985). Change in nursing: The application of change theory to practice. *Nursing Practice, 2,* 85-91.

1984

Byers, M. (1984). Getting on top of organizational change: Part 1. Process and development. *Journal of Nursing Administration, 14*(10), 32-39.

Gawlinski, A., & Rassmussen, S. (1984). Improving documentation through use of change theory. *Focus on Critical Care, 11*(6), 12-17.

Ingersoll, G. L. (1984). Implementing primary nursing in a surgical outpatient department. *Nursing Management, 15*(5), 32-36.

Kemp, V. H. (1984). An overview of change and leadership. *Topics in Clinical Nursing, 6*(1), 1-9.

Williams, D. D., & Davis, J. H. (1984). Change and persistence: A paradox in promoting health behaviors. *Journal of Community Health Nursing, 1*(1), 21-26.

Young, M. S., & Lucas, C. M. (1984). Nursing diagnosis: Common problems in implementation. *Topics in Clinical Nursing, 5*(4), 68-77.

1983

Bailey, B. J. (1983). Using change theory to help the diabetic. *Diabetes Educator, 9*(3), 37-39, 56.

Green, C. P. (1983). Teaching strategies for the process of planned change. *Journal of Continuing Education in Nursing, 14,* 16-23.

1982

Greaves, F. (1982). Innovation, change, decision-making, and the key variables in nursing curriculum implementation. *International Journal of Nursing Studies, 19*(1), 11-19.

Holloran, S. D. (1982). Teaching male catheterization: An application of change theory for an entire nursing staff. *Nurse Educator, 7*(1), 11-14.

King, E. S. (1982). Coping with organizational change. *Topics in Clinical Nursing, 4*(2), 66-73.

Sheridan, D. R. (1982). The season for collective bargaining. *Nursing Administration Quarterly, 6*(2), 1-7.

Sullins, M. L. (1982). Staff nurses can inspire OR changes. *AORN Journal, 36,* 672-678.

D.2. Bennis, Benne, and Chin
Literature in Nursing Periodical Articles

1992

Bushy, A. (1992). Managing change: Strategies for continuing education. *Journal of Continuing Education in Nursing, 23,* 197-200.

Ehrenfeld, M., Bergman, R., & Ziv, L. (1992). Academia: A stimulus for change. *International Nursing Review, 39,* 23-26.

Haynes, S. (1992). Let the change come from within: The process of change in nursing. *Professional Nurse, 10,* 635-638.

Swan, J., & MacVicar, B. (1992). The rough guide to change. *Nursing Times, 88*(13), 48-49.

1991

Aliberti, L. C. (1991). Managing change: A practical perspective for the gastroenterology laboratory. *Gastroenterology Nursing, 13,* 162-165.

Degerhammar, M., & Wade, B. (1991). The introduction of a new system of care delivery into a surgical ward in Sweden. *International Journal of Nursing Studies, 28,* 325-336.

Gish, B. A., & Campbell, J. (1991). Introducing standardized care plans in an intermediate care setting. *Focus on Critical Care, 18*(1), 51, 53-57.

Harris, M. G., & Bean, C. A. (1991). Changing the role of the nurse in the hematology-oncology outpatient setting. *Oncology Nursing Forum, 18*(1), 43-46.

Harrison, N., & Calvey, H. (1991). A change for the better. *Nursing Times, 87*(24), 49-51.

Pillar, B. (1991). The introduction of new technology on the nursing unit. *Nursing Economic$, 9,* 50, 51, 63.

1990

Gibbs, A. (1990). Curriculum innovation and the management of change. *Nurse Education Today, 10,* 98-103.

Sheehan, J. (1990). Investigating change in a nursing context. *Journal of Advanced Nursing, 15,* 819-824.

Stevenson, D. (1990). The energy crisis of change. *Nursing Practice, 4*(1), 15-17.

Tierney, M. J., Grant, L. M., Cherrstrom, P. L., & Morris, B. L. (1990). Clinical nurse specialists in transition. *Clinical Nurse Specialist, 4,* 103-106.

Williamson, N., McDonough, J. E., & Boettcher, J. (1990). Nurse faculty practice: From theory to reality. *Journal of Professional Nursing, 6,* 11-20.

1989

Bushy, A., & Kamphuis, J. (1989). Rogers' adoption model in the implementation of change. *Clinical Nurse Specialist, 3,* 188-191.

Cashman, J. (1989). Effecting change through the stream analysis process. *Journal of Nursing Administration, 19*(5), 37-44.

Littlefield, V. M. (1989). Creating an administrative structure to support faculty governance: A participatory process. *Journal of Professional Nursing, 5,* 336-344.

Ouelett, L. L., & Rush, K. L. (1989). Forces influencing curriculum evaluation. *Nurse Education Today, 9,* 219-226.

Schwartz, L. A., & Lowe, D. (1989). Applying a theoretic framework for reducing medication errors in intensive care units. *Focus on Critical Care, 16,* 438-443.

1988

Knollmueller, R. N. (1988). Reshaping supervisory practice in home care. *Nursing Clinics of North America, 23,* 353-362.

1987

McDougall, G. J. (1987). The role of the clinical nurse specialist consultant in organizational development. *Clinical Nurse Specialist, 1,* 133-139.

Noone, J. (1987). Planned change: Putting theory into practice. *Clinical Nurse Specialist, 1,* 25-29.

Stephenson, P. M. (1987). The process of change in intensive care nursing. *Intensive Care Nursing, 2,* 148-156.

1986

Everden, J. J. (1986). Preparing for change: An investigation into the attitudes of assessors to ward-based assessments as a preliminary to continuing clinical assessments. *Journal of Advanced Nursing, 11,* 713-718.

Filkins, J. (1986, February 12). Introducing change. *Nursing Times,* pp. 26, 29-30.

Haffer, A. (1986). Facilitating change: Choosing the appropriate strategy. *Journal of Nursing Administration, 16*(4), 18-22.

Harkness, J. C., & Porras, J. I. (1986). Stream analysis: A method for planning and directing care. *Perioperative Nursing Quarterly, 2*(1), 20-31.

Hollefreund, B., Clark, N. L., & Wadsworth, N. S. (1986). The human resource consultant in nursing. *Journal of Nursing Administration, 16*(7-8), 21-25.

1985

Loomis, M. E. (1985). Knowledge utilization and research utilization in nursing. *Image: The Journal of Nursing Scholarship, 17,* 35-39.

Partridge, B. (1985). The change process: A N.S.W. reflection. *Australian Journal of Advanced Nursing, 2*(2), 45-50.

Pearson, A. (1985). Nurses as change agents and a strategy for change. *Nursing Practice, 2,* 80-84.

Schramm, C. (1985). The clinical nurse specialist: The role in the OR. *AORN Journal, 41,* 579, 581-583, 586-587.

1984

Byers, M. (1984). Getting on top of organizational change: Part 1. Process and development. *Journal of Nursing Administration, 14*(10), 32-39.

Hope, M. (1984). Suggestions are welcome. *Nursing Mirror, 158*(19), ii-iii, vi-viii.

Llewellyn, J., & Holm, K. (1984). Implementing changes in critical care. *Dimensions of Critical Care Nursing, 3*(1), 37-41.

Ward, M. J., & Moran, S. G. (1984). Resistance to change: Recognize, respond, overcome. *Nursing Management, 15*(1), 30-33.

Williams, D. D., & Davis, J. H. (1984). Change and persistence: A paradox in promoting health behaviors. *Journal of Community Health Nursing, 1*(1), 21-26.

Young, M. S., & Lucas, C. M. (1984). Nursing diagnosis: Common problems in implementation. *Topics in Clinical Nursing, 5*(4), 68-77.

1983

Bailey, B. J. (1983). Using change theory to help the diabetic. *Diabetes Educator, 9*(3), 37-39, 56.

Green, C. P. (1983). Teaching strategies for the process of planned change. *Journal of Continuing Education in Nursing, 14,* 16-23.

Miller, L. E. (1983). Resistance to the consultation process. *Nursing Leadership, 6,* 10-15.

1982

Greaves, F. (1982). Innovation, change, decision-making, and the key variables in nursing curriculum implementation. *International Journal of Nursing Studies, 19*(1), 11-19.

D.3. Rogers Literature in
Nursing Periodical Articles

1992

Bushy, A. (1992). Managing change: Strategies for continuing education. *Journal of Continuing Education in Nursing, 23,* 197-200.

Haynes, S. (1992). Let the change come from within: The process of change in nursing. *Professional Nurse, 10,* 635-638.

1991

Gibbs, A. (1991). Cultural and political limitations within a rational approach towards educational change. *Journal of Advanced Nursing, 16,* 182-186.

1990

Barker, E. R. (1990). Use of diffusion of innovation model for agency consultation. *Clinical Nurse Specialist, 4,* 163-166.

Bircumshaw, D. (1990). The utilization of research findings in clinical nursing practice. *Journal of Advanced Nursing, 15,* 1272-1280.

Coyle, L. A., & Sokop, A. G. (1990). Innovation adoption behavior among nurses. *Nursing Research, 39,* 176-180.

Geis, M. J. (1990). Diffusion of associate degree nursing programs among US community colleges. *Journal of Nursing Education, 29,* 176-182.

1989

Brett, J. L. L. (1989). Organizational integrative mechanisms and adoption of innovations by nurses. *Nursing Research, 38,* 105-110.

Bushy, A. (1989). QA: Behavioral responses to change. *Journal of Nursing Quality Assurance, 3*(4), 1-8.

Bushy, A., & Kamphuis, J. (1989). Rogers' adoption model in the implementation of change. *Clinical Nurse Specialist, 3,* 188-191.

Delaney, C. W. (1989). Nurse educators' acceptance of the computer in baccalaureate nursing programs. *Computers in Nursing, 7,* 129-136.

Polfus, P., & Bigbee, J. (1989). Innovation-diffusion theory and the evolution of the nurse practitioner role: How a good thing has caught on. *Journal of the American Academy of Nurse Practitioners, 1*(2), 38-43.

1987

Brett, J. L. L. (1987). Use of nursing practice research findings. *Nursing Research, 36,* 344-349.

Hall, B. A. (1987). Strategies of persistence in a professional bureaucracy: A field study of a psychiatric hospital. *Archives of Psychiatric Nursing, 1,* 183-193.

Holbrook, N. J. (1987). Learning to be change makers. *Kansas Nurse, 62*(3), 3, 4.

1986

Horsley, J. A., & Crane, J. (1986). Factors associated with innovation in nursing practice. *Family and Community Health, 9*(1), 1-11.

1985

Crane, J. (1985a). Research utilization: Nursing models. *Western Journal of Nursing Research, 7,* 494-497.

Crane, J. (1985b). Research utilization: Theoretical perspectives. *Western Journal of Nursing Research, 7,* 261-268.

Loomis, M. E. (1985). Knowledge utilization and research utilization in nursing. *Image: The Journal of Nursing Scholarship, 17,* 35-39.

1984

Fine, R. B. (1984). Changing expectations in the workplace: The clinical career ladder. *Nursing Administration Quarterly, 9*(1), 21-24.

Kemp, V. H. (1984). An overview of change and leadership. *Topics in Clinical Nursing, 6*(1), 1-9.

Mercer, R. T. (1984). Nursing research: The bridge to excellence in practice. *Image: The Journal of Nursing Scholarship, 16*(2), 47-51.

Milne, D., & Turton, N. (1984). Making the nursing process work in mental health. *Senior Nurse, 5*(5-6), 33-34.

1982

Barnard, K. E. (1982, Summer). The research cycle: Nursing, the profession, the discipline. *Communicating Nursing Research,* pp. 1-12.
Greaves, F. (1982). Innovation, change, decision-making, and the key variables in nursing curriculum implementation. *International Journal of Nursing Studies, 19*(1), 11-19.
Kirchhoff, K. T. (1982). A diffusion survey of coronary precautions. *Nursing Research, 31,* 196-201.
Puetz, B. E. (1982). The occupational health nurse and the process of change. *Occupational Health Nursing, 30*(2), 9-12.

D.4. Bhola Literature in Nursing Periodical Articles

1985

Loomis, M. E. (1985). Knowledge utilization and research utilization in nursing. *Image: The Journal of Nursing Scholarship, 17,* 35-39.
(Also see Bhola, H. S. [1994]. The CLER model: Thinking through change. *Nursing Management, 25*[5], 59-63.)

Name Index

Subject Index

About the Authors

Constance Rimmer Tiffany is Professor Emeritus of Nursing, Andrews University, Berrien Springs, Michigan, where she taught for 24 years. Half this time she spent teaching courses in the Master of Science in Nursing program in the College of Arts and Sciences. She also taught a course in the Masters in Business Administration program (hospital administration emphasis) for the School of Business. After retirement, she served as a contract teacher at Indiana University-Purdue University at Fort Wayne. She earned a PhD in education with a major emphasis on the diffusion and adoption of educational innovations at Indiana University, Bloomington. Doctoral minors include management in the IU School of Business and medical-surgical nursing in the IU School of Nursing. While at IU, she was included in one of the first groups of women inducted into membership in Phi Delta Kappa. She holds membership in Phi Kappa Phi, the Indiana State Nurses Association, the Nursing Research Consortium of Fort Wayne, and the Eta Zeta and Xi Nu chapters of Sigma Theta Tau. Her research interests include pay equity for nurses and the development of procedures for the evaluation of planned change theories. She has published professional articles on pay equity issues, the professionalization of nursing, and planned change theory. She is one of the few nurses in the United States with doctoral preparation in the field of planned change theory.

Louette R. Johnson Lutjens is a Nursing Research Consultant at the Cook Institute for Research and Education, Grand Rapids, Michigan. She also holds an Adjunct Associate Professor position at Grand Valley State University (GVSU), Allendale, Michigan. Before joining the Cook Institute in 1995, she was Associate Professor at GVSU, where she taught nursing theory, nursing administration role courses, and health care delivery systems at the graduate level. Her position also entailed serving as chairperson and committee member on thesis committees. She has held positions in nursing administration in nursing service

407

organizations and faculty positions in academic institutions. She holds certification in nursing administration, advanced (CNAA), by the American Nurses Association. She earned a PhD in nursing from Wayne State University, Detroit, Michigan. Her minor is in management and organizational sciences. She also holds a master of science degree in nursing and a post-master's certificate in nursing administration from Wayne State University. She is active in many professional nursing organizations including the North American Nursing Diagnosis Association, the Lambda chapter of Sigma Theta Tau International, the Midwest Nursing Research Society, and the Michigan Nurses Association. She has written books on nursing theory and many articles in refereed journals. Her research interests include client outcomes, use of nursing theory, and systems.